Good Night, Sleep Tight

Good Night, Sleep Tight

Gentle, Proven Solutions to Help Your Child Sleep Well and Wake Up Happy

Kim West LCSW-C
with Joanne Kenen

piatkus

The anecdotes included in this book are based on the real experiences of individuals and families. In all cases, names and identifying characteristics have been changed to protect the privacy of individuals.

The information and advice presented in this book have been reviewed by a qualified pediatrician. It should not, however, substitute for the advice of your family doctor or other trained health care professionals. You are advised to consult with health care professionals with regard to all matters that may require medical attention or diagnosis and to check with a physician before administering or undertaking any course of treatment.

PIATKUS

First published in the US in 2004 by Vanguard Press,
a member of the Perseus Books Group
This edition published in 2010
First published in Great Britain in 2010 by Piatkus

5 7 9 10 8 6

A CIP catalogue record for this book
is available from the British Library.

ISBN 978-0-7499-4221-2

Typeset in Bembo by Palimpsest Book Production Limited,
Grangemouth, Stirlingshire
Printed and bound by CPI Group (UK) Ltd, Croydon, CR0 4YY

Papers used by Piatkus are from well-managed forests
and other responsible sources.

MIX
Paper from
responsible sources
FSC® C104740
www.fsc.org

Piatkus
An imprint of
Little, Brown Book Group
100 Victoria Embankment
London EC4Y 0DY

An Hachette UK Company
www.hachette.co.uk

www.piatkus.co.uk

To Denise Drake, who helped
me expand my vision of my work
and encouraged me years ago
to become The Sleep Lady.

—Kim West

To Ken, Zach, and Ilan,
who make my dreams sweet.

—Joanne Kenen

Contents

16 Routine Busters: Dealing with Travel, Illness, and Life's
     Other Disruptions   413
17 Problem Solving and Taking Care of Mums and Dads   435

     Appendix: Safe Sleeping Recommendations for Babies   459
     Resource Directory   463
     Photo Credits   473
     Index   475

Acknowledgments

I want to thank Joanne Kenen for the thousands of hours she put into this book, for hearing and conveying my voice, and for believing in The Sleep Lady program. I couldn't have done this without her expertise, encouragement, and commitment.

Each of the families who have laughed, cried, and celebrated their struggles and progress with me is central to this book. Thank you for letting me into your lives and for allowing me to learn along with you.

My entire family has offered me extraordinary support, endless encouragement, and a willing ear even when they were tired of hearing about sleep. A special thank-you to my wonderful daughters, who were my first teachers of the gift of sleep and who continue to teach me new things to this day.

Finally, thank you to Roger Cooper, David Wilk, Lottchen Shivers, and all of the Vanguard team who believe in me and my message. Thank you to our editors, Mary Bahr and Francine LaSala, for their patience, time, and enthusiasm for this book.

—*Kim West*

Acknowledgments

I would like to thank Kim West for sharing her 'Sleep Lady' secrets and including me in this book project. In addition, my friends and colleagues – including Deborah Zabarenko, Michael Arkus, Nancy Zuckerbrod, and my mother, Regina Kenen – read and helped me improve sections of this manuscript, as did our editor, Mary Bahr. Sylvia Stein and Andrew Nibley were also great sounding boards. My husband, Ken, and my sons, Zach and Ilan, graciously endured having a book-writing mum in the house. Finally, I want to thank the dozens of mums and dads who found time in their busy lives to share their stories and insights with me. We changed their names to protect privacy, but I hope I remained true to their voices and experiences, and that through them, other parents and children will find their own path to good nights.

—*Joanne Kenen*

Preface

Since the first edition of *Good Night, Sleep Tight* was published in 2004, I've heard from thousands of grateful families from all over the world who have used my Sleep Lady system to get their babies, toddlers, and preschoolers – as well as themselves – to sleep. In this revised and updated edition, my goal is to make it even easier for you.

I've updated the book to include the latest pediatric research on sleep safety, dummy use, and breastfeeding guidelines (and yes, you can breastfeed for as long as you want and still have a family that sleeps at night). I've expanded sections that parents have told me were the most difficult, including phasing out nighttime feedings and that tricky transition when toddlers go from two naps to one. I've given you more information on dealing with siblings' sleep and added some intriguing new finding on interpreting your newborn's cries. I've included new tips to help both Mum and Dad confidently bond with their baby and help the baby form a healthy secure attachment to them. And I'm pleased that Helen Garabedian let me share some bedtime poses from 'Itsy Bitsy Yoga,' which I think you'll love as much as your children do. I've also added a section on postnatal depression, which I hope all mums and dads and grandparents read. It can help you recognize the warning signs of depression not just in yourself but in friends and family members. And it tells you how to get help.

As I've worked with families over the years, one of the topics that always comes up is whether to 'cosleep' or 'bedshare,' and if so, for how long. I'm supportive of bedsharing, if it's what you want and you do it safely. But I also know a lot of families who end up with a baby in the bed not because they've chosen to cosleep but because they just can't figure out what else to do. So I give you plenty of help if and when you want to stop bedsharing, and I also talk a lot (and recommend to many of the families I work with one-on-one) about a middle way, roomsharing. That means you'll keep the infant in your room but in a separate bed, literally at your fingertips if you want, for the first three to six months. It makes night feeding easier, and may make you sleep better too if your new little baby is right by your side.

If you've looked at other parenting sleep books, you'll find that they usually cover just the first few months or maybe the first year of life. You have to buy a second book to cover the toddler and preschool years. I thought that was a little silly. First of all, many of you have more than one child: I didn't want to make you buy two books! Also, you may discover that even good sleepers may face different sleep challenges as they move through childhood – when they switch from two naps to one, or when they move from a cot to a bed, when you travel, and when a baby brother or sister is born, to name a few common examples. And not all children do everything on a precise schedule. One baby might hit a developmental milestone at eleven months, and another baby who is just as bright may hit it at thirteen months. Both are normal. But I didn't want you flipping through two books trying to figure out which one had the answer to your particular problem. Of course, that means this book is long! With this edition, I tried to make it easier for sleep-deprived parents to find the information they need. You'll find some easy reference boxes, tips, and lists – as well as some adorable pictures from my readers! I hope it helps.

Even though I do cover ages from newborn to five years all in one volume, the Sleep Lady system does have two distinct phases. In the first few months of life, we concentrate on soothing techniques and establishing basic rhythms and routines to help babies learn to sleep. It's subtle but effective. For many infants, this foundation will enable them to start going to sleep by themselves and staying asleep all night between ages four and six months. Other babies may need more intervention, and my Sleep Lady Shuffle provides a sleep-shaping system that is structured but gentle. But the Shuffle is not designed for newborns. Usually we don't introduce it until about six months. Some parents have had success with the Sleep Lady Shuffle with a healthy baby as early as four months, but if it doesn't work that early, please don't give up. Keep following the steps I recommend for four- or five-month-old babies, and try the Shuffle again if you need to at six months. Always check with your baby's doctor before beginning any sleep-training system.

One last – absolutely essential – thought. You know how in property it's all about location, location, location? Well, in parenting it's all about consistency, consistency, consistency. That's especially true for sleep. Take a little bit of time to familiarize yourself with my philosophy and my system. And when you are ready to start putting it into action, you need to do so consistently. Inconsistency is not kinder to your child; it is confusing to your child. Instead of minimizing tears, you risk maximizing tears if your child does not know what to expect or what is expected of him. That's not what we want. If you can't be consistent at certain times, have your spouse or partner take over. Find another parent to be your sleep buddy, and get on the phone every morning and keep each other on track, the way you might if you were starting a diet or exercise program. Research has shown that whatever sleep system you choose – and although I hope you choose mine I know you have a lot of alternatives – consistency is the single biggest factor in success.

Sleep tight,
Kim West, LCSW-C
'The Sleep Lady'
www.sleeplady.com

Foreword to the First Edition

My favorite part of the title to Kim West and Joanne Kenen's book *Good Night, Sleep Tight: Gentle, Proven Solutions to Help Your Child Sleep Well and Wake Up Happy* is the word *gentle*. The book is gently worded, gentle on the reader's heart, and gentle to implement. For all the parents who have lost countless hours of sleep trying the tough-love approach of letting the baby cry it out, this book comes as a wonderful, informative reprieve.

My own son, who is now eighteen years old, had colic as a baby. I nursed him to sleep, and either my husband or I held him all the time. During the first few years of his life I wondered what I was doing wrong. Dr Richard Ferber had just written *Solve Your Child's Sleep Problems*, and I was persuaded to try his cry-it-out approach. My son cried so long and hard the first night that he lost his voice. After a week, he did sleep better, but I was wracked with guilt. I wish I had been able to use Kim West's approach back then.

I have been in private pediatric practice for eighteen years, during which time I have noticed that the pace of daily life for most parents has dramatically increased. Not coincidentally, I have seen a marked rise in sleep difficulties in babies and children as the pressures of their parents' busy schedules impact their routine. While there are many books on this issue, most of them take a very firm cry-it-out approach that, in my experience, leaves parents emotionally exhausted and filled with guilt. I have been looking for a definitive how-to book on sleep that I can recommend without reservation. *Good Night, Sleep Tight* is that book – one that will serve as a manual to both parents and medical practitioners.

Good Night, Sleep Tight addresses a wide range of sleep issues for children through to age five. Each age-specific chapter provides guidelines for creating a schedule and implementing change but also invites the parents to tailor the program for their child and their lifestyle. Real-life examples from families helped by Kim West illustrate the program's practical steps and offer encouragement to the reader. And, unlike most authors of books on sleep, Kim West and Joanne Kenen are mothers who share not only their professional expertise but their personal experiences as well.

As a community pediatrician, I give advice about feeding, development, safety, immunization, and behavioral issues at each checkup. Many of the concerns parents want to discuss stem from their child's need for sleep. A parent recently came in with a ten month old who was teething and up all night for nights on end. The mother was fearful that her baby was in severe pain. After a full exam, it was clear that the infant needed a regular sleep schedule. I discussed Kim West's approach and explained why many of the crying spells were related to sleep deprivation. She was relieved to learn how to effectively soothe her baby and delighted to discover that the cry-it-out approach was not her only option. I have sent many families to see Kim West in her private practice and am looking forward to recommending this book to many more.

—Faith A. Hackett, M.D.
Fellow of the American Academy of Pediatrics
Courtesy Staff Physician, Johns Hopkins Hospital
Staff Physician, Anne Arundel Medical Center

Part One

Introduction

Meet the Sleep Lady

O f all the questions new parents face, none is more common than 'Does your baby sleep?' If the baby sleeps well, the answer all too often is 'Yes, she's a good baby.' By implication, those who don't sleep are bad babies. The mother and father, already overwhelmed by exhaustion, must also deal with feelings that they are failing their first test as parents.

Of course, the millions of babies who don't initially sleep through the night are not moral failures. They are just new little people who have not yet learned to put themselves to sleep. *Learn* is the key word. We all know that the need for sleep is biological, but we don't always realize that the ability to sleep is a learned skill. All children can learn it. All parents can teach them. But like everything else in life, some just need a little more help than others.

> We all know that the need for sleep is
> biological, but we don't always realize that
> the ability to sleep is a learned skill.

I'm Kim West, also known as the Sleep Lady, and I have spent more than a decade providing help to thousands of weary and bleary families. I won't promise you no tears, but I do aim for fewer tears, and I never tell you to just shut the door and let your baby bawl alone in the dark.

My gentler method depends on step-by-step changes in bedtime, napping, and overnight routines so that your child can develop sleep independence, go to sleep on her own, and sleep more soundly and longer while feeling confident that Mum and Dad will be nearby and responsive. A well-rested baby is usually an easier, less cranky baby. A well-rested parent (in case it feels like it's been so long that you can't remember) is an easier, less cranky parent, able to show the child more joy and love, and less of the irritability and frustration that are inevitable when they are up with him ten times a night.

About eighteen years ago, I moved to the Annapolis, Maryland, in the United States, where I later opened a general therapy practice as a clinical social worker. At the time I had no particular interest or expertise in childhood sleep. But I did have a personal stake in the topic. I need a fair amount of good, solid, uninterrupted sleep myself, and as I began to think about having children, I began to worry. I saw my friends start families and lose sleep. I saw the rings under their eyes, heard the strain in their voices, witnessed the brittle irritation with their spouses. Sometimes it seemed like their only topic of conversation was what a bad night they'd just had, and I could discern a growing sense of guilt and anxiety on their part.

Convinced that there had to be a better way, I began to research everything available to me about the physiology and psychology of pediatric sleep. I began to interweave what I was learning about sleep cycles, arousal states, and the physical need for sleep with what I already knew about child development and behavioral psychology, especially the need for parental consistency as we try to teach and mold our children's behaviors.

Neither of my own two daughters was an 'angel baby' who just drifted off into peaceful slumber. The second one, in particular, was fussy and had reflux, putting my theories to the test. Still, I had Carleigh sleeping for an eight-hour stretch at night by eight weeks, Gretchen at ten weeks – and, yes, I breastfed both of them. Gradually, I began helping my friends to teach their babies and toddlers to sleep, and then friends of friends. Word spread, and soon I had a growing number of sleepy parents with sleepless babies knocking on my door.

Given how common sleep problems are – affecting up to one in four children under the age of five – finding practical help is surprisingly difficult. The field of sleep medicine has grown in recent years, but specialists are still relatively few and far between. Not all sleep clinics treat very young children, or they accept only those pediatric cases involving breathing disorders such as apnea. You do need to rule out any medical conditions that hamper sleep. Talk to your doctor about your baby's sleep problems and feeding patterns, and be sure to mention any digestive difficulties, allergies, noisy breathing, or snoring.

But most childhood sleep problems are behavioral, not physical, and some pediatricians receive amazingly little training about sleep, often only an hour or two during their residency. You may find that even caring and competent doctors might not have much to offer regarding behavioral sleep problems. That leaves many parents with the mistaken notion that they have no alternative to enduring sleep deprivation indefinitely, that they just have to wait and hope that the child will somehow, someday, outgrow it on her own.

One in four children under the age of five has sleeping problems.

To the extent that you do get advice, whether from doctors or well-meaning friends or relatives, it usually falls into one of two categories. On one hand are the variants of 'crying it out.' On the other are the 'attachment theorists' who promote cosleeping and nursing on demand well past the early months of infancy. Either of those approaches is fine – *if* they feel right for you and right for your kids. They aren't fine if they don't feel right, if they strain your marriage, if they don't fit into your adult needs – or if they don't help your child learn to put himself to sleep and stay asleep.

The most common advice is to let your child cry it out, an approach popularized in the mid-1980s by Dr Richard Ferber, the famed Boston Children's Hospital sleep expert. Simply put, 'Ferberizing' means leaving a baby to cry but having a parent go in to briefly check on the child at regular but less and less frequent intervals. The theory is that if a child can learn to fall asleep on his own, without being rocked, nursed, stroked, or serenaded, he will be able to go back to sleep on his own during the frequent but brief awakenings that everyone experiences, awakenings that a good sleeper doesn't even remember by morning.

An even starker method, promoted by Dr Marc Weissbluth of Northwestern University's Feinberg School of Medicine and known as *extinction*, has the child cry it out as long as it takes without Ferber's frequent parental checks. Research has shown that, while neither approach works all the time, both do have respectable success rates – if parents can turn off their ears and heartstrings long enough to tolerate the screams. Anecdotally, I know many families who use Ferber's or Weissbluth's approach find it improves their children's sleep – but they absolutely dread the process. (In one case the husband was the enforcer, letting the kids cry at bedtime while the more tenderhearted wife drove around in fierce snowstorms until she knew it was safe to come home.)

My Sleep Lady approach is a gentler alternative for families who emotionally or philosophically resist letting their babies cry it out, for families who tried Ferber and it didn't work, and for families who let their child cry it out when she was three or four months old but found it didn't help later. I have also worked with families who believe in cosleeping but find that their children aren't really sleeping all that well, even nestled snugly with Mum and Dad. And I've helped guide many families who did bedshare for a few months or a few years but now want the family bed to revert to a marital one.

Sleep Lady Tip

Children may need a little sleep help as they cope with big changes in life, like the start of preschool, Mum's return to work, or the birth of a baby brother or sister.

Much of my work is with babies aged six to eighteen months whose pediatricians agree should be able to sleep through the night. I also run Right Start workshops for pregnant couples or families with newborns, including many couples whose first child had sleep problems and who want less of an ordeal with the second. But if your child is older, don't worry; it's not too late to improve her sleep, although it may take a little longer to break habits that are more deeply ingrained. I have helped numerous toddlers, many sets of twins, and more than a smattering of school-age children.

This book contains age-specific advice for the first five years, and I'll give you a glimpse into the sleep challenges ahead in the school years. Even if your child is basically a sound sleeper, you might turn to this book periodically as she enters new developmental stages requiring some minor sleep adjustments. You might need advice, for instance, on how to help her consolidate two naps into one, or when to move her from the cot to a bed. A child may need a little sleep help as he copes with big changes in life, like the start of preschool, Mum's return to work, or the birth of a baby brother or sister.

A Word About Attachment Parenting

Many families I work with tell me they have been influenced by *attachment parenting* or *attachment theory*, so it's worth spending a moment thinking about a *secure attachment*. We all want our children to have a secure attachment to us, a cornerstone of emotional health. But parents, particularly inexperienced new parents, often misconstrue what a secure attachment is and how to encourage it. Some of the popular child-rearing and parenting books, even if they have some insights on how to be loving and effective parents, add to the confusion, particularly regarding cosleeping and how much we should rely on nursing to soothe our babies. Instead of the books' teaching confident parenting, mums and dads have told me they often promote even more insecurity, second-guessing, and guilt, particularly if the approaches don't allow their child to be upset even briefly – as they inevitably will. We end up constantly worrying that we will emotionally damage our children, and we may decide to go through months or years of exhaustion rather than use even gentle methods to help our children learn to sleep on their own.

> Attachment between parents and children is a cornerstone of emotional health. But parents, particularly inexperienced new parents, often misconstrue what a secure attachment is and how we should encourage it in our children.

Attachment theory is not new. It dates back to the 1950s, when research by psychologist Mary D. S. Ainsworth and famed child psychiatrist John Bowlby laid the scientific groundwork for understanding how babies form healthy, secure attachments. A securely attached child feels loved, nurtured, safe, and protected in his relationship with his parents. And a secure attachment forecasts healthy social, emotional, cognitive, and motor development as the baby becomes a child, as the child becomes an adolescent, and as the adolescent becomes an adult.

In Chapter 6, 'Newborn to Five Months,' I'll share some more tips on how mums – and dads – can support their baby's emotional security, drawing from the excellent research reviewed by Lisa Berlin and her colleagues at the Center for Child and Family Policy at Duke University. Basically, as the Duke experts reassuringly remind us, we don't have to be perfect parents, even if we get all sorts of messages that make us feel guilty if we aren't perfect. We just have to be, as Ainsworth framed it years ago, 'good enough' at doing what comes naturally: providing warm, sensitive, positive, and responsive care. As we feed, soothe, hug, smile at, and look into the eyes of our babies, as we meet their needs and express our love, we cultivate a sense of trust. As they get older and begin to joyously and curiously navigate their expanding world, we encourage them with clear, consistent, developmentally appropriate expectations and protect them – but not overprotect them – with emotional and physical supervision. We don't want them to stray so far that they get lost or panicked or are at risk in any way, and we don't want them to get excessively frustrated. We do want them to crawl, toddle, or stride away from us to try out a new toy at playgroup, or to chase a butterfly in the park. We don't have to go get the new toy for them; we don't have to force them to be curious. We want them to feel confident in going forth, knowing they can return to us, the secure parental base.

> We want to strike that balance between security and support, confidence and freedom. We need to let our children learn, slowly and gently, to deal with emotions such as frustration, excitement, and anger and with behaviors such as sleep, to self-regulate. We can't do this for them, any more than a coach can get out on the field and play for his team.

In *A Secure Base: Parent-Child Attachment and Healthy Human Development* (1988), Bowlby cites studies that found that nursery schoolers 'who are most stable emotionally and making the most of their opportunities are those who have parents who, whilst always encouraging their children's autonomy, are nonetheless available and responsive when called upon.' In other words, we don't want to tie our children to us, nor do we want to cut them loose. We want that balance between security and support, confidence and freedom. We need to let our children learn to deal with emotions such as frustration, excitement, and anger, and with behaviors such as sleep, to self-regulate. We can't do this for them, any more than a coach can get out on the field and play for his team.

Families I work with like that coaching analogy. A coach teaches, directs, and supports the players, but he doesn't play the game for them, make the goal for them, swim faster for them. Even when the team loses, the coach can give strategies for doing better next time, but he still can't play the game for them. It's the same with sleep. We can help our children learn how to fall asleep, but we can't keep doing so much of it for them, not beyond the newborn stage. When they have trouble sleeping, we can empathize, we can reassure, we can guide, we can support – and like the coach, we can help them acquire the skills to do it better next time. But then we have to let them do it themselves.

Parents tell me that they are hesitant about providing structure and direction; they are nervous about enforcing rules or confronting negative behaviors. I often hear a parent say, 'I don't want my child to feel bad about himself' or 'I don't want to crush her spirit' or 'I don't want my child to not like me.' As my colleague Peter Grube, a clinical social worker, noted to me, 'Parents want to be loving, but unfortunately the term *loving* is often interpreted as meaning no boundaries for the child or parent.'

Countless studies tell us that our children do need structure, consistency, and clear boundaries, at bedtime and during the day. Setting limits does not mean that we don't give our children some choices or autonomy. Rather, it means giving age-appropriate choices within healthy boundaries. For instance, you might let a young child decide which pajamas he wants to wear to bed, or choose which dolls she wants tucked in with her at night. But you should not let her decide whether to brush her teeth or what time to go to bed. Alternatively, some parents go to the other extreme, never letting their children make any decisions for themselves for fear they might make a wrong choice and experience emotionally damaging frustration. My own sleep-coaching methods promote a secure attachment, a secure base. Aside from those first three months or so when our newborns do need us to create the magic of sleep, we aren't taking over their sleep indefinitely. I advocate letting them explore how to sleep for themselves, but I do not advocate letting them do it all on their own, or just shutting a door and letting them yell and scream. Gradually and gently, the baby learns to fall asleep on his own. His confidence grows as he learns that even if he can't always see us, we are right there, being loving and responsive parents.

Before we go on to talk briefly about crying and tears, let me share a wonderful quotation from Robert Karen's *Becoming Attached: First Relationships and How They Shape Our Capacity to Love* (1998): 'There is something simple and life-affirming in the attachment message – that the only thing your child needs in order to thrive emotionally is your emotional availability and responsiveness. You don't need to be rich or smart or talented or funny; you just have to be there, in both senses of the phrase. To your child, none of the rest matters, except inasmuch as it enables you to give of yourself.'

Setting limits does not mean that we don't give our children some choices or autonomy. It means giving age-appropriate choices within healthy boundaries.

Understanding Tears

Parents often tell me they can't stand hearing their child cry, that they fear crying will scar a child or cause emotional damage. I don't like forlorn, hysterical babies any more than you do, and I certainly couldn't have let my own babies wail in the dark. But there is no such thing as a tear-free childhood. The Sleep Lady system is designed to *minimize frustration and maximize reassurance*. By being present, by offering physical and verbal caresses and reassurances, we reduce the stress on ourselves and on our children, but we won't eliminate every single tear. However, it's easier for us as parents to tolerate the tears if we understand that they are a form of communication, and if we think about what our children are trying to tell us through their cries.

When a young baby or toddler is crying, he is telling you that he wants or needs something. And that's all his brain can concentrate on at that moment. When you calm him by helping him meet that need, his brain can focus on other things. But if you don't respond to that need, if you repeatedly ignore the cries, it can lead to overstimulation and lay the groundwork for later difficulties. Some research suggests that a pattern of unattended crying can actually affect the 'wiring' of the brain. A baby whose brain becomes used to chaos may seek out chaotic situations later in life. Now please note that I'm talking about *a pattern of prolonged unattended crying*. I don't mean that a little bit of crying will destroy your child's psyche or prevent him from forming a secure attachment. You will not scar your child for life if he fusses (safely) in his swing while you are right nearby taking a shower. Naturally, we are less tolerant of crying with a newborn than we are with an older baby. That's one reason I recommend only the gentlest of sleep-coaching techniques in the first few months of life, and I don't introduce my Sleep Lady Shuffle until a baby is six months old. (Sometimes a modified version can work at four months, with a pediatrician's approval, but more on that when we get into the age-specific chapters.)

Through my Sleep Lady system, you will learn when and how to put your child to bed when he is still awake – drowsy but still awake. And yes, you may well have some tears. But you will be able to respond to them, which is exactly what your heart and brain (not to mention all that attachment research we just reviewed) tell you to do. Hearing those cries can be hard on parents. It's easier if you remind yourself that the cries are his way of saying, 'Why did you put me down awake? I don't know how to go to sleep! *You're* supposed to put me to sleep. I am tired! What are you doing? Why have you changed things? This is frustrating, and *I don't like it one little bit!*' This is where you have to remember that you are the coach, not the player. You are giving love and support and comfort and reassurance – being that secure base. But you aren't fixing, rescuing, or doing it all for him. You aren't erasing every scrap of frustration (even if your heart aches to) at the price of his learning and sleeping. And once you give him that safe and secure space from which to learn, from which to explore, sleep isn't all that different from venturing out at that playgroup or chasing that butterfly.

You are the coach, not the player. You are giving love and support and comfort and reassurance – being that secure base. But you aren't fixing, rescuing, or doing it all for him.

Watch your baby. You will see him work through that frustration. You will see him discover what helps him go to sleep, what feels good, what is soothing. You will see him learn to suck his thumb, or rock his body, or rub a soft blanket against his cheek. Once children gain confidence, when they know they own this skill, going to sleep isn't so hard anymore; it isn't so mysterious. And there's no longer a need to cry. By teaching your child to sleep, you have not damaged him emotionally. You have helped him grow.

'We thought we were bad parents if he was crying,' said Megan, whose son, Bruce, you will meet in Chapter 8, 'Nine to Twelve Months.' 'We thought crying made him feel alone and abandoned; we thought crying was torturing him. But we learned that we were hurting him by not letting him sleep. Sleep was so important to his growth and development. You have to keep telling yourself that over and over again. He needs to sleep; what you are doing is right.'

Tess, who vividly recalled her own childhood fears and who had slept in her parents' bed until she was eight, was almost phobic about letting Jason cry, even when she was bone-tired and emotionally drained after being up all night with a ten month old who nursed every hour or two and spending all day in the hospital helping her mum get through chemotherapy. When Tess finally decided Jason needed to learn to sleep better, even if that meant some tears, she handed Jason over to her husband, Ron, and went to a hotel. 'I told a friend of mine I was convinced I was going to ruin Jason; she told me she knew a lot of messed-up people, but she didn't think it was because they had cried when they were ten months old,' Tess recalled with a laugh. The next morning, Tess approached her front door with her own tears flowing, convinced that she was going to find emotional wreckage within. Instead, Jason and Ron were happily playing on the living room floor. Jason had done some crying, and he would cry for two more nights — but only two more nights. He was learning to give himself and his parents some badly needed sleep.

Parents often ask me how long their child will cry. The answer is usually a lot less than you expect. However, older toddlers and preschoolers may cry and protest more than young babies simply because their problematic sleep patterns are more ingrained. Exceptionally aware and alert babies, like Ari in Chapter 6, 'Newborn to Five Months,' might cry a bit more than other children because they have a harder time shutting out the world so they can sleep. Children whose parents have been inconsistent about sleep may also cry more as you begin sleep coaching. But throughout this book, you will be able to see how more consistent parenting makes life – and sleep – easier both for ourselves and for our children.

Parents often ask me how long their child will cry.
The answer is usually a lot less than you expect.

Your Child's Sleep Success

When I work with a family, I explore their values, lifestyles, and approach to parenting as I develop an individual sleep plan. I never suggest anything that would make anyone feel like a horrible parent, nor do I believe in miracle cures. Changing sleep patterns can take time, and it definitely takes consistency. Most families solve their bedtime problems within two weeks, even if poor napping, early rising, and occasional night wakenings take a little longer.

Some of the families you will meet in this book experienced extremely rapid improvement. But more often I've chosen to include hard cases, families who faced challenges and setbacks, because I wanted this book to illustrate as many scenarios and solutions as possible. Don't be discouraged if it goes slowly, especially if your child is older and has been sleeping poorly for a long time. (My coauthor Joanne Kenen's son fell into that second category. A smart little guy who was able to stay remarkably cheerful on far too little sleep, Ilan was actually a difficult case, but with time, patience, and consistency he reached the point where he would go to bed and declare, 'I sleep great.')

Most families solve their bedtime problems within
two weeks, even if napping, early rising, and
occasional night wakenings take a little longer.

You will see progress quickly, but give it a few weeks to consolidate the gains, to see the old patterns fade away. Sometimes you'll
accomplish 90 percent of your goals in a matter of days, meaning
your life should be much more bearable. But it can then take longer
for you to get that last 10 percent in place. Be patient and remember
that learning a skill – whether sleeping, walking, handling a fork,
or using the potty – takes time. Disruptions of routines, including
illness, moving, travel, or a parent away on business, can also cause
temporary setbacks. If you stick to the routine, your child should
absorb those minor shocks and get back to his normal schedule in
a reasonable period of time. Eventually, his sleep skills will be so
secure that he can take them anywhere – on vacation, to his grandparents' house, later to slumber parties, summer camp, and even off
to college.

Before you turn to the chapter on your child's age group, please
read the remaining chapters in this section, where I outline my
methods and review a few simple essentials about sleep science that
will help you understand and interpret your child's natural rhythms.
My system works, and it can work for you. May you enjoy many
peaceful nights of sleep ahead!

1

The Sleep Lady System

As a loving and responsible parent, I believe we have five essential obligations to our children. We need to take care of their emotional health and their physical health. We need to give them good nutrition and a good education. And we need to make sure they know how to sleep. It's that simple and it's that important.

The Sleep Lady system gives you a framework for understanding your child's sleep and provides tools for modifying her sleep behavior. I give a lot of age-specific and problem-specific advice throughout the book, but in this chapter I'll give you some essentials that apply across most age groups. I always tell parents I need three things from them: patience, a united front, and consistency. We'll address all three of these in this chapter, particularly consistency, a cornerstone of behavioral psychology. In the next chapter, I will also give you some practical tips, steps that will help you get started and help you stay on track. Always, I will encourage you to mix the knowledge you gain with your own parental insights and instincts to develop sleep-enhancing solutions for your children and yourself.

The Sleep Lady Shuffle

In the first months of life, we concentrate on soothing techniques and establishing some basic rhythms to help babies learn to sleep. We aren't doing a lot of very active 'sleep training,' but we are laying the groundwork for good sleep, and for many babies these gentle steps will be enough to enable them to learn to fall asleep and stay asleep by themselves sometime between the age of three and six months. From about six months on, a central aspect of my program is the Sleep Lady Shuffle. Think of it as a kind of weaning for sleep. To give the child a consistent response, we use the Shuffle at bedtime, for middle-of-the-night wakenings, and, in many cases, for naps, too. The Shuffle varies subtly from one age to the next, and I'll walk you through it with a lot more detail in the age chapters.

Briefly, the Shuffle goes something like this: You, or your spouse or partner, will start out seated right by your child's cot or bed, where you can easily comfort and reassure her. Every three days, you are going to move a little further away, across the room, to the doorway, right out in the hall, but you will still be able to soothe her. Sometimes I advise parents to sleep on a mattress or sleeping bag in the baby's room for a few nights, as a reassuring prelude (although it may be the parents who need the reassurance as much as the child!). Sometimes if a baby is responding very quickly to the changes, I have the parent move through the Shuffle more rapidly.

Finally, you will be able to leave her alone for five minutes at a time so she can fall asleep on her own. This sounds like a huge leap for you, but it's not so huge for her. Through the Shuffle, you've given her nearly two weeks of preparation. As you have soothed her less, she's learned to soothe herself more, sucking a finger, twirling her hair, nestling into her blanket, or snuggling up to a teddy bear. You have slowly and gently moved away at bedtime and during the night, while letting her build confidence that you are still nearby and responsive. She has learned 'Mummy is there for me even though I can't see her,' and 'Daddy is nearby and loves me.' She will be ready to sleep on her own, if you let her.

In all probability you will still face some tears during the Shuffle, but generally much less than the hours parents commonly report in the crying-it-out and extinction methods. And usually you are close by and comforting her when she does cry, which is far less stressful for the parents.

> She has learned 'Mummy is there for me even though I can't see her,' and 'Daddy is nearby and loves me.' She will be ready to sleep on her own, if you let her.

Patience

You might be very tired the first few nights you embark on this program because in the short run you might get even less sleep. That's because as you modify your baby's sleep behavior, you are going to have to give up some of the middle-of-the-night crutches known as *negative associations* that may get her back to sleep in the short run but won't prevent her from popping up again in an hour. She may resist the change. The behavior may even get worse before it gets better as she adjusts to new routines, to new positive associations. Try to find some time to nap, or try to get to bed a little earlier than usual. Each morning, give yourself a pep talk and a reminder that it is worth it, that soon you all will be sleeping through the night.

A unique aspect of my private practice that parents find extremely helpful is frequent morning telephone calls. We speak every morning for the first five days, and then about every other day for the next two or three weeks. These intensive calls are part fine-tuning and part pep talk. They help a lot during those first draining days when it can be hard to keep perspective, to be patient and consistent, particularly if you've already gone months or years without a decent night's sleep.

As you aren't going to have me on the phone, find a sympathetic soul, a buddy, to talk to each morning. A spouse who is also familiar with the Sleep Lady approach. Another mum who has been through it all. Another sleep-starved parent who can be a partner as you go through the program together, critiquing, cheerleading, and supporting one another. You may find that every mum in your playgroup wants to take part! The point of these morning calls is to rehash the previous night, talk about what adjustments you need to make, whether it was great or whether you caved and did something you probably shouldn't have. Parents tell me they feel more accountable and stay on track when they have to report to someone every morning. They also like having someone to commiserate with during the hard parts and someone with whom to celebrate each bit of progress.

Parents tell me they feel more accountable and stay on track when they have to report to someone every morning. They also like having someone to commiserate with during the hard parts and someone with whom to celebrate each bit of progress.

A United Front

Before you decide exactly where you want to go with your child's sleep, take a good look at where you are. Get both parents involved, and, where relevant, other caretakers and grandparents.

Parents need to talk about their goals, and make sure they agree. For instance, if Mum wants the child to sleep in the family bed and Dad wants the baby in her cot, it is just not going to work. Similarly, if a mum's head is telling her that Junior should be in his cot, but her heart still yearns to have those sweet-smelling baby curls snuggled up next to her chin at night, it's a problem. Think it through. Talk it through. Discuss how much crying each of you can tolerate, and what your parenting styles are regarding limit setting and consistency.

Think about your child's temperament, history, and ability to self-regulate. What soothes him? What does he do to soothe himself? How can that be incorporated into his bedtime routine? You can't cleanly separate sleep from everything else in life in terms of parenting. If you make a plan but as parents you can't follow through together, it won't work and it's unfair to your child. If you are first-time parents, of course you may not yet know what your parenting style is, or what aspects of parenting are most challenging for each of you. Keep talking about it, and look for common ground.

Inconsistency is a big problem for children of all ages, right up through those teen years, and disagreement about child rearing can be a problem in marriages if you don't keep communication open. Shared responsibility and decision making about children promote happier marriages.

Parents need to talk about their goals
and make sure they agree.

Consistency

One of the most damaging things we can do as parents, whether we are dealing with sleep or other aspects of child rearing, is to be inconsistent. Psychologists call it *intermittent reinforcement*, and it means that sometimes you give in, and sometimes you don't, giving such a mixed message that a child, particularly a baby or toddler, can't make any sense of it. He can't figure out what behavior he must change and what behavior will be rewarded if he screams, whines, or wheedles enough. *Inconsistently reinforced behavior is the hardest type to modify or extinguish. It takes the longest to change, and it often provokes even more of the tears we are trying to avoid.* This is particularly true if the child is more than a year old. Sometimes it is okay for us as parents to bend rules, make exceptions, give treats. We all do it. But breaking rules hither and thither, responding in different ways all the time, is counterproductive, and that's doubly true for sleep.

> Inconsistently reinforced behavior is the hardest type
> to modify or extinguish. It takes the longest to
> change, and it often provokes even more of the tears
> we are trying to avoid.

An obvious example, one we've all seen and most of us will experience, is the toddler in the supermarket checkout line demanding sweets. Usually Mum (or Dad) says no, and the kid stops whining fast – or reasonably fast. But one day, for whatever reason, Mum gives in. Maybe she's tired. Maybe he's making a bigger scene than usual and Mum just wants to spare the other hundred sets of eardrums in the store. Whatever the reason, he smells blood – or at least he smells chocolate. The next time they are in the store, when he asks for sweets and Mum says no, he's not going to stop whining. He knows that she gave in once, and if he makes enough of a fuss, she may give in again. And he won't really understand if she doesn't. He'll be asking himself, quite legitimately, 'How come I can't have the sweets now if I had it last time? What can I do to get my way?' He's going to try everything he can think of, and it's not going to be pretty.

Now, if it's that hard to deal with lollipops with a well-rested child in a nice, bright supermarket, think about how painfully difficult it is to deal with a tired child in the middle of the night who doesn't know how to sleep. Consistency is absolutely crucial. *If you aren't consistent, you aren't just making it harder for yourself. You are making it harder for your child.* If you are trying to move a child out of your bed and into a cot, you need to keep him in the cot every night, not most nights. If you are trying to stop pacing up and down the hallway with him from 3:00 to 4:00 a.m., you need to resist the urge to pace every night, not most nights. He can't understand why you bring him into your bed on Tuesday but you let him scream for ninety minutes on Thursday, or why you won't take him to your bed at 1:00 a.m. but are too wiped out to resist at 4:00 a.m. *Babies can't tell time!* He's going to cry. It's his way of saying, 'Hey, what's going on here? It's late and I'm tired and I need to go back to sleep, and why can't I get into your bed now when you let me yesterday?'

> If you aren't consistent, you aren't just making it harder for yourself. You are making it harder for your child.

Decide on a response to his awakenings and then stick with it. You'll get some tears at first, but remember, you don't have to turn your back on those tears. Soothe him, help him, show and tell him that you love him, and the tears will stop.

Ellen, the mother of two, knew that it wasn't going to be easy to follow the Sleep Lady's advice in the middle of the night. She was softhearted and didn't like tears – and she was just so very, very tired. Sometimes it was so tempting to just give in and let James have one more bottle or let him snuggle in her bed. But Ellen knew she had to be consistent or she was going to be exhausted for the long haul – and her kids would end up with more of the tears of exhaustion, frustration, and confusion that she had hoped to avoid. Since I couldn't be there by her side cheering her on all night, she did the next best thing. She made herself cue cards and taped them by the cot. Here's what she wrote:

1. *Good sleep is good for the whole family. All deserve it and all benefit from it. We will be better parents, partners, friends, workers with enough sleep.*
2. *Good sleep habits are learned. I, as a good parent, must teach them to my children.*
3. *Husband and wife can sleep together. Their healthy relationship is very important to family life. A happy marriage helps kids be happy.*
4. *My child will grow and develop better with good sleep.*

I'm going to end this section with advice that may surprise you: I don't care what sleep system you use. Obviously, I have faith in the Sleep Lady approach. I know from my private practice, from the talks and workshops I've given, and from the response to the earlier editions of this book that tens of thousands of families have found it a workable, attainable, realistic system that starts showing benefits in just a few days. I think it provides the right balance by giving you clear rules and structure but also letting you adapt it to fit your own family. But if it's not right for you, try something else.

You've probably noticed that there is no shortage of sleep systems and books out there for you to choose from. Whatever method you choose, give it a chance. Don't follow my advice (or anyone else's, for that matter) for only twelve hours and then give up! Some studies have shown the 'extinction system,' where you let the baby cry and cry alone in his room, is fast and successful – for parents who can endure that many tears. *Whatever approach you choose, the key is consistency. If you don't follow it, it won't work.* And if you do follow it, research by the American Academy of Sleep Medicine has shown, it probably will work. Not 100 percent of the time, but you've got an excellent chance of success. But only if you are consistent.

Remember that when you start changing how you respond to your child's sleep and wake patterns, he may resist and for a couple of days (or nights) it may get worse before it gets better. Then if you remain consistent the tears will stop. Children actually crave consistency, and not just at bedtime. Our predictability reassures

Why Consistency Is Key

Intermittent reinforcement does make it harder for your child to learn to self-soothe and sleep. Here are three examples:

Parent #1 nurses her baby to sleep at bedtime. When he wakes up during the night, sometimes she nurses him back to sleep, and sometimes Dad rocks him to sleep. Usually at some point he's crying in confusion and frustration. Too tired to deal with it, Mum or Dad ends up taking him into their own bed, only to go through the whole mess again the next night.

Solution: Work toward putting your child down to bed drowsy but awake (which we'll learn more about in the next chapter). Respond to the baby consistently each time he wakes at night.

Parent #2 lets the baby cry – sometimes – for fifteen or thirty minutes because Mum or Dad is desperate and was told it might work. But Mum or Dad can't take the tears, and one of them ends up picking up the baby and rocking him to sleep. Without realizing it, Mum or Dad is training the baby that if he cries long and hard enough, his parents will do whatever they can to get him to sleep, and he will never learn to do it himself.

Solution: Don't embark on a cry-it-out system if you can't stand the tears! Try my gentler approach, or a cry-it-out variant where you can go in and check on the baby. Stick to it for more than a half hour!

Parent #3 brings the baby into her bed, but only after 5:00 a.m. This is a problem, as I've yet to meet an infant who can tell time. They will wake up earlier and earlier, not understanding why it's against the rules to go into Mum's bed at 2:00 a.m. or 3:00 a.m. or 4:00 a.m. but perfectly okay at 5:00 a.m. What the heck is a clock anyway?

Solution: Follow the advice for early risers in the chapter corresponding to your child's age. It's a particularly tough challenge, as we adults are not at our best at 5:00 a.m., but consistency is imperative.

them, and helps them know what to expect and what is expected of them. It helps them feel safe and sound. The more consistent you are, the faster he'll respond. The more mixed signals you give him, the longer and harder it will be for him to adapt. So consistency is truly a gift to your child. It's the key to success.

Cosleeping

Numerous studies and surveys have shown that cosleeping is on the rise, partly because more women are breastfeeding and many nursing mothers find it easier to have the baby right alongside them. Some families make a conscious decision to cosleep, either for the first few months or for several years, because they believe the family bed is the most emotionally satisfying approach, or it's most in tune with their parenting style. Others just sort of end up with the baby in their bed as the path of least resistance.

I devote a whole chapter to cosleeping (Chapter 12, 'Whose Bed Is It Anyway?') and encourage you to think it through before the baby is born, or at least in the first few months. Ask yourself where you want your child sleeping at age two, or four, or six. Think about changes in your lifestyle – another baby, a new partner if you are a single parent – that could alter the composition of the family bed or the dynamics of the family. Consider roomsharing as an alternative – keeping the baby in a cot or Moses basket right by your bed. If you want to keep the baby next to your bed for the first three months, which is a common choice, I'll help you transition at around twelve weeks. If you want to cosleep longer but want the child to be in her own bed by age two, I do recommend you begin the transition much earlier. What two year old willingly abandons her parents' bed to start sleeping alone in her own room? Since birth she has been under the impression that your bed *is* her bed!

If you like the idea of cosleeping but everybody is tired all the time – if it's all 'co-' and no 'sleep' – I would ask you to think it through once more.

If the family bed is the right choice for you emotionally and philosophically, if it's the right match for your parenting style, and if you follow all the cosleeping safety rules (see 'Safe Sleeping Recommendations' on page 495), I understand and support that decision. My family-bed chapter will show you how to help your baby strengthen her sleep skills, particularly while napping, even in a bedsharing family. But if you find that you like the idea of cosleeping but everybody is tired all the time – if it's all 'co-' and no 'sleep' – consider whether it's time to make a change. Don't feel like you have failed an early parenting test if you set out to cosleep and it just didn't work for you. It's hard to be a wonderful, responsive, cheerful parent if you are constantly fighting to keep your eyes open, and prolonged exhaustion can be a risk factor for depression.

The Sleep Lady System Works

One reason I believe so strongly in my approach is that I've seen it work over and over again. I can't tell you how many times I've had parents tell me that their child was impossible, that I wouldn't be able to help them, only to hear them declare a few weeks later that I had wrought a miracle: The baby was sleeping. In some cases, particularly with older children, a brief period of night wakening might persist for a while, but if you stick to the program, he'll eventually drop that one, too. Occasionally your child might regress, either because his routine has been thrown off or because he's entering a new developmental stage or just because he's having a few 'off' days. Don't despair. You will now have the tools to get him back on a good sleep schedule.

Nicole

When people ask me for a real-life example of how this works, I often think of Nicole. When Cory and Alan consulted me, Nicole was eleven months old and still getting up once or twice every night to nurse. Although she took two ninety-minute naps, her schedule was unpredictable, as was her morning wake-up time. Earlier Nicole had had several health problems

– reflux and dairy sensitivity, frequent ear infections – and Cory and Alan were not willing to let her cry too much at night. 'She was crying from pain, not behavior,' Cory said. 'Letting her cry that way just wasn't in me.'

By the time I met the family, Nicole's doctors had corrected or controlled her physical ailments. But her discomfort had left its mark. It had robbed her of the chance to learn to self-soothe and fall asleep on her own. Months later, the whole family was still paying the price. Cory later confided that when she logged on to my Web site, she burst into tears, so relieved that help was at hand. She recalled feeling, 'I just can't function like this anymore. I'm going to lose my mind.'

While Nicole was very little, she had slept in her parents' bed. 'We enjoyed that,' her mother said. 'I was nursing, and it was easy for me to have her there.' This was particularly true after Cory went back to her accounting job part-time when Nicole was three months old. At six or seven months, they moved her into a cot in her own room, but it wasn't easy to get her to sleep, and she still ended up in their bed a lot.

Even before they started working with me, Alan and Cory did have the beginnings of a good bedtime routine. At around 7:15, they would put on a classical CD, and Cory would nurse. They would put the baby into her cot with a dummy and Kitty the bear, her lovey. Sometimes she would drift off quickly, if a parent stayed in the room. But often she would need a few sessions of back rubbing. When they – intermittently – tried leaving her alone for ten minutes to see if she could fall asleep without them, she would scream and cry. Either Alan or Cory would return to her, rub her back, and sit by her side until she slept. Even then, she used to rouse herself the minute she heard one of the floorboards squeak as her parents tried to leave. 'I used to wish I could fly,' Cory recalled thinking as she tried to tiptoe out without making a sound.

Once they finally got her to sleep, it didn't last long. Sometime between 11:30 p.m. and 1:30 a.m. she awoke, wanting to nurse. Occasionally they tried to break her of the habit, but they never stuck to it (inter- mittent reinforcement!), and as far as Nicole was concerned, nursing was a nonnegotiable demand. After a few minutes, one of the sleepy parents would surrender, bringing her into their bed, where Cory would nurse and they would all try to sleep. 'It was the path of least resistance,' Cory said.

When I met Cory and Alan, we agreed on a few immediate changes.

Cory nursed Nicole a half hour before bedtime, not right at bedtime, to blur her association between nursing and sleep. They put a night light in her room and gave her more time to wind down in her room before they put her in her cot. And they would talk to her about their expectations. 'We would have a conversation: 'Now it's time for bed. We're putting on your night light. We're pulling down the shades.' They understand a lot more than you think they do, and we got her to sleep at night without a whole lot of crying,' Cory said. They began the Shuffle but never got past the first step, sitting by her cot. Nicole began falling asleep and staying asleep on her own almost immediately.

Though thrilled with the quick bedtime progress, Cory and Alan were apprehensive about her nighttime awakenings. That too went more smoothly than any of us anticipated. When they'd tried to stop nighttime nursing in the past, Alan would let her fall asleep in his arms. But no matter how delicately he handled his 'little package,' she woke up the instant he put her down. With my help, he learned how to soothe her while she stayed in the cot. He responded as soon as he heard her stir, trying to reach her before she was sitting up and moving much in her cot. He tried to soothe her back to sleep, without picking her up or bringing her to their bed. Instead, he rubbed her back sporadically and whispered to her just as he did at bedtime.

The first three nights were rough, but by the fourth night there was peace and quiet. Nicole had got the message and quickly decided that if she wasn't going to get nursed in the middle of the night, she wasn't going to bother getting up anymore. 'It's amazing how quickly it went. She almost knew we were trying to do something that was helpful to her,' Alan said. 'We had been artificially doing things she needed to learn on her own. But she was really ready for us to stop it.' She needed her parents to change their behaviors so she could learn to change hers.

As Nicole matured, her bedtime routine changed. She listens to more bedtime stories, and now she puts both Kitty and her baby doll to bed before her parents put her to bed. But by setting rules and sticking to them, Cory and Alan have kept bedtime a warm and cozy time, not a tug-of-war. They have also remained vigilant about keeping her bedtime steady, even on weekends. 'We work ourselves around her bedtime,' Cory said. 'We don't work her bedtime around ourselves.'

Looking back, Cory realizes how anxious she and Alan had been about

Nicole's bedtime, and how they may have transmitted that anxiety to their daughter, making it even harder for her to sleep. 'We used to think, "Oh, no, it's bedtime."' Now Cory and Alan listen to Nicole murmur herself to sleep, look at each other, and say, 'Oh my goodness, she's asleep. It's that simple.'

2

Getting Started and Tips for Success

Now that you know about my philosophy, my method, and the importance of consistency, let's go over some concepts and practical tools that will set you up for success.

Sleep Crutches

We have a lot of ways to help our newborns fall asleep. We nurse them, rock them, walk them, swing them, sing to them, rub their backs, grip their tiny fingers in their cots, take them into our beds. But as they get older – past three or four months, and definitely after six months – if we continue these behaviors until they fall sleep at bedtime and each time they wake up at night, they become *negative associations* or, as I prefer to call them, *sleep crutches*. Not because they are 'negative' or bad behaviors in and of themselves. They aren't. Rocking, snuggling, and singing are all wonderful behaviors. But they become a problem, or a crutch, when they are so closely linked in the child's mind with slumber that he cannot drift off without them. Throughout this book we'll be learning how to replace *negative* associations with *positive* ones that help babies and children go to sleep, stay asleep, and wake up happy.

Drowsy but Awake

If your baby falls sound asleep in your arms for every nap, every bedtime, every time he wakes up at night, he isn't going to have a clue about putting himself to sleep. I want you to put your baby down when he is 'drowsy but awake' so he can learn to do that last part of falling asleep on his own. We start doing this at bedtime when they are about six to eight weeks old (for healthy full-term babies) as we begin to gently shape our young babies' sleep. And it's essential that we do it as we go on to follow the Sleep Lady Shuffle. 'Drowsy but awake' takes on a different dimension as children get older. With toddlers and preschoolers, we rely on the calming routine of bedtime songs and stories to prepare them for slumber.

If you have trouble visualizing what 'drowsy but awake' means, imagine a scale of 1 to 10, 1 being wide awake and 10 being deep sleep. You want to put the baby down at about 7 or 8. He should be quite sleepy but awake enough to know that he is going into the cot. *If he falls asleep too quickly, in less than five minutes or so, he was probably too drowsy; put him to bed when he is a tad more alert the next night.*

If he's still waking up a lot at night, you may need to put him to sleep a little more awake at bedtime so he gets better at resettling himself when he stirs at night. Even when you put him down at the right point on the drowsiness scale, he might wake up a bit and protest and fuss as you lay him down. Don't worry – but don't get him out and start the whole routine over again. Instead, stay nearby and use your Sleep Lady comforting techniques to soothe and reassure him, and he will learn to transition from drowsiness to sleep.

If you rock, swing, or walk your baby to sleep, you may want to try cutting down the minutes. You want to reach the point where he is very calm and drowsy but not sound asleep. Watch your baby to see how he responds and adjust the timing accordingly. Every once in a while, a baby from about six to eighteen months will get really mad if you give him only ten minutes of, for instance, rocking when he's used to twenty minutes. He feels like you are teasing him. If he gets worked up, he isn't getting drowsy. Either limit the rocking to just one minute, or eliminate it completely. Give him a kiss, put him down, and incorporate other soothing techniques in a new bedtime routine. Remember, if you have to choose between too drowsy or too awake, choose awake and then work on soothing him to a drowsier point in the cot.

If you were nursing or bottlefeeding to sleep – by far the most common pattern I see with newborns and infants – shorten the last feeding before bedtime and feed him with a light on so you can pay close attention to him. When he stops sucking energetic-ally and swallowing, and instead is suckling gently, a sort of flut-tering motion on your breast (or bottle), he is past the 'drowsy' target. In fact, if you look, you'll see his eyes are probably closed. He's asleep or almost asleep. Unlatch him, put him down, and try to catch him a little earlier the next time.

Sleep Lady Tip

Try nursing with a dim light on. It will help you monitor his behavior and see where he is on that drowsiness scale. The dim light will also help lessen that association in his mind between nursing and falling asleep after the first few months.

If he wakes up as you are unlatching him and still seems hungry, giving you that look that says, 'Hey, I didn't mean to fall asleep on the job,' give him one more chance. Help him latch back on or give him the bottle. If he starts eating, fine, let him finish, because he's still hungry. But if he goes back to that fluttery suckling, you've been duped! He isn't hungry, he wants to suckle himself to sleep. Do either of the following:

1. Unlatch him, burp him, give him a kiss, put him to bed, and try for drowsy but awake the next night.
2. Arouse him just a bit – maybe through a diaper change or some minor adjustment to his clothes. Then put him in his cot, a bit more awake, and soothe him.

Experiment with both the timing and the lighting. You might want to feed him earlier, a bit before bedtime, so he isn't going directly from eating to sleeping. For example, maybe you bathe him and then feed him. See if reversing that order, feeding and then bathing, helps you reach 'drowsy but awake.' Try keeping a light on while you feed him, both to keep him from crossing that 'drowsy' point and to monitor his behavior and see where he is on the drowsiness scale. Having a light on will also help lessen the link in his mind between nursing and falling asleep. (During middle-of-the-night feedings, you want the light to be quite dim, enough for you to see him but not enough to make him more alert.)

If your child just doesn't get drowsy, if he's really good at fighting sleep to keep you close by and engaged, you will have to put him into his cot or bed anyway. But make sure you have an appropriate bedtime and a really good, relaxing evening routine to help prep his mind and body for sleep and give him some of that time with you. Once he's in bed, use your repertoire of soothing techniques to help him transition to sleep.

Choose the Right Time

Choose a time to start sleep coaching when you can expect about three weeks without any disruptions or major changes, including travel, moving, or having a new baby. If something unexpected occurs once you're in midprogram, such as illness, do the best you can to stick with it. Some families try to make these transitions during the summer or during the winter holiday season because the adults won't have to juggle so many work responsibilities. That often works well, but be very careful to keep the child's schedule consistent even if yours is not. For instance, don't introduce a sensible 7:30 p.m. bedtime the very week you plan to let her stay up until 10:00 with grandparents on Christmas Eve or are going to have a horde of entertaining young cousins camping out in your living room at half term.

When you choose a time to begin sleep shaping, start waking up your child at a consistent time for four or five days before, preferably around 7:00 or 7:30 a.m. Also make sure the child naps well for a day or two before you start, even if you have to bend all my napping rules or rely on the sleep crutches that we're about to phase out. You don't want to start sleep shaping with a baby who is already frustrated, cranky, and overtired.

> When you do pick a night to start sleep shaping,
> make sure the child gets a good nap that day – even
> if you have to bend my napping rules.

Keep a Log

Keep a log for a week or two as you familiarize yourself with this book. Some parents find it easiest to keep the log right next to the baby's bed so they can groggily scribble notes even at 3:00 a.m. Having a record in writing, instead of relying on scrambled mental notes in your sleep-deprived brain, will help illuminate your child's patterns and your own responses.

Here are some things to note in the log:

- Where and when the baby or child goes to sleep, naps, wakes, nurses, eats, and so on.
- When, how long, and how intensely he cries (for example, is it a whimper or a full-out scream?).
- The timing and frequency of night awakenings. How long does it take you to get him back to sleep? Do you rock him, walk him, nurse him, sing to him, rub his back, or take him into your bed?

Compare your child's daily schedule with the typical routine I suggest in the chapter corresponding to his age. If you are pretty much on track, terrific – part of your sleep-training work is already done. If not, don't worry, I'll walk you through it when we get to the chapter on your child's age. Babies adjust pretty easily because you'll be shifting to a schedule that corresponds to what their little bodies need.

Tracking your child's sleep patterns will help you better
read the cues he sends when he is tired and know
when to seize a sleep opportunity before that lethal
second wind of infant or toddler energy kicks in.

Once you start my program, continue your log. Keep it simple
enough so that it is manageable for you but detailed enough so
that you can see the patterns. Tracking his sleep patterns will help
you better read the cues he sends when he is tired and know when
to seize a sleep opportunity before that lethal second wind of infant
or toddler energy kicks in. The log will help you detect what situations or circumstances throw your child off so you can figure out
how to avoid them or compensate for them in the future.

The log will also help you see much more vividly those little
steps of progress that might not be so clear to you from day to day
– or night to night. And seeing progress helps keep *you* consistent.

*'I took a lot of notes. I looked at it like a prescription. 'This is the
routine. This is what I have to do.' I had to just try to stick to it as
strictly as I could,' said Linda, whose daughter was nearly one year
old. Adele, the mother of a toddler, found that keeping a rather detailed
log helped her stick to the program, although she had tried and failed
a half-dozen other sleep systems before. 'I would look at my log and
spend all day telling myself over and over this is what I had to do
at 3:00 a.m. If I had thought about it only before I went to bed, I
would never have remembered in the middle of the night. You have
to coach yourself.'*

As you learn about your child's routines and body clock, pay
attention to your own routines as well, particularly from about 6:00
p.m. to bedtime. Are you missing your baby's sleep cues because
you are so busy cooking dinner, washing dishes, checking mail or
e-mail, paying bills, or talking to your spouse about which one of
you has time to go to the cleaners, the chemist, and the school rota
the next day? Are you focused on an older child, or children, who
are also tired and need your attention in the evening? You may

need to postpone some of your evening tasks until after the kids are asleep, divvy them up differently with your spouse, or make some temporary modest tweaks to the older kids' routines until you get the baby sleeping. But please don't let them zone out in front of the television for hours!

Routines

When I talk about routines, I don't mean rigid, inflexible worship of the schedule gods. I mean a degree of predictability and stability, which many studies have shown children need. I will give you detailed suggestions of what an age-appropriate daily structure should look like for a newborn, an infant, a toddler, and a preschooler. If you are wildly off (and your log will be helpful), start adjusting. Eleven p.m. is not a suitable bedtime for a baby or even a school-age child, and 6:00 p.m. is not a wise time for a nap. Although I usually recommend making these adjustments gradually, thirty minutes or so at a time, sometimes with a child under the age of three you can make the changes quite quickly if you learn to recognize her natural patterns. (The log can help you see the patterns. For instance, if your twenty month old is used to going to bed at 10:00 p.m. but you can see he is drowsy at 7:30, you don't need to spend days gradually adjusting. Just put him to bed at 7:30 p.m. and make sure you do so, consistently, the next night and the night after that.)

Children also need consistent wake-up times. If your child wakes very early one day and very late the next (and 8:30 or 9:00 a.m. is very late for a baby), it throws off their internal clocks, making bedtime and especially naptime even more difficult. By about the age of five months, you should be waking her at a consistent time, usually around 7:00 or 7:30 a.m. Early rising is a whole different problem, and we'll spend a lot of time on it in the age chapters.

Sleep Lady Tip

A lot of parents ask me about sleep training two or more children, or how older children react when you are sleep training their baby brother or sister. Once you familiarize yourself with my system, please see Chapter 13, 'Helping Twins and Siblings Sleep.' I like holding 'family meetings' so the older children understand what's going on and buy into it. One crucial point: If you anticipate needing the cot for a new baby, make the older child's transition to a bed at least two months before or four months after the birth to avoid feelings of displacement. Better yet, if your toddler or preschooler is not ready to give up the cot, do not push it. Borrow a cot for the new baby or buy a secondhand one until he is ready. I address the move from cot to bed in Chapter 10 ('One and a Half to Two and a Half Years Old') and Chapter 11 ('Two and a Half to Five Years Old'), and I also talk about sleep-related adjustments to a new sibling in Chapter 16, 'Routine Busters.'

Bedtime

If there's one thing that just about every childhood sleep expert agrees on, it's that all children need a comforting and predictable bedtime routine. They need it from early infancy right up through the school years. A few quiet activities like books, songs, or prayers help the baby throw that switch in his brain from 'alert' to 'sleepy.' My bedtime motto is 'Bore them!' It's not the time for tickling, wrestling, pillow fights, scary stories, or anything else that stimulates him or makes him fight sleep. I also encourage attachment to a 'lovey,' a favorite stuffed animal or blanket that he can use to comfort himself when he sleeps (once he's old enough to have one safely, usually around six months). The whole tone of bedtime should be calm and reassuring as you prepare him to separate from you all night.

If your child hates some aspect of bedtime, get that part over with first. For instance, if she can't stand having her pajama top pulled over her head, do it right after her bath, not after you've nursed her, read three books, sung two songs, and got her all snug and cozy. If she can't stand brushing her teeth, even if you spent good money on a purple and pink vibrating enchanted-mermaid toothbrush, brush them as soon as you get her upstairs, not when she's drowsily saying her prayers. The point of your bedtime routine is to calm your child, not to get all those stubborn little toddler juices flowing.

Bedtime also has to be a sensible time, of course. Keeping a log and watching your baby, learning to see his natural sleep cues, will help you figure out his natural 'sleep window,' when he's ready to sleep. If you aren't confident that you are 'reading' him well, or he doesn't seem to have a consistent time yet, you'll find suggestions in the age-specific chapters. For example, a two year old needs eleven hours of sleep. Your two year old wakes up at about 7:00 a.m. That means she needs to be asleep – asleep, not getting ready for her bath – at 8:00 p.m. Add on whatever time you need for bed and bath routines. If you need forty-five minutes, start her evening routine at 7:15 p.m. If you need an hour, start the routine at 7:00. Better to leave a little extra time for a calm, relaxing bedtime than cutting it short and having everyone feel rushed, tense, and upset.

Dummies (Pacifiers)

Research and recommendations have changed over the years on dummy use, and they may well change again, so I suggest you discuss the issue with your doctor or health visitor. The current thinking, however, is that dummies not only satisfy a baby's instinct to suck but may also reduce the risk of sudden infant death syndrome (SIDS) in the first six months.

I usually tell parents not to use the dummy for the first three or four weeks, until breastfeeding is well established. (Some doctors and lactation consultants say six weeks. Ask yours.) You don't have to use it 24/7. If it falls out, don't feel you have to constantly replug it. If the baby doesn't want it, don't force it. Because of the SIDS research, some parents use the dummy quite a bit for the first six months. Others, after going in thirty times a night to replug it, decide to do without. We'll talk about how to stop dummy use in the relevant age chapters.

Some Other Helpful Hints

- Most sleep problems are behavioral, not medical, *but check with your doctor to rule out any physical causes or undetected disease.* Make sure medications, including over-the-counter remedies, aren't disturbing her sleep.
- Babies exposed to bright lights in the early afternoon often sleep better at night. This is pretty natural for most of the year, but you may have to work on it during the winter.
- Leave a dim night light on. (A few kids I've worked with did better in total darkness, but you'll probably be able to figure it out quickly.) Besides, you'll probably want a bit of light while you are sleep training so you aren't bumping around in total darkness. Some researchers recommend avoiding exposure to light at night – both for babies and for parents, because it interferes with melatonin and the biology of sleep. Lights that are amber, orange, or red may be less disruptive than your conventional white lightbulbs that have blue rays. If you are a parent who has a lot of trouble getting back to sleep after being up with the baby or who had trouble with postnatal depression, you might want to try amber glasses (see www.lowbluelights.com) to screen out certain parts of the light spectrum at night.

- Consider using a white-noise machine or a fan if you live in a particularly noisy home. I particularly like the Marpac Sleepmate 980, but there are plenty of good, small, inexpensive models on the market (including some small enough to travel with, which can help). Children can and should learn to sleep through routine household sounds, but some places are just really loud, and some kids are really sensitive. Go ahead and block the noise from heavy traffic, rumbling trucks, nearby construction, barking dogs, noisy neighbors, or siblings and the like.
- If you will worry less – and sleep better yourself – when you can hear *and* see your baby stir at night, you may want to buy a video monitor. That way you won't be tempted to rush in and wake your baby even more just as she is learning to self-soothe herself back to sleep, and you may find that you fall back to sleep more easily yourself if you don't get up and walk (or run!) around. On the monitor, you'll see that she's all right – and know if there's a problem that really does require your presence. It's not a necessity, but it's something that makes some parents feel better; it's your choice.

Sleep Lady Tip

Some families like to use lullabies to mask sounds, but I prefer playing lullabies during the bedtime routine, not while he's falling asleep, so he doesn't get so accustomed to the music that he needs you to come in and press 'rewind' five times a night.

- Install room-darkening shades, particularly if your child is an early riser or a problem napper.
- Many young children wake too early – before 6:00 a.m. – and we'll talk a lot about Sleep Lady techniques for early risers throughout the book. A wake-up light or music can signal your child when he needs to try to go back to sleep or at least stay in his bed, and when it's okay to get up and start his day. First you can try a wake-up light. Get an appliance timer from a hard-

ware store and attach it to a lamp in his room. If he sleeps through it sometimes, fine, but you can teach him (as he develops the necessary language skills) that he can't get up before his light goes on. Set it for about 6:00 a.m., and once he sleeps pretty consistently until 6:00, you can gradually set it later. The wake-up light can work right through the preschool years. At around age two and a half, if you choose to, you can use a wake-up sound instead of a light – a clock radio or an iPod or CD player with a timer. Keep it out of reach for safety, or if he has learned how to turn it on himself. Some families stick with the light because it's less likely to wake the child, but it's your choice. With either the light or the music, be consistent. If you allow your child to get out of bed and start his day even fifteen or twenty minutes before the wake-up music or light comes on, she will not take the music or light seriously the next day. Why should she be consistent about it if you aren't?

- You might be astonished to learn how many babies and toddlers have televisions in their bedrooms. I strongly recommend against this. TV is a common sleep crutch for adults; it's why companies manufacture sets with timers. Watching television puts the brain into a light trance, similar to the first stages of sleep. You want this to occur in a cot or bed, without the television as a sleep crutch. Also, as children get older, they learn to put the television on themselves, and if it's in their room, it becomes harder for you to monitor what they are watching and when they are watching it. Ditto for computers. I don't like them in kids' bedrooms, and you really are going to want the computer in a place where you can monitor it when they get older.

- If you live in a one-bedroom flat, you can still sleep coach, but you'll have to be a bit more creative as you preserve the concept of gradually fading away from the cot. The beginning of the Shuffle, through night 3, will be the same. Starting on the fourth night, if the baby wakes up in the middle of the night, go to the cot and do a quick reassurance check. Then go to your own bed and use your voice to keep soothing him. You can sit up in your bed if you want so he can see you. Some parents have reversed the process, starting the cot next to the adult bed and gradually moving it further away. Mum is just where she always was! You could also try a room divider, either buying a screen or hanging a sheet if you think it's too hard for your baby to see you sleeping close by but not with him.

- If your child gets soaking wet at night, or goes through an occasional phase when he gets soaked, use a larger-size nappy with an insert or find extra-absorbent overnight nappies. Not all stores carry the overnight varieties anymore, but if you look around you will find them. Nappy inserts, or 'doublers,' are an extra pad that you can stick in the nappy and use overnight, or when the child is sick. They can be very handy when you are taking a long car or plane trip as well. If you are a good quick-change artist, you might be able to remove the soaked nappy quickly while he is in a deep sleep. Try to do this without taking him out of his cot or bed.

- Some children dirty their nappy just as you put them to bed at night or naptime – and some parents become convinced that it's intentional, that the child knows you will pick him up and get him out of the cot. Obviously, you need to change the child, but do it as quietly as you can, in light as dim as possible. If you can manage it, slip a travel changing pad under him and change him in the bed or cot instead of picking him up, taking him out, and having to get him back into bed all over again. If this happens while you are doing the Sleep Lady Shuffle, just change him, hand him his lovey, and return to your Shuffle position.

  If this happens at naptime, view it as a too short nap and follow the nap-training advice in the appropriate age chapter. If it happens at 5:00 a.m., follow the advice for early risers. Children often find it difficult to go back to sleep after a thirty-minute nap and then a nappy change, or after a 5:00 a.m. nappy change. You may see some crying here, but stay consistent and reassuring. If you feel your child needs a little more reassurance than normal to go back to sleep after his nappy change, then it is okay to sit closer that night if you feel it will help. On the following night return to your usual routine.

- A lot of parents worry that if they let their babies cry too long, they will vomit, particularly if the child has or had reflux. This may be the case if you leave the child to cry extensively on his own, but I have found it is extremely rare when parents use my gentler, more gradual method and stay in the room to comfort their child. If your child is prone to vomiting, for reflux or other reasons, avoid feeding him right before bed so he has time to digest. (For tips on handling reflux, see Chapter 15, 'Medical Problems.')

Occasionally, a young child, or even a baby, vomits intentionally because he knows Mum or Dad will take him out of his cot and fuss over him. If you see your child trying to make himself gag (and they can do this without using fingers), firmly say 'No!' but immediately follow up with soothing reassurance. If he does throw up, keep the cleanup as quick as possible, and try not to talk to him or engage him too much. Use wipes or a nappy or a washcloth, if you can, rather than getting him completely up for a bath. Don't turn the lights on, if you can help it. Some parents leave an extra sheet on the floor to use for cleanup so they can just roll it up and toss it in the hamper. You may want to offer a sip of water, if they have started taking water, but I don't recommend feeding them again. Reassure your child back to sleep. Remember, you don't want to give the message that if he throws up, he will get out of the cot and not have to go to sleep. This isn't very common, so don't worry too much about it.

Obviously, this doesn't apply to a child who is sick. In that case, you need to comfort him and follow your doctor's timetable for giving him fluids. In the past, some sleep experts told parents not to worry if the babies cried until they threw up, to just ignore it. I never agreed with that, and I don't think many of the leading experts out there today would endorse that attitude, even if their systems tolerate more tears than mine does.

• To the extent possible, work with babysitters and child care centers to develop consistent, or at least not wildly incompatible, sleep rules and schedules. But if your otherwise warm, loving, and reliable sitter can't handle any aspect of sleep coaching, particularly nap training, which can be hard, do your best to work around her and improvise where you have to. For instance, focus on nights and weekend naps if you can't get the sitter to do weekday naps. Ditto for child care centers, which may or may not have the flexibility to work with you. Quality child care is too hard to find to risk losing it. (For more details on napping at a child care center, see Chapter 16, 'Routine Busters.')

Sleep Lady Tip

Children need morning rituals just as much as they need bedtime rituals. These rituals help reinforce their understanding of wake-up time versus sleep time.

- If your child has a particularly rough night while you are doing the Shuffle, don't stop the sleep training. Keep going. But you may need to let him nap more for a day so he doesn't get impossibly overtired and make the next night even more of a challenge. Provide the extra naptime within the sample timelines I give in the age chapters. Let's say that your eight month old has been up since 5:00 a.m. On a normal day, he would start his nap at around 9:00 a.m., but on this day he'll be too tired to stay awake until 9:00. Don't force it. Let him nap at 8:00 – but don't throw his schedule completely out of whack by letting him nap at 6:30. If he takes a third little nap in late afternoon, that's fine. Or if he sleeps a half hour longer than usual for a nap, that's fine, too. Similarly, if your preschooler normally naps from 1:00 p.m. to 3:00 p.m., it's okay to let him sleep until 4:00 if he needs it after a rough night or a too early morning – but don't let him snooze all the way until dinner. Another way of handling a temporary sleep deficit is to put the child to bed a little earlier than usual for a few nights. In short, watch your child, trust yourself, and make some commonsense adjustments, but keep them within the basic framework of an age-appropriate schedule.
- Do a 'dramatic wake-up.' Throw open the blinds, switch on the lights, sing some cheery good-morning songs, and start the day.

A lot of families like having morning be 'Daddy playtime,' especially for fathers who come home on the late side from work and get little or no evening time with their child. Dads also tend to like to play games that are very active, maybe a little rambunctious, and it's far preferable to play helicopter or rocket ship in the morning than right before bed.

- I will often remind you to avoid picking up or snuggling your baby at certain times of night, or after the first night of the Shuffle (although I do believe in plenty of soothing and physical affection). *If your child is crying very hard, go ahead and pick him up briefly to reassure him, but don't let him fall asleep in your arms.* The no-snuggles edict does not apply to a child who is sick or who has had a nightmare or scare. Just try not to do so much snuggling that he will expect it even when he is feeling better. In general, I'd rather have you sleep in a makeshift bed next to a sick child than to allow him in your bed if you've just ended cosleeping. But I know a lot of parents who do bend this rule. Just make sure to get back to your usual routine as soon as possible.

- Once your child can speak, avoid power struggles but encourage them to 'buy into bedtime.' You want win–win cooperation, not win–lose confrontation. For instance, don't say, 'Mary, would you like to take a bath now?' If she says 'No!' (and some toddlers might say no even if they do want a bath!), you have set up a confrontation. Better option: 'Mary, it's time for your bath. Why don't you pick which of these three toys you want to play with?' (or 'which of these two pajamas you want to wear' or 'a song you want me to sing'). You are respecting and encouraging her growing autonomy and sense of self – but still getting her into that bathtub on time.

- If you are working on stopping or reducing breastfeeding at night, it's often best to put the father in charge of that aspect of sleep training. If the baby sees Mum, he will naturally hope and expect to be nursed, and he's going to be even more upset when those hopes are dashed by Mum. Also, Dad may or may not have a better tear tolerance than Mum, but he definitely can't cave in, lift his shirt, and nurse.

- Both parents should be able to put the child to bed. They don't have to have absolutely identical routines, but they need to be similar, and they need to have similar responses to tantrums, stalling tactics, and the like. It's generally a good idea to have one parent in charge at each bedtime when you are doing sleep training. In other words, if you are on night 5 of the Sleep Lady Shuffle, and Dad is positioned in his chair at bedtime or for a night wakening, Mum shouldn't switch places with Dad after ten minutes. This just stimulates and confuses the child. It's also often a good idea to have one person 'on duty' per night for middle-of-the-night wakenings. Some couples do, however, trade off because of their own sleep needs and body rhythms, with, say, Mum taking midnight to 3:00 a.m. and Dad taking 3:00 to 6:00 a.m.

Special Tips for Very Alert Children

Often in my practice I've found that unusually alert, bright, and aware children tend to have a little more trouble learning to sleep. These children often reach their physical milestones, like walking, on the early side, and they tend to have slightly disturbed sleep. Temperamentally, they may be the kind of children who know what they want and when they want it and are willing to hold out until they get it. That's a great quality in an adult, but it can be a little daunting to parent such a determined little person.

Make sure you don't fall into the trap of thinking that an alert child needs less sleep than average. He needs just as much sleep as any other baby – maybe even a little *more* than average – but he has a harder time shutting out the world in order to get to sleep.

Room-darkening shades are essential for these babies and children; sound screens can help for naps. These babies may also need to be nursed in a dim, quiet environment because they are easily distracted. Be extremely vigilant about watching their sleep windows, as their sleep clues are often difficult to read. These children tend to be less flexible sleepers for several years, so they can be extrasensitive to disruptions of routine or travel. My suggestions in Chapter 16, 'Routine Busters,' can help.

These kids are a bit temperamentally different from other children. But that does not mean they can't learn to sleep; I've seen them learn, and you'll read about a few success stories with children like this later on in this book. It might take them a little longer. They may test you a bit more. And you are going to have to be extrasuper patient and consistent. But it can and will work if you stick to it. My second child, Gretchen, was very alert, as was Joanne's son Ilan. Both learned to sleep – and their alertness and inquisitiveness have been assets, not liabilities. High alertness as a baby is not an early warning sign of attention deficit/hyperactivity disorder.

3

Lessons from Itsy Bitsy Yoga

Parents from all over the world, from vastly different cultures, ask me for ways to strengthen the bond with their children while helping them calm their bodies and minds before naptime and bedtime. A few years ago, I discovered Helen Garabedian and Itsy Bitsy Yoga® (www.itsybitsyyoga.com). I've experienced the benefits of yoga personally, on my own and with my daughters. And I've seen how much her Itsy Bitsy Yoga program (or you may be able to find baby-parent yoga classes near your home) can help parents and young children. I'm very grateful that Helen has allowed me to share some poses that you can do with your child (or children) at home. They dovetail beautifully with my Sleep Lady system.

Helen is a mother, author, certified Hatha yoga teacher, infant-massage instructor, and infant developmental movement educator. Her Itsy Bitsy Yoga blends yoga postures, developmental movement, and parent-child bonding.

We all know that healthy physical activity helps us sleep more soundly. You probably shouldn't do your vigorous, blood-pumping aerobics routine right before bed, but gentler activities like yoga or stretching routines are terrific evening rituals. Yoga can be beneficial for small children, too. As Helen says, 'Yoga and mindful relaxation help calm the mind and body before bed. Parents who practice

Itsy Bitsy Yoga with their children notice their children sleep longer and more soundly on days that yoga is practiced. Naps double in length and they sleep longer through the night too!' For mums, yoga can be a great way of easing ourselves back into a regular exercise routine after pregnancy, and some of the stretches can open up those shoulder and back muscles that we may tense as we get used to breastfeeding and caregiving.

In this chapter you'll learn five Itsy Bitsy Yoga poses that you can easily incorporate into your naptime and bedtime routines. You can start them anytime, even with a newborn and include them in the bedtime routine right up through to the age of four. With young babies, the poses can help get them ready for that calm and contented 'drowsy but awake' stage we strive for at bedtime. If you are doing the Sleep Lady Shuffle with a toddler or young child, the poses can create a calm prelude.

Practice the poses in a calm, relaxed environment free of distractions. Your child's bedroom with the shades down, or after a bath, is perfect! Use a yoga mat or a favorite blanket. The routine is a mutually rewarding presleep ritual that takes as little as five minutes (but you and the baby may love it so much you'll want to take longer). Mix and match the poses as you wish, doing any combination or all five. It's helpful to make the poses a consistent part of the bedtime and naptime routine, as predictability helps babies sleep easier and faster. But if you skip once in a while, it's nothing to worry about – although once you see how much your baby loves this, you probably won't skip very often.

Heart-Warm Touch

A baby can lie on either his back or his tummy. Toddlers can be in any stationary position. Rub the palms of your hands together above your child to generate warmth and love. Imagine loving energy pouring out from your heart and into your hands. Place both your hands on your child's shoulders and slowly move your Heart-Warm Touch all the way down his body to the tips of his toes. Caress his body with this firm and predictable Heart-Warm Touch for up to one minute. Sweetly singing your child's name as you perform the Heart-Warm Touch can enhance the experience.

Heart-Warm Touch Benefits: Similar to the feeling your baby enjoyed while in a cozy womb. Deepens the parent-child bond through skin-to-skin contact. If a baby is failing to thrive or was born prematurely, this pose may help him establish a healthier weight. Builds muscle tone and body awareness.

Corkscrew

Let your child rest on her back with your thumbs holding the back of her thighs and your forefingers resting on top of her thighs. Circle her thighs clockwise with both your hands as you sweetly say (and sing) the word *corkscrew*. If your child is mobile, you may wish to give her a toy to hold while engaging her in Corkscrew. Continue for five to sixty seconds, keeping your voice and movement fluid and rhythmic.

Corkscrew Benefits: Relieves gas, eases constipation, builds lower digestive tone, and promotes sleep.

Rolio

Position your child on her back with her feet nearest you. Using both of your hands, bring your child's two hands together above her chest. While continuing to hold your child's hands together with one hand, use your dominant hand to bring her feet up into your hands one at a time. Now your baby's hands and feet are held with your two hands. Place both of your thumbs behind the heels of her feet. Position your baby's wrists between your middle and index fingers. Your remaining fingers rest gently on top of her wrists. Roll your child's body from side to side as fast or as slowly as she would like as you emphasize the three syllables found in the word *Rolio* with your sweetest voice.

Rolio Modifications Based on Age

- *Younger babies* – Until a baby starts to bring his feet into his hands, at five or six months, Helen Garabedian recommends a developmentally appropriate modification that does not include gathering the baby's feet to hands. Place your first two fingers on your baby's cheeks and use your lower palms and hands to embrace your baby's shoulders so as to keep his head aligned with the spine. Encourage a slow forty-five-degree roll to alternating sides as directed. Holding feet with hands occurs naturally at about five to six months, shortly after the baby learns to roll over, and that's when it's okay to include the baby's feet in Rolio.
- *Toddlers* – Invite your toddler to wrap his hands and feet around an oversized stuffed animal so it makes it easier to roll in Rolio.
- *Preschoolers* – Encourage your youngster to do Rolio beside you or on her own.

Rolio Benefits: Builds hand-eye coordination. Soothes the central nervous system. Increases the circulation of cerebrospinal fluid. Relaxes your child.

I Love You

Place your child on his back on a blanket with his feet nearest you. Place your thumbs into the palms of your child's hands. Wrap your fingers around the outside of his hands. Mindfully repeat the words *I love you* s-l-o-w-l-y as you and your baby perform the following movements together:

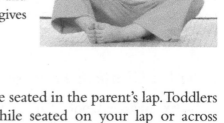

I: Guide his fists to his heart.

Love: Guide his fists and arms out to the side.

You: Guide his fists to his heart and wiggle him side to side as he gives himself a hug.

Repeat three to five times.

Mobile babies can do this while seated in the parent's lap. Toddlers and preschoolers can do this while seated on your lap or across from you. You can ask him what he loved about his day or what his favorite animal is. Be creative.

I: Bring both fists to your heart.

Like or *Love*: Open both arms out to your sides.

Their Answer: Bring your arms in and hug yourself (or hug both of you if she's on your lap) as you wiggle side to side.

Invite toddlers to say the words and practice this activity more independently with each repetition.

This is a great way to wind down or recap the day's activities.

I Love You Benefits: Crosses the body's midline, which helps integrate the right and left parts of the brain and body, allowing for better focus today and in the future. Expands breathing capacity. Increases spatial, organizational, and bodily awareness. Soothes children and helps to regulate their vestibular system (which controls balance). Deepens parent-child bond.

Special-You Song

This easy song and exercise combination is similar to the tune 'If You're Happy and You Know It.' Practice this activity with your baby in his cot or with a toddler lying in bed. As a toddler begins to identify his own body parts, invite him to place his own hands on the suggested body parts (eyes, head, and so forth) while mimicking the parent.

Sing and Do

If you're special and you know it, touch your head!
(Your hands touch the top of your baby's head.)
If you're special and you know it, touch your eyes!
(Your hands touch your baby's eyebrows.)
If you're special and you know it, touch your throat!
(Your hands touch your baby's throat.)

Continue this pattern for the heart, tummy, belly button, legs, and feet and finish with 'You're special and you know it 'cause your body is here to show it!' Caress her with a steady, smooth stroke of your hand from head to toe. Your toddler can rub her hands together.

'You are special and you know it – Namaste!' (which means 'The light in me honors the light in you.')

Share the Heart-Warm Touch you learned earlier in this chapter with your baby. Have your toddler give herself a soft huglike massage down her arms and legs.

Finish by placing the palms of your hands together in front of your heart. Gaze lovingly and bow to honor yourself and your child.

Special-You Song Benefits: Builds body awareness, increases self-esteem, deepens the parent-child bond, provides loving and gentle tactile stimulation.

If you have a hard time imagining your child sitting still for yoga, or you feel your baby is too overtired and fussy to do this before bed, visit www.itsybitsyyoga.com/sleeplady.html to download several additional poses to calm your fussy or active child. Try a little bit at a time as you and the baby get used to it and see and feel the benefits.

4

Sleep Basics

Physical Basics

Sleep Cycles

Sleep is divided into two basic types, REM (rapid eye movement, also known as dream sleep) and non-REM. REM sleep is active sleep, and it's also a lighter sleep. It's the sleep in which we dream and organize our memories. During REM we have limp limbs, irregular breathing, twitching, and rapid eye movement.

Non-REM has several stages of its own. They are called *light sleep*, *true sleep*, and *deep sleep*. As we pass through these non-REM stages, we move from a gentle drowsiness to that state of deep, deep sleep where, if awakened, we feel groggy and a little disoriented. During non-REM sleep our breathing is slow and regular. Our muscles are a little tense, and not as floppy as in REM sleep.

Children also have both non-REM and REM cycles, although their sleep cycles differ from adults'. For the first four months their sleep, particularly daytime napping, is not very organized neurologically. About half of their sleep is light REM sleep, when they are quite active and easily aroused. For a newborn, that's about eight hours of REM sleep and eight hours of non-REM sleep a day. At around four months, REM sleep begins to slowly drop off, and by age two a child's sleep cycles more closely resemble those of an adult. REM constitutes about 20 to 25 percent of adult sleep, or about two hours a night.

We all go through these sleep cycles, and as we switch from one phase to another, the change in our brain activity often wakes us up a little bit. This is called a *partial arousal*. Sometimes we are more awake than at other times. For instance, about every 90 to 110 minutes (50 minutes for infants), while we are still in a fairly light sleep, we have a partial arousal. We don't wake up completely, but we may mumble or roll over, for example.

Nobody 'sleeps through the night.'

Every three to four hours, we experience a partial wakening that is a little more pronounced. Maybe we notice that our pillow is on the floor, or we want a sip of water, or we need to adjust the blanket. Usually we get right back to sleep and scarcely remember the awakening in the morning. But that's because we know how to get ourselves back to sleep. Babies don't – until we teach them.

When babies experience these partial arousals, they may cry out, thrash around, become startled. If they have negative sleep associations or sleep crutches, if they need us to get them back to sleep, the partial arousal will become a complete arousal. They are basically saying to themselves, 'Hey, I'm sort of awake and I'm in my cot. I'm tired and I don't know how to go back to sleep without Mum nursing me or Dad walking me up and down the hallway, or someone helping me find my dummy. So now I'm going to do the only thing I can do. I'm going to cry.'

Once we help our children give up these associations, they will still have the partial awakenings, but they will no longer need to let you in on them. They can open their eyes for a second, recognize that they are safe in their own room, and then suck their thumb or reach out for their favorite stuffed animal or special blankie and get themselves back to sleep. The partial arousal stays partial.

Clocks and Windows

We all have a circadian rhythm, an internal clock that tells us when to be awake and when to be asleep. Falling asleep when our body clock is set to 'wake' is challenging, as is staying alert when our clock says 'sleep.' Sleep is not as restorative – meaning we don't feel as rested – when we sleep off our clock or when our clock is on a 'wake' mode. For example, people who sleep all day and work the graveyard shift, from midnight to 8:00 a.m., often don't get quality sleep because they are not in sync with their internal clocks. Or, for a two year old, a nap from 1:00 to 3:00 in the afternoon feels better than a nap from 4:00 to 6:00 in the evening. The clock is mostly set by light, although social cues such as noise and temperature can affect it, too. This is one reason that I recommend room-darkening shades for children, particularly those who wake up very early or who have trouble napping.

As adults we know how to compensate, at least in part, when our circadian clock is upset. If we have to go to sleep one night well before our usual bedtime, to catch a plane or attend an unusually early meeting, we know how to prepare ourselves, to cue our brains to sleep at the unaccustomed hour. We try a hot bath, a good book, a relaxation tape, or maybe just a mental image of a warm, palm-fringed beach. Babies don't know all those tricks. They need us to protect their sleep by paying attention to the clock – both the external time and the baby's internal rhythm.

> We sleep better, and we feel better, if we go to sleep at about the same time each night and wake up at the same time each morning.

To keep ourselves 'ticking' well and protect our sleep, we should regulate our sleep. We sleep better, and we feel better, if we go to sleep at about the same time each night and wake up at the same time each morning. We can vary our routine on weekends, but only by an hour.

> A well-rested child can handle variations in a sleep
> schedule better than an overtired child.

Babies are even more sensitive, especially if they are already overtired. A well-rested child can handle variations in a sleep schedule better than an overtired child. We all know they need routines and predictability for their emotional well-being, for that sense of order and security in their new world. But they also need routines to keep their internal clocks correctly 'wound,' and to cue their brains to start preparing for sleep by secreting melatonin. Production of melatonin, a hormone that promotes sleep by relaxing our muscles and making us drowsy, begins at about three months. Secretion levels are linked to darkness, another aspect of our circadian rhythm.

If you miss your child's 'sleep window,' that natural time to sleep, his body won't be pumping out calming melatonin. Precisely the opposite will occur. His adrenal glands will send out a rush of cortisol, a stress-related hormone that will overstimulate your baby, make him 'wired,' and create a second wind. To him, it probably feels like you slipped a double shot of espresso into his bottle. He will be more agitated, more difficult to console, more likely to need a lot more of your time and energy to help him wind down again and get to sleep.

So if, by natural rhythm and habit, he is ready for sleep at 7:00 but you keep him up until 8:00, he is going to have a hard time getting to sleep. And even after he does get to sleep – often with a lot more tears and resistance than normal – the cortisol and over-tiredness team up to make it harder for him to stay asleep. He is more likely to wake up at night and to wake up too early in the morning, before he is truly rested.

This cycle can then lead to poor naps the next day, which will lead to an overtired baby at bedtime, which leads to poor night-time sleep. We've all seen this pattern in our children at some time – I know I've seen it in mine, and they are good sleepers. Our task is to correct this cycle before it becomes a self-perpetuating downward spiral.

Sleep Window Signs

Recognizing your child's sleep windows so that you can get him down before the cortisol rush is key. What should you look for?

- eye rubbing
- yawning
- slowed activity
- listlessness
- limpness
- zoning or staring blankly into space
- whining and fussing
- loss of interest in people and toys

It takes a little practice to spot the signs because not all kids are the same, and some may have their own unique signals, like asking to read stories or to snuggle with a special stuffed animal. But the end result will always be 'Put me to bed right now or you'll regret it.' If you have trouble detecting your child's signals, keep one eye on him and another on the clock. Try going into a quiet, dimly lit room and engaging in a very gentle activity when you think naptime or bedtime is approaching. The signs may then appear.

At two, my coauthor's son Ilan would rub his eyes and ask for his special songs when he got sleepy, even if he was proclaiming loudly that he didn't want to go to bed. From monitoring the eye rubbing and his general activity level, Joanne would usually know whether to speed up or slow down the bedtime routine to calibrate exactly when his head should hit the pillow. But some nights he was able to mask his tiredness. If he began leaping up and down, shouting gleefully, 'I jump on bed like monkey, Mummy,' she knew she had miscalculated and that the window was slamming shut.

Sleep Lady Tip

If your child always falls asleep in the car, she's probably not getting enough sleep.

Quality and Quantity

When it comes to sleep, parents sound like they all hail from the dreamworld equivalent of Lake Wobegon. Everybody thinks his or her child needs less sleep than the average. Wrong. Sleep needs do vary somewhat, but the natural variations are a whole lot less than most parents think. These babies may be *getting* less sleep than average, but they *need* a lot more than they are getting. Remember, sleep begets sleep. To help you accurately gauge your child's needs, I provide average sleep requirements at the start of each age-related chapter.

Children need to get the right amount of sleep, and they need to get the right kind of sleep. Quality counts along with quantity. Good sleep should be largely uninterrupted. If your child is getting up a lot, she isn't getting all the sound sleep she needs. As we've all experienced on nights when we've slept poorly, fragmented sleep or interrupted sleep just does not make us feel as rested and refreshed as uninterrupted sleep.

After a newborn's first eight weeks, good sleep also means sleep in a cot, bed, or Moses basket – not in a car, stroller, or swing. Motion lulls us to sleep, but it also keeps us in a lighter, more fragmented sleep; our brains never reach the level of full restorative sleep if we're moving. Sure, your baby will occasionally fall asleep in a car. But make it the exception, not the rule, and even if you occasionally resort to using the car to get him to fall asleep, don't keep driving around. Either transfer him back to his cot as soon as possible, or park and sit in or next to the car so he can sleep without movement. I know one mum who brought her laptop and a pile of blankets into the car. Another would park in the driveway, and if the weather was nice, she would leave the car door open and weed the flower beds that had otherwise been neglected since the birth of her first child.

> After a newborn's first eight weeks, good sleep also means sleep in a cot, bed, or Moses basket – not in a car, stroller, or swing.

Quality sleep also means sleep that is not interrupted by medical conditions such as asthma, allergies, obstructive sleep apnea, reflux, or other disorders. See Chapter 15, 'Medical Problems,' and of course consult your doctor.

5

The Right Start for Newborns and Infants

When our doctors and nurses hand us our brand-new babies in the hospital, they make sure we know how to hold them, nurse them, swaddle them, change them, and swab that umbilical cord. But they seldom say a word about how to put our babies to sleep, or even help us define realistic expectations about sleep. They don't tell us that sleep is a learned skill, that we have to teach our babies to develop healthy sleep habits. In fact, we may get precisely the opposite advice. They may sympathetically cluck about how exhausted we will be during the first few months, about how it's normal to feel overwhelmed.

But it doesn't really have to be that way – at least not for too long. Of course, a newborn is a lot of work, and you won't get eight hours of uninterrupted sleep. But there's a difference between being tired – even very tired, for six or eight or even twelve weeks – and being so drained and besieged month after month that you can barely function, let alone coo at your own son or daughter or be civil to your spouse.

As I told you earlier, sleep coaching has two distinct phases. In the first few months of life, we concentrate on establishing basic rhythms and routines that will help babies learn to sleep better. We also learn a repertoire of soothing techniques that will help us become more confident parents, able to help our babies feel calm and secure, without relying exclusively or constantly on the breast or a bottle. That's what we'll focus on in this chapter and the next.

These early sleep–shaping techniques are subtle but effective. But they won't have your baby sleeping through the night at two, four, or (in most cases) even twelve or fourteen weeks. Babies just aren't wired to sleep all night in the first few months, although some will sleep six or eight hours at a stretch after the newborn period, or around the end of the third month. But these early sleep–shaping steps do lay a foundation, and for many infants that will be enough. They will start going to sleep by themselves and staying asleep all night between four and six months. Other babies may need more help from you to learn to sleep. We'll talk more about my Sleep Lady Shuffle and other aspects of sleep coaching in subsequent chapters.

Here, I will help you get your baby off to the right start. If you follow the Sleep Lady's Eight Rules of Infant Slumber your baby will have an easier time learning to sleep and will sleep longer. If you learn nothing from me except these eight steps, your life will be simpler. You will discover during the next few years that babies and children go through numerous sleep stages – learning to sleep through the night, changing nap schedules, separation anxiety, and the like – and laying a good foundation will help your baby and your entire family travel down these developmental paths. I will describe some tricks to help your baby learn to self-soothe so he doesn't need you to spend all night every night rocking, walking, nursing, or bouncing him.

The First Two Weeks

Before we get started, I want to offer a few reassuring words about the very beginning. Don't worry about schedules and rules during the first two weeks – and don't beat yourself up if you make a mistake, because there aren't any mistakes to be made. Just focus on healing and recovering from delivery, establishing your milk supply and learning how to breastfeed, and, most delightfully, getting to know your new baby. Accept as much help as you can get from family and friends, and grab as much sleep as you can whenever you can. Don't worry about the dirty dishes or that linen closet you tore apart during your 'nesting' moments but never had a chance to reassemble before you went into labor. None of that is important.

Your baby will probably sleep most of the time at the beginning, but she won't sleep very deeply. Newborn sleep is not well organized neurologically, which means it's a very light slumber. Hold her, rock her, swing her, do what feels right and comfortable for the first ten to fourteen days. Then, at the start of the third week, gradually start applying the Sleep Lady Slumber Rules and establishing patterns.

You aren't seeking a huge, dramatic transition. Just start weaving these routines and patterns into your baby's life. Keep your expectations realistic. This is a process. You won't see enormous overnight changes in her sleep patterns in the third week, but you will be laying the groundwork for improvement in the coming weeks and months.

The Sleep Lady's Eight Rules of Infant Slumber

1. Create a flexible feeding and sleeping routine.
2. Encourage soothing techniques other than nursing.
3. Offer a dummy for soothing and sucking.
4. Feed your baby when he wakes up after a nap.
5. Put your baby down drowsy but awake at least once a day.
6. Introduce one bottle a day – *even if you are committed to breast-feeding, as I was with my own children* – around the third or fourth week if breastfeeding has been established. You can, of course, used pumped breast milk. I'll explain more about this later.
7. Create a sleep-friendly environment.
8. Carefully think through bedsharing (or cosleeping) and roomsharing.

Bonding with Your Baby

Some of us feel an intense bond the minute our baby is born. For many other parents, that passionate connection isn't that immediate – and they feel guilty. Be kind to yourself; it often takes days or weeks for those feelings to well up, and it can take as long as seven months, an ongoing process of positive give-and-take, for parents and babies to form a secure attachment. If persistent sadness interferes with the bonding, please seek an evaluation for postnatal depression (see Chapter 17, 'Problem Solving and Taking Care of Mums and Dads').

You don't have to be a supermum or -dad to create the bond as you get acquainted with your baby. But here are some ways you can nudge the process along. Some may be intuitive for you.

1. Create routines that your child can expect and count on – not just at bedtime, mealtime, and bath time. Have a special toy for nappy changes, or a favorite song as you start your daily walks.
2. Respond to his needs quickly. If he cries because he's wet, change him. If he makes hungry noises, feed him. If you can't address his need immediately, acknowledge him clearly, let him know you heard him and will be there as soon as you can. If possible, give him a toy to hold and talk to him while you finish whatever you're doing (such as taking care of another child!). You can't spoil a child by being 'too responsive' in the first nine months or so of life.
3. Cultivate predictability. To feel safe and secure, babies need to know they can count on you. Your routines and prompt responses will help meet this need for predictability.
4. Hold him! Physical skin-to-skin contact is vital. Strap him onto your chest or use a sling rather than always plopping him in the stroller. Hug him, cuddle him, look into his eyes, and when he coos at you, coo back! On the other hand, you don't have to 'wear' your baby every minute, and it's not a crime to use a stroller some of the time. Remember that babies need and enjoy stimulation from playing on mats, baby gyms, and the like, too, so you don't need to hold him all the time.

5. Let go of your guilt and perfectionism. The less guilt-filled and
    self-critical you are, the more emotionally available you will
    be to your child. It's great for toddlers to start learning that
    everyone, even parents, may make mistakes and that they are
    loved anyway.

Remember that both parents should bond, and if the two parents
have slightly different approaches, that's fine as long as you are both
providing warmth, responsiveness, touch, and consistency.

For more on bonding and attachment, I highly recommend the
Circle of Security website (www.circleofsecurity.org) and their free
handout, 'Building a Secure Attachment for Your Baby.' I have also
posted the handout on www.sleeplady.com.

Sleep Lady Slumber Rule #1: Create a Flexible Feeding and Sleeping Routine

A lot of parents nowadays cringe at the word *routine*, but by *routine*
I don't mean a rigid, minute-by-minute regimen. I mean a
commonsense framework with time mapped out for eating,
napping, sleeping, playing, and awake time – a framework that
you can adapt as you grow more adept at reading your baby's
signals and cues.

Many new parents fear a routine will constrain them or tie them
down excessively. To the contrary, you will find that a flexible
routine for your baby means more options for you. You can't do
whatever you want whenever you want, but you will be able to
better plan your day. You'll know when you can get out of the
house, run errands, meet a friend for coffee, or walk off that baby
fat. And you can invite the grandparents over when your baby is
going to be at his cooing and adorable best, not his tired and
crankiest worst.

Sleep Lady Tip

Even very young babies like predictability. They find it calming; they sleep better, and they are more capable of soothing themselves.

A routine makes parenting easier. If your baby is crying, a routine helps you figure out what he wants. You can ask yourself, 'How long has he been awake? When did he last eat?' If you know by his schedule that he is well fed and well rested, you can then go through a list of questions to figure out what's bugging him. Is it too hot or cold? Are his clothes scratchy? Is his nappy soaked? Is he sick? Is he overstimulated? Does he need to be in a quieter environment (dimmer lights, less noise, fewer people)? If you have a completely unstructured, haphazard day, you won't be able to answer the basic questions about whether he is hungry or tired because you won't know. The lack of a routine makes it harder for you to interpret what he is trying to tell you and to respond to his needs.

Sleep Lady Tip

A darker, quieter room often helps with those late-afternoon fussy periods.

As you work on developing a routine, keep a simple log. Jot down when he eats and for how long. Do the same for his sleep. Don't obsess over it; your life doesn't need any more complications with a newborn in the house. But it will help you to detect his natural patterns and establish your own.

Carol and Daniel had had a terrible time with their first child, Joshua, and worked with me when he was about fifteen months old. With Deborah, their second child, they tried to build on what they had learned the hard way. 'I tried to think more about having a schedule – not a rigid schedule but a schedule. That way if she cried, I would be able to ask myself, 'Is she hungry?' and know that she wasn't, that she ate just an hour ago,' Carol recalled. 'It wasn't just that she was an easier, mellower baby, and she wasn't so colicky. It was also that I more easily recognized the signs of tiredness. And I think I created some of Joshua's sleep problems myself. If Joshua cried, I would give it about one second before I grabbed him and fed him. With Deborah, my instinct is still to rescue her, but I have more awareness; I know that I can let her try to get to sleep on her own.'

A routine means a modified approach to cue feeding (also sometimes known as demand feeding). Sure, you should feed on demand the first few weeks, and I certainly believe in feeding a baby when he is hungry. The problem is that we as new parents often don't really understand when our child is hungry. We think every cry is a hunger cry, and we end up feeding them and feeding them, turning ourselves into human dummies, or becoming, as one mother who nursed her four month old five times a night called herself, 'the boobie lady.'

I have worked with thousands of youngsters with behavioral sleep disorders, and by far the most common problem is that they never learned to fall asleep without a breast or bottle in their mouth. At the beginning, when we are nursing novices, it's very hard to tell how much they are ingesting – whether they are eating or just sucking, and whether they really want to be eating or they are eating simply because we placed them at our breast. (See 'Tips for Successful Breastfeeding' on page 71.)

We as new mothers and fathers worry and worry so much about whether they are eating enough and growing enough, whether we are producing enough milk, whether we need to supplement. When in doubt, we feed. If you are having these concerns, a visit to the doctor for a quick weight check can address those questions. It is also wise to arm yourself with knowledge about how often babies need to eat and how it changes in these early months (I give you a month-by-month breakdown in the next chapter). If you are routinely nursing your baby more frequently, you need to stop and think about why. Is it his hunger or your reflex? What else could he need?

Dr William Sammons, in *The Self-Calmed Baby: Teach Your Infant to Calm Itself – and Curb Crying, Fussing, and Sleeplessness* (1991), has a great bit of advice: 'We use feeding to help our baby go to sleep thinking that satisfying hunger accomplishes this when it is sucking, body contact, warmth and body motion, and the parents' attempt to calm the environment' that help our babies go to sleep. We're going to learn several techniques, other than the breast, for soothing babies. Keep in touch with your doctor or health visitor about your infant's growth and your dietary concerns (particularly if your child was premature, is not gaining weight, or has other health issues that could require a more frequent feeding schedule).

Sleep Lady Tip

Your newborn may have to eat every two to two and a half hours, but if you are routinely nursing more frequently, you need to stop and think about why. Is it his hunger or your reflex? What else could he need?

Remember that nursing has stages, which can also affect sleep. First the baby gets the *foremilk*, which is higher in lactose. Then she starts getting the *hindmilk*, sometimes called the *cream*. The fattier hindmilk balances out that high lactose, and it also makes babies feel drowsy. But babies who feed more than every two hours often nurse for just a few minutes at a time. That means they may be getting too much lactose and not enough cream, missing out on the components that enhance drowsiness. The disproportionate amount of lactose can make them gassy and fussy – which certainly doesn't help them sleep. And you may respond by nursing them even more, aggravating the problem.

Sleep Lady Tip

While some people say it's an old wives' tale, many nursing mums swear that if they eliminate caffeine – coffee, tea, fizzy drinks, chocolate – and cut back on dairy products, their infants are less fussy and sleep better. If you do remove certain foods from your diet, don't expect to see a difference overnight. Give it two or three weeks for the change to have a sustained impact on your baby.

Try to help your baby take a complete feeding, by nursing longer on one side so he can get to the hindmilk. (As they get a little older they become more efficient at eating so they will get to the hindmilk faster.) Between feedings, if he wants to suck, try offering a dummy if he is more than six weeks old and breastfeeding is well established, meaning you feel comfortable and it's become second nature. Also, although some people say it's an old wives' tale, many nursing mums I have worked with swear that if they eliminate caffeine (coffee, tea, fizzy drinks, chocolate) and cut back on dairy products (including the 'hidden' dairy ingredients in many foods – read labels), their infants are less fussy and sleep better. If you do remove certain foods from your diet, don't expect to see a difference overnight. Give it two or three weeks for the change to have a sustained impact on your baby. Ask a lactation consultant for specific suggestions of what to eliminate, or ask your doctor or health visitor at your next checkup.

Sleep Lady Slumber Rule #2: Encourage Soothing Techniques Other Than Nursing

If you give babies a chance, they will develop a host of ways to soothe themselves, but in the first few months they do need our help. Our challenge is to find soothing techniques other than nonstop nursing, which becomes a problem if the child always needs to nurse to get to sleep. Dr Harvey Karp's helpful book, *The Happiest Baby on the Block: The New Way to Calm Crying and Help Your Newborn*

Baby Sleep Longer (2002), recommends the 'Five *S*'s' – swaddling, side holding, 'sh-sh-sh,' swinging, and sucking – to get the baby through the first few months, sometimes called the *fourth trimester.*

Tips for Successful Breastfeeding

When I had my first baby I was very worried about how long she needed to nurse – and how to tell whether she was hungry or full. I'll give you some specifics about how often an infant needs to eat in the first weeks and months. Remember that these are general guidelines and averages – and while guidelines are useful, not every baby will be a perfect fit, and not every book or expert will give you precisely the same answer. (Much of the material here is drawn from the American Academy of Pediatrics and La Leche League.) Ask your doctor or a lactation consultant if you need more help, and don't stress out if your child's pattern varies a bit once in a while as long as she's growing and gaining weight. Following are some tips to help you feel confident and competent about breastfeeding.

1. How can I tell when my newborn is hungry?

At the very beginning she is going to be hungry a lot, needing to eat at least eight times in twenty-four hours until breastfeeding is established. Frequent nursing also helps to stimulate mum's milk production. Use this time to start recognizing her hungry cues:

- Waking and becoming alert
- Putting her hands toward her mouth
- Making sucking motions, or moving her little fists to her mouth
- Flexing her arms or hands
- Fidgety body movements
- Trying to find your breast when you hold her

You'll get better at 'reading' your baby quickly. As you learn her hunger cues, try to nurse before she starts crying. She'll latch on better when she isn't fussing.

2. Is she really eating?

For starters, you need to know if your baby is latched on correctly so she can suck properly. If not, she won't get the full 'letdown' of milk, and she'll miss important nutrients. Take a peek at her.

- Is her mouth all the way open?
- Can you see her ears wiggle when she swallows?
- Can you hear her swallowing?
- Are her eyes rolling around in a 'milk drunk'?

You may not detect all of these clues, but if you can't see any of them, she's not eating; she's 'sucking around' for pleasure. You are not a human dummy, and if you let her keep doing this, you will have sore nipples. That's unpleasant for you and can make breastfeeding difficult.

3. How do I know when my newborn is full?

You may find that your baby takes long feedings at certain times of the day but is quickly satisfied at others. She'll usually let you know when she's done by letting go or drifting off to sleep (maybe with spurts of sucking for comfort but not for food). She may have a 'limp noodle' feel to her arms. As you get more experienced, you'll get better at feeling and seeing the difference.

4. Is she getting enough to eat?

Here are some ways to tell during the first month:

- She has at least six wet and three dirty nappies each day
- She looks happy and full when she leaves your breast
- Your breasts feel full before nursing and empty afterward
- Her color is good, and her skin is firm
- She appears satisfied for a couple of hours after a feeding
- She is gaining weight

5. What is cue feeding?

Cue feeding is what we used to call 'demand feeding.' Basically, it means feeding babies when they signal that they are hungry. I certainly believe in feeding a hungry baby, but we don't feed them all the time. We shouldn't assume that every cry or bit of frustration means she is hungry or that the breast is our sole means of comforting her.

As your baby gets a little older, you can begin to regulate feeding (which also helps him get longer stretches of sleep). It goes without saying that if your baby's cues tell you that he is hungry outside his 'regular' or scheduled time, you feed him, just like you'd eat yourself if you were truly hungry outside a regular mealtime.

6. What do I do if she keeps falling asleep on my breast, but I don't think she's had enough to eat?

Wake her up – gently! Rub her back, loosen her clothing, ever so softly blow on her face, change her nappy, do something that stimulates her just enough to stay awake long enough to fill her tummy (and empty your breast). Read tip 4 to determine if she's getting enough to eat. Don't forget to pause briefly during the feeding to burp her, or otherwise she will be awake but not too happy.

If you need help, you can find a lactation consultant through the hospital or birth center where you had your baby, by asking your doctor or obstetrician, or by checking the International Lactation Consultant Association (www.ilbc.org) or Lactation Consultants of Great Britain (www.lcgb.org). I also give you breastfeeding resources in the back of this book.

Swaddling

The pressure of swaddling, similar to what babies felt in utero, comforts babies and lengthens their sleep – and it often works well along with white noise. Wrap him snugly in a thin receiving blanket, making sure the blanket is not near his face, and his ears and toes are not too hot. Usually, babies like their hips to be slightly bent.

For the first three months, they usually like having their arms inside the blanket. Parents tell me they love the Miracle Blanket for swaddling. At about twelve to sixteen weeks, start leaving the arms out. Or try leaving one arm out. If your baby seems unhappy – Dr Karp says a baby will sometimes hit himself – go back to swaddling and test again in a few weeks. (For preemies, Dr Karp suggests swaddling with the arms up, as it helps their neurological development and alertness.) Experiment a little, and you'll be able to tell when he's comfortable. Halo makes a blanket sleeper I like that has 'wings' so the body is swaddled but the arms are out. I swaddled my own daughters tightly, with their arms at their sides or across their chest during that fussy evening period in the first six to eight weeks. For bed, I tended to wrap lighter around the arms so that they could move a little bit. Ask a nurse to show you how to swaddle your baby in the hospital, and take a newborn-baby care class at your local hospital to go over the basics before you give birth.

Side Holding and Sh-Sh-Sh

Babies should sleep on their backs to reduce the risk of sudden infant death syndrome, or SIDS, but not all of them like it. It's not a position they experienced in utero, and it may trigger their *Moro*, or *falling reflex*. Sometimes it helps ward off that falling sensation if you hold the baby at a little bit of an angle as you put him down, so his feet are a bit lower than his head.

They don't have to be on their backs when they are awake or when you are holding them. Many find it comforting to be on their sides, particularly their left side. You can hold him on his side in your arms or on your lap, swaddled if you like, and make a

Soothing Techniques

I often remind you to use your repertoire of soothing techniques, so you don't rely exclusively on nursing or feeding to calm your baby. Much of this is instinctual, but sometimes our anxieties and all the conflicting advice we get drown out our own instincts. Here's a quick checklist to remind you that you do have quite an extensive repertoire. Some, like swaddling, we use for only the first several months, but others, like gentle massage, are terrific through much of childhood.

Remember to respond to your newborn quite quickly, because once the baby gets hysterical, he's harder to soothe. Later on we try to strike a little more of that balance we discussed between immediate response and letting babies learn to self-soothe, but in the first few months, it's our job to create their calm.

If one technique doesn't work after about ten minutes, try another. If you get to the point where you are even more frustrated than your baby, let another adult take over and give yourself a break. If you are alone and have reached a breaking point, it's better to let the baby cry for a few minutes in a safe place (i.e., his cot or bouncy chair) while you take a few minutes to calm yourself.

Here are some of the common strategies:

- Carrying your baby
- Swinging or rocking your baby
- Swaddling
- Repetitive soothing sounds or music
- Offering a dummy
- Massaging the baby (I recommend some massage books in my resource list at the end of this book)
- Offering loveys or security blankets (after about age six months when they can have them without danger of suffocation)

gentle, rhythmic 'sh-sh-sh' noise to remind him of your heartbeat in utero. Swing or sway your body a little for comfort. Holding him on his side helps with that fussy evening period or with colicky babies who cry more than average – which believe it or not is three hours a day. The swing or sway should be in a slightly upright position, which lessens reflux and allows a burp to jiggle out, according to Karp. However, remember that there's a difference between holding a baby on his side and putting him to sleep on his side. Holding is wonderful; side sleeping is dangerous.

The American Academy of Pediatrics and the U.K. Department of Health advises against side sleeping for young babies. If you think your baby is more comfortable on his side, do not make a change without discussing side-sleeping safety with your doctor. When he gets old enough to sleep safely on his stomach or side, usually when he can roll over consistently in both directions, you may find that he suddenly begins to sleep more soundly if that's naturally more comfortable for him.

Swinging

Gently rocking and swinging our babies is so instinctive that I scarcely have to mention it, but it does calm newborns. It's also fine to let your baby nap in a swing during the day for the first two months. After that, he'll still like being in the swing, and you can use it for fun and comfort, but don't use it as a bed.

To gently ease out of the swing–sleep habit, go ahead and put him in the swing at his customary speed, and then slow it down. Stop it when he's asleep. At about two months, start to move him into his cot for his morning nap. Start his prenap routine in his room, and swing him a bit in your arms if it helps the transition. Then put him in the cot. Stay by him; pat, stroke, or gently rock his body, if that helps until he drifts off to sleep. He should make the adjustment in a few days. Start this with one nap a day, usually the morning, and add the second nap whenever you think he's ready.

Sleep Lady Slumber Rule #3: Offer a Dummy for Soothing and Sucking

The final *S* is the sucking reflex. Babies do need to suck, especially during the first few weeks. It's not just about food; babies suck on their fingers, their hands, their dummies. Recent research suggests that dummies may also help protect babies against SIDS, but as I noted, the medical advice on dummies has changed frequently over the years, and it may well change again. Please check with your doctor, and check in again as your baby gets a little older. If you are nursing, wait four to six weeks until nursing is well established before you introduce the dummy. Bottlefed babies can start earlier.

If your baby spits out the dummy, don't automatically replug it! If you keep plugging up his mouth all the time, you may be hampering his early attempt to communicate with you, and interfering with your ability to differentiate between his cries. Sometimes he will want the dummy back – and he'll let you know it. But if you don't assume it's the dummy he wants, you may realize he's trying to tell you something else. You'll be surprised how many times babies spit out the dummy parents stick it in, babies spit it out, the parents stick it back in, never stopping to think that maybe the baby is spitting it out for a reason. If, after the first few months, he's taking the dummy more than you would like, try other soothing techniques and reduce stimulation to lessen the need for sucking. Also, dummies don't help very gassy babies because they tend to swallow more air as they suck it.

Why dummies may protect against SIDS isn't yet completely clear. The First Candle organization, dedicated to preventing infant deaths, cites several possible explanations, among them that dummies may discourage babies from turning over onto their tummies during sleep. The sucking reflex may also keep them from falling into a deep sleep or position the tongue to keep the airways open.

Even if you use the dummy when the baby sleeps, you may choose not to use it all the time when he is awake and fussy. You can reconsider how and when you want him to continue with the dummy when he gets to be about six months old. When babies get older, they may start sucking their thumbs, which is a perfectly good way of self-soothing and satisfying that instinct to suck. Some parents prefer it. Unlike a dummy, you can't lose a thumb, you don't have to worry about its falling on the floor, and you can't forget to pack it in the nappy bag!

A lot of children outgrow thumb sucking on their own, but my daughter Carleigh didn't. When she was five we found the perfect behavioral modification technique, although it meant we had to adopt her kindergarten class's hamster! You'll hear about that adventure when we get to preschoolers.

Sleep Lady Slumber Rule #4: Feed Your Baby When He Wakes Up

Most mothers breast- or bottlefeed at bedtime for many months. A nice, long nursing, including the hindmilk, does tend to encourage sleep – which is exactly what you want at bedtime. But you want to avoid too strong an association between nursing and sleep because it will cause problems later.

Some of the time, nurse when he is getting up, not only when he is going to sleep. This comes naturally when he wakes up in the morning, but try to get in the habit of nursing *after* naps, not *before* naps, at least once or twice a day. Most mums find it's easiest to do this first thing in the morning and at the first morning nap. It doesn't work as well in the late afternoon or early evening when they are tired and fussy and nursing can help them calm down and get ready for bed.

> Get in the habit of nursing after naps, not before
> naps, at least once or twice a day.

Sleep Lady Slumber Rule #5: Put Your Baby Down Drowsy but Awake at Least Once a Day

In the first weeks, we usually do nurse our babies to sleep at bedtime and when they are hungry during the night. But once he is about four weeks old, get in the habit of putting him down drowsy but awake at least once in each twenty-four-hour period. He doesn't have to be wide awake, but he shouldn't be out cold from being fed, rocked, or swung each time he goes to sleep. He may fuss a little, but give it a moment or two. Don't pick him up again at the first squeak; let him surprise you. Between six and eight weeks, try to make this the norm at bedtime.

Sometimes he will fall asleep nursing, and then of course you shouldn't wake him. What you want to aim for is nursing him until he has had enough to eat and is getting drowsy. Then unlatch him gently before he falls fully asleep. It may take a little practice, but you'll figure it out within a few days, and if it doesn't work one night, just try again the next. (See Chapter 2, 'Getting Started and Tips for Success,' for more help with 'drowsy but awake.')

Sleep Lady Slumber Rule #6: Introduce One Bottle a Day

No matter how committed you are to nursing for the long haul – and I breastfed both of my daughters – introduce a bottle once a day around the third or fourth week if breastfeeding has been established. It's up to you and your doctor whether you use expressed breast milk or formula, but get your baby used to a bottle early. It's a commonsense preparation for unforeseen circumstances, be it a huge traffic jam that prevents you from getting home by nursing time or an emergency appendectomy.

Sleep Lady Tip

Because formula takes longer to digest, some parents find that a bottle of formula at bedtime lets the baby sleep slightly longer before he wakes up hungry again. It doesn't work for everybody, but go ahead and try it if you want and your doctor approves.

Although some babies adapt easily to a bottle later, others will refuse the bottle once they differentiate between breast and bottle. Since you have no way of knowing how your baby will respond six months from now, do yourself and him a favor and familiarize him with the bottle now. Some couples also like to use occasional bottles so Dad can share in the feeding. That gives Dad some wonderful bonding time. And it gives Mum a little break, and a chance to get a badly needed stretch of at least a few hours of uninterrupted sleep. For instance, Mum might want to pump and let Dad do the 10:00 p.m. feeding with a bottle. In my family, we occasionally used formula, because I wanted the peace of mind of knowing my girls could take formula if they ever needed to.

Some families fear that if they give a baby a bottle, he will then reject the breast. This form of nipple confusion is actually a lot less common than people think, and it tends to be more of an issue if you give a bottle at the very beginning, before he has learned to latch onto the breast and before you have learned to nurse. One bottle a day *after* nursing has been established for several weeks shouldn't be a problem.

Sleep Lady Slumber Rule #7: Create a Sleep-Friendly Environment

I strongly believe that the baby's environment affects his sleep. I like room-darkening shades and calm, soothing colors in the baby's bedroom. I don't like bright or stimulating mobiles in the cot. Let him enjoy the mobile somewhere else, where he spends awake time.

At bedtime, the message to the brain is 'Slow down,' not 'Stay up and watch your bright-colored mobile spin.'

I also want the cot to be a place for sleep and maybe for a few minutes of quiet play right after waking as he gets a little older. It's not a place to park the baby while you wash dishes, nor is it a place to pen a baby in when he begins to scoot and crawl.

Sleep Lady Tip

Some mums worry about whether to turn the phone off during naptime. Do whatever makes sense for you. My own approach was to turn off the upstairs phone, which was near the girls' rooms, but leave it on downstairs. That way I could hear it, but the noise would be muted for them.

White Noise and Music

White-noise machines, fans, or sound screens can be useful during the first few months, or even longer for naps. Babies who are extremely alert also do well with white noise, because it helps them shut the world out. I have found that a white-noise machine or a fan is more effective than music in screening out sounds, but many parents understandably prefer lullabies, and that's fine.

By around two to three months, take care to use the music to set the mood before you put her down. If you let music become a sleep crutch, you'll spend the night running in to turn it on each time she stirs. Play music as she gets ready for bed, but don't keep it running as she is falling asleep, and don't keep putting it back on during the night when she wakes up. Let it wind down at bedtime, or turn it off or turn the volume down very, very low. When it goes off, it goes off – that's it.

Cheryl and Gary's four-month-old son, Ari, was, as Cheryl put it, 'hyperalert.' 'He's always exploring; he's a distractible, active kid.' To help him tune out the world enough to sleep, they created a prenap routine that was quite similar to his bedtime ritual, just a bit shorter. They started downstairs, where they spent ten minutes watching a quiet video. Then they'd go upstairs and read to him in his room. After that they'd say good night to various objects in his room – the mirror, Noah's ark, and so forth. Cheryl would play a short lullaby, lay him in his cot, say 'Night-night,' and walk out of the room.

Motion Sleep

Motion sleep can trip up parents. Babies are very portable. They can sleep wherever you put them – car seats, strollers, swings, bouncy chairs, noisy cafés, shops, at your best friend's house when her three kids are all bouncing off the playroom walls. But even though they can do this, it doesn't mean they should do this. It's okay some of the time (like in the late afternoon and early evening), but try to have them nap in a nice, quiet cot or Moses basket most of the time, starting at about six to eight weeks.

Sleep Lady Tip

If your baby does fall asleep in the car seat, remove it from the car and put it in his bedroom or at least in another quiet, sleep-conducive place.

Also, nobody ever tells us that babies shouldn't nap on the go forever – so we keep doing it, particularly letting them sleep in cars. Motion sleep keeps the brain in a light sleep, and as babies mature, they need deeper sleep as well. Think about it. When you doze off in a car, do you feel as refreshed as if you had slept in a bed? The same is true for your baby, especially after the first two to three months.

Getting him out of the car and into the cot may mean that you will be more housebound for a few weeks – not forever – until your baby develops more predictable nap patterns. If you go stir crazy, get a sitter for a few hours a week, make a deal with your spouse so you can get some time off, invite your mum to visit for a week, or find a friend to join you in some co-op babysitting. Again, you don't have to go overboard with rigidity here. Sure, he'll fall asleep in the swing, stroller, or car seat once in a while. Don't worry about it. Just don't make it a habit.

> *At five months, Lydia was still on the same schedule – or nonschedule – she had as a newborn. Nina and Lydia were often on the go, feeding on the run, grabbing a nap in a car seat or stroller. But Lydia didn't eat well, and she didn't nap well. Nina learned that Lydia needed more structure and less stimulation. She needed to nap in her own home, in a quiet place, with no lights, no noise, no distractions. 'She became more aware of her surroundings; she couldn't just nurse anywhere, sleep anywhere,' Nina said. 'I realized I needed to be home for naps.'*

Bedtime Routine

Developing a bedtime routine early, by about six weeks, is essential. It will be very simple at first. You'll probably start with a warm bath, then move into his dimly lit room. Maybe you'll do a few minutes of infant massage (take a class!). Nurse him or maybe let Dad give him a bottle. Swaddle, snuggle, or rock him, and then lay him in his cot or Moses basket. You'll add little games and stories and other rituals of your own as he gets older. But you'll always need a bedtime routine. Predictable routines not only soothe babies but also cue the brain

to slow down and get ready for sleep, just like a good book can help an adult wind down. If an infant is tired but doesn't get to sleep, he gets a cortisol rush, which then makes it even harder for him go to sleep – a downward spiral.

Bonding Tips for Dad

Mums have built-in bonding opportunities, particularly if they are breastfeeding. But dads don't have to feel left out. Here are some ways fathers and babies can get closer:

- Feeding. A breastfeeding mum can pump during the day, and Dad can bottlefeed the baby once at night. This gives Mum a chance to get one good stretch of sleep during the night.
- Bath time. This intimate activity is a great opportunity for Dad and baby, plus it gives Mum a bit of a break in the evening (or time to focus on older children). Dads may want to learn a bit of infant massage or baby yoga.
- Carry the baby. Buy a front carrier and take a walk every day with the baby on Daddy's chest.

Sleep Lady Slumber Rule #8: Carefully Think Through Bedsharing (or Cosleeping) and Roomsharing

I devote a whole chapter to bedsharing (or cosleeping) and roomsharing (Chapter 12, 'Whose Bed Is It Anyway?'). A lot of families want to keep the baby either in bed with them or right near them for the first three to six months for bonding, nursing convenience, and parental anxiety control. That's fine, but if you opt for the family bed, make sure you know all the safety rules and think about where you want the baby to be sleeping a few months or a year or two from now. Also read the cosleeping chapter for napping tips, which can help a baby develop sleep skills that he will need as he gets older.

Sleep Lady Tip

If you want your baby close by but don't want him to be actually in your bed, there are various 'cosleepers' available. Among them are cots that attach to your bed like a sidecar so the baby is next to you but in his own space.

I recommend that he make the transition to the cot in his own room at about three to six months, when an established presleep routine becomes so essential. It's a little harder after that, and much harder a year or two later. Some parents keep the baby with them for a few months and then sleep on a spare bed or mattress in the baby's room for a few days or weeks when they move him to the cot. Either is fine; just make sure you have a plan for getting yourself out of the room, because he'll get more accustomed to it than you realize.

Some parents start to cosleep but find that, for them, it's uncomfortable, no one is getting any sleep, and it's distracting or noisy. Don't feel guilty. You need your sleep as much as the baby needs hers, so put the baby in a Moses basket or cot in your room, or go ahead and move her to her own room if that's the best solution. I know my own kids made a huge racket at night. As a new mum I was very surprised by all the grunts and squeaks that came out of those tiny throats at midnight. If you need a little help with this transition, read Chapter 6, 'Newborn to Five Months.'

Many families end up doing what's called *reactive cosleeping*. That means the baby starts out the night in his Moses basket or cot but ends up in the parents' bed because that's the only way they can get him back to sleep. Or they wanted to cosleep for three months, and here it is the fourth or fifth month and they haven't figured out how to stop it. Cosleeping by choice is one thing; cosleeping by default is another. If you follow my Sleep Lady Slumber Rules you'll find alternative ways of getting your baby back to sleep and getting him to sleep through the night so the problem doesn't arise.

Part Two

Part Two

6

Newborn to Five Months

Parents often wonder how early they can start shaping children's sleep. I say, the sooner the better. Naturally, we are very gentle at first, just nudging them to start distinguishing between day and night, light and dark. Later, we'll start teaching them to fall asleep with less assistance from us, to sleep longer intervals at night, to lengthen their naps. I break this advice down month by month, but of course it's an estimate. Phases overlap, and changes unfold over days and weeks, not overnight. A baby eating every two hours at thirty days is not likely to jump to every three hours on the thirty-first day just because he arbitrarily crosses that 'one month old' threshold. But this is a useful guideline.

Please keep in mind that my feeding advice is for healthy full-term babies. Preemies will catch up, but you may have to supplement and feed more frequently until they reach their adjusted birth-age weight. Then, with your doctor's approval, follow these timelines. If your baby is not gaining weight as expected or has other health problems, please consult your doctor or health visitor about feeding.

Many parents are ambivalent about sleep coaching in these first months. On one hand, the mums and dads want to sleep and know that their babies need to sleep, too. On the other hand, infants fuss and cry enough as it is. They wonder why they should endure any more tears or force the child to shed them. In fact, there are a lot fewer tears than you would imagine. In these first few months, we shape sleep ever so gently, and your baby will get plenty of soothing, holding, and snuggling.

Nina, who worked on her daughter's sleep habits at five months, found attachment-parenting practices very attractive, and she was loath to let Lydia cry or to be apart from her very much. But her baby fussed and cried anyway, and the sleep portion of attachment parenting just didn't work for her family. As Nina gently modified her parenting style to introduce more structure and independence, she was thrilled to discover that Lydia thrived. The baby who used to be so tired, who fussed even when riding in her stroller, now smiled all the time, slept all night — and hardly ever cried.

After four months of dealing with an overtired baby who had reflux, Tracy reluctantly decided to address Lucas's sleep problems. She knew that postponing the inevitable wasn't going to make the situation any easier. 'Many of my friends are embarrassed to admit that their kids still aren't sleeping now that they are two or three years old,' said Tracy. 'When friends confessed that to me, it really helped me. I knew that my husband and I couldn't live that way. I couldn't function. I needed to sleep. I didn't want to be so tired that I couldn't enjoy my baby.'

Once babies get to around four or five months, we'll be a little more directive, helping children sleep through longer without a night feeding, or perhaps with one night feeding. In most cases, we don't get to full 'sleep training' with my Sleep Lady Shuffle until a baby is six months old. Some families have done it earlier, at four months, successfully. If you want to try it, and your doctor says it's okay, then go ahead at four months and focus on the nights primarily. Don't worry about the Shuffle for naps with a four month old; fill the daytime sleep tank any way you can. But please understand that the Shuffle, though gentle, is a behavioral modification technique designed for slightly older children. If it works at four months, and it can, that's terrific. Enjoy your sleep. But if it doesn't, rather than giving up on my system, I recommend that you follow the slower approach I outline in this chapter, and then try the Shuffle again when your baby is a little bit older, around six months. Occasionally, I have encountered a family that has tried the Shuffle with a baby who is only a few weeks or months old. The Sleep Lady Shuffle is neither designed for nor recommended for such young babies. But the steps I outline here can help improve infant sleep.

How Infants Sleep

'Sleeping like a baby,' as the saying goes, is not all that it's cracked up to be. Newborns sleep a lot, about fifteen to eighteen hours a day, but their sleep is not organized, not well developed. For the first four months, about half their sleep is REM (rapid eye movement) sleep, the most active kind of sleep. That means they are sleeping lightly, and are more easily aroused than an older child or an adult who spends much less time in REM. Young babies also cycle between the two sleep states, REM and non-REM, much more than adults or even older children do.

Each time they switch, they have a *partial awakening*. For us as adults, a partial awakening may last only a few seconds, and we may scarcely remember it in the morning. But that brief moment of semiawakeness can startle babies and make them wake up even more. They then cry – and we rush in and frantically try all sorts of things to rescue them from their tears.

I strongly believe in responding to a child's cry, both for his sake and for our own peace of mind. As parents, we need to make sure that they are okay, that they haven't been sick or got tangled in something, that their nappy hasn't leaked, that sort of thing. But we shouldn't overdo it. Remember that balance between comforting our children and allowing them to learn to comfort themselves. That's an essential component of sleep shaping.

Sleep Lady Tip

Creating sleep crutches by teaching our babies that they must always be held, rocked, nursed, or bottlefed, to get to sleep and back to sleep, means they will never learn how to get themselves back to sleep after partial arousals and never learn how to sleep through the night.

Feeding

When you do feed your baby at night, keep the lights off and don't interact much. Feed him, burp him, give him a few hugs, and then put him right back in his Moses basket, cot, or wherever he began the night. It isn't playtime, and it isn't time for musical beds. If he wakes up between feeding times, make sure he's truly awake before you run in and wake him even more. Sometimes they stir during a partial awakening, make a few strange baby noises, and then go right back to sleep.

> 'With Holly, our first child, with one whimper we'd jolt out of bed and rush into her room,' said Marianne, who had three children in three years and became quite a skillful sleep coach out of necessity. 'We learned that making noise doesn't mean they are awake. When Holly made a noise, we were actually waking her up by barging in.'

If he's definitely awake, go in and stroke him, pat his back, sh-sh-sh him, swaddle him, or use other soothing techniques to get him back to sleep. Don't overdo it, though. Maybe all he really needs is to be reswaddled and put back down. Sit right by his cot until he dozes off if you think it makes him – or you – feel better. Follow this advice not just in the first month but until he outgrows night feedings.

I know that there's a lot to absorb in this chapter and following all this advice isn't easy, especially when you are tired and overwhelmed by all the emotional, logistical, and marital changes that accompany parenthood. Some mums who consulted me for sleep problems with their first child vowed to do everything differently with the second child – and ended up calling me sheepishly a few months later to help them undo all the things they failed to do differently!

> *'My first child was adopted, and we didn't get him until he was six months old,' said Ellen, the mum who wrote those cue cards I shared with you in Chapter 1, 'The Sleep Lady System.' 'My second child, Vanessa, was my biological child. I had her from birth, and I had big ambitions of starting good habits with her from the beginning. After all, I was a veteran! But she was so strong-willed and she had horrible reflux, and I didn't even try. We both fell over into bed together, and I nursed her every two hours.'*

The reflux subsided at six months, and Ellen finally called me at eight months. The good news is that we got her little girl into her cot and off all that nursing in just three nights. Looking back, Ellen realized she could have spared her whole family a lot of sleepless nights if she had not let herself get so overwhelmed and been more consistent.

> *Lisa had a different experience. Her son, Teddy, had many sleep difficulties that we addressed when he was about seven months old. But when her daughter, Brittany, was born, Lisa began shaping her sleep from the start. She paid more attention to when she nursed, worked on putting her down drowsy but awake, and was careful not to hold her to sleep all the time. And she didn't panic quite so much if the baby cried sometimes. Her consistency, and her more confident parenting, paid off, and Brittany slept very well from early on.*

You'll read more about her experience in a moment. But whether you are more like Ellen or Lisa, the important thing is this – don't beat yourself up over things you could have done differently. Just focus on making it better from now on.

The First Month (0–4 Weeks)

For the first week, babies typically sleep a total of sixteen to eighteen hours, about half during the night and half spread out over four daytime naps. By the end of the first month, they sleep an average of fifteen and a half to seventeen hours total, about eight and a half to ten hours at night and six to seven hours during the day spread over three or four naps. They will still wake up two or three times at night for feedings but should go back to sleep quickly.

According to the American Academy of Pediatrics, once the mother's milk comes in, newborns may feed as often as every hour and a half, and they shouldn't go more than three hours without eating – for a total of around eight to twelve feedings in twenty-four hours. Formula fed babies will eat a bit less frequently, about two to three ounces every three or four hours, for a total of six to eight feedings a day.

Even during these first few weeks, your baby is beginning to pick up on your cues and feelings and to realize that he can affect the world around him. He will recognize the scent of your breast milk, will prefer soft sensations to coarse ones, and will like to be handled very gently. Abrupt or rough moves can frighten or startle him.

Although he won't fully distinguish day from night for six to eight weeks, he will develop this ability faster if you expose him to light now. You don't want to shock him with bright, glaring lights in his eyes, but you can open the blinds when he gets up in the morning and keep him in brighter rooms when he's awake and in dimmer ones when he is going to sleep.

Be careful not to overstimulate him, either by letting him stay up too long without a nap or by exposing him to too much noise or activity. Sometimes more is less – you could inadvertently stimulate when you are trying to soothe. If you spend thirty minutes trying to soothe a newborn and he's still fussing, try swaddling him and putting him down in a dimly lit room. He may then calm down on his own. When newborns have had too much stimulation, they may *habituate*. That means they go into a state that looks like sleep but is actually just a way of shutting everything out. It's a form of self-soothing they use until about six to eight weeks, when they begin to develop other ways of coping with stimulation.

It's sometimes hard for parents to distinguish dozing from habituating. A sleeping baby tends to wake up alert and responsive. After habituating, a baby is not so alert; in fact, he may be fussy and irritable. You want to avoid a lot of habituation because if he shuts down during the day, chances are he will be up a lot more during the night. Newborns need a certain amount of tranquillity when they are awake, and if they can't get that peaceful awake time during the day, they will seek it out at night.

I remember taking my first daughter, Carleigh, to a wedding when she was five weeks old. Much to my distress, she cried much more than usual during the ceremony when of course I most wanted her to be quiet – and then she appeared to sleep through the very loud reception, complete with Greek music and dancing. But then she stayed up and cried all night long. Much later, as I learned more about infant sleep, I remembered that wedding. I realized Carleigh had responded to overstimulation at the ceremony with tears, and then habituated during the reception to protect herself from even more sensory overload. She was then so overtired and out of kilter by nighttime that she cried. By the time my second child was born, I was more protective of her sleep and knew better than to take her to a Greek wedding!

Sleep Lady Tip

Cluster feeding, meaning feeding in more frequent intervals, can help in that hungry, fussy, overstimulated-and-getting-tired part of the day – from roughly 3:00 p.m. to 7:00 p.m. – and may also help your baby sleep longer stretches in the evening.

The feeding guidelines are just that: guidelines. They're goals, not a straitjacket. If she's really sobbing and you already tried other soothing techniques, then feed her, particularly if you're getting pretty close to the next feeding time. But if you feed her more frequently, pay close attention to her response. If she stops sucking after just a few minutes or she dozes off quickly on the breast, that's your clue that she wasn't really hungry or a sign that you may have a milk-supply problem. Review the breastfeeding information in Chapter 5, 'The Right Start for Newborns and Infants,' for help on recognizing your baby's hunger signs and for some alternative soothing techniques if you find yourself always nursing and are too quick to offer the breast as her main means of comfort.

During the day, he should sleep two, sometimes three, hours at a time. But just like you can't let him sleep too long without feeding, you can't let him stay awake too long, either. The limit is about two hours. He may look alert, he may seem fine, but as countless mothers have learned the hard way, the reality is if we wait until they don't look fine anymore, we're too late. He will be hungry, overstimulated, and overtired, and all that cortisol now rushing through his bloodstream will make it hard to get him to sleep.

Plan his last feeding and bedtime to coincide with your bedtime, sometime between 10:00 p.m. and 11:00 p.m. (His bedtime will be earlier in a few months.) Keep him awake for the two hours before that bedtime. A lot of babies stay up easily during those two hours, and it can become a nice family time, particularly a good time for Dad to be with the baby if Mum has had him all day.

Some newborns have trouble staying awake until 10:00. If your baby is tired, fussy, and unable to feed well at 10:00, then move the bedtime to an earlier time. It may take a little trial and error to find the right time, but watch for his sleep cues; they will tell you more than the clock. Usually an adjustment of just an hour or a half hour does the trick, but I've worked with a handful of newborns whose natural sleep window was as early as 8:00 p.m.

A consistent bedtime and some rudimentary bedtime rules, even at this tender age, are important. It's how we start to regulate sleep. These first few weeks he may well need you to hold, rock, or nurse him to sleep in your arms, but at least once a day try to use those tools only to the point of drowsiness, not until he's fully asleep. Then very gently lower him into his cot, swaddled, and let him finish falling asleep.

If you find yourself tensing up at the thought that he might cry, take a few deep, calming breaths before you put him down. If he does cry, you'll be right there to comfort him. At this early age, you can pick him up to soothe him again if you need to; just try not to let him fall asleep in your arms all the time.

If he nursed shortly after waking up, as most babies do, he won't need to nurse again before napping. Use the other soothing techniques (see Chapter 5, 'The Right Start for Newborns and Infants'). Even if you are cosleeping in these early weeks, have him nap in his cot or Moses basket. You don't want him to need to sleep curled up next to you all the time; it will make napping harder in the coming months.

Sleep Lady Tip

Remember to take care of yourself and sleep whenever you can.

Tummy Time

You've heard the rule 'Back to Sleep' for safety. But our babies need time on their tummies too for healthy motor development. So the safety slogan version 2.0 is 'Back to Sleep. Tummy to Play.' For tummy time, they need to be awake, and properly supervised, particularly in those early months before they can roll over.

Tummy time is essential for motor development – and for sleep safety. Good strength and control of the head and upper body reduces the risk of sudden infant death syndrome or suffocation. It helps babies develop the muscles they will use to roll over, scoot, and eventually crawl.

The American Academy of Pediatrics and the NHS in the U.K. recommend that we start with a little bit of tummy time as soon as you get home from the hospital. Try three to five minutes, two or three times a day, and gradually increase the time as the baby indicates he likes it more. Good times to try it are after a nappy change or when he wakes from a nap, when he's been in a bouncy seat or a car seat, or even when you've been holding him in a sling or carrier.

Sleep Lady Tip

If your baby doesn't seem to like it, make it fun. He can lie tummy to tummy on you; you'll see him start learning how to lift his head to see your face. You can put a toy nearby and encourage him to reach. When he's a little older, put toys in a circle around him, which is a great way of developing muscles and coordination. Properly supervised, an older child can gently play with the baby on the floor, in which case you'll have two happy children.

Tummy time comes more naturally once infants start to roll over, and some research suggests that infants start sleeping better at that point, too. By rolling over, they have a self-soothing tool because they have a bit more control over their bodies and their comfort. Of course, it's hard to figure out cause and effect here. Babies tend to start rolling over at about three or four months – and that's the time when their sleep cycles are lengthening anyway as their brain chemistry matures a bit. But encouraging the tummy time in the early weeks and months helps the baby develop those early motor skills that help him learn to roll over and back safely.

The Second Month (5–8 Weeks)

Babies sleep on average fifteen and a half to seventeen hours total, eight and a half to ten hours at night and six to seven hours during the day, spread over three or four naps. By the end of this month some will wake only once a night to be fed, although others will still need two overnight feedings for a few more weeks.

Breastfed babies will still need to eat about every two to two and a half hours, although some will go three hours.

The normal range is anything from eight to twelve feedings in twenty-four hours. By around six weeks they can sleep for one four- or five-hour stretch at night. Formula-fed babies will probably take about four ounces per feeding, about every three to four hours. They too can sleep for about five hours by six to eight weeks.

During the second month, your efforts to help her distinguish light and dark will start to bear fruit as she begins to recognize day and night and establish her natural circadian rhythms, her body clock.

Hallmarks of the second month are those adorable first smiles — and intense fussiness, particularly in late afternoon and early evening. At six to eight weeks, babies are too old to *habituate*, to just shut down and shut out stimulation. But they have not yet mastered self-calming. In this section, I will give you some tips on how to get through these difficult fussy weeks, and some advice on how to start helping your baby take the first steps toward sleeping longer and deeper. Always remember to use your whole repertoire of soothing techniques, not just the bottle or breast.

At this point, the maturing brain starts organizing nighttime sleep, and babies sleep up to four hours at a time, sometimes longer toward the end of the second month. During this month, your efforts to help her distinguish light and dark will start to bear fruit as she begins to recognize day and night and establish her natural circadian rhythms, her body clock.

During the day you still want to wake him after three hours so he keeps his best sleep for later. Aim to keep him awake from about 8:00 p.m. to 10:00 p.m. so he can have a final feeding around 10:00 and go to bed. He should then be able to sleep until about

2:00 a.m., wake to eat briefly, and then sleep again until about 6:00. (A common and acceptable variation is an 11:00 p.m. final feeding, a 3:00 a.m. middle-of-the-night feeding, and a 7:00 a.m. morning feeding.) Although babies get up between 6:00 and 7:00 a.m., they will nap again within the next two hours. Remember to get yourself to bed as early as you can.

By six to eight weeks, start being more conscious of sleep habits and patterns. Focus on bedtime, when you cue the brain to fall asleep and begin working on putting him down drowsy but awake. *In fact, drowsy but awake at bedtime is your big sleep goal for this month.* Stay nearby and soothe him as he finishes falling asleep. Make sure he doesn't always fall asleep with a breast or bottle in his mouth. If you are using a dummy, you may need to put it back in for him a few times, although you can also wait a bit and see if he can settle himself without it. (In the middle of the night at this age, don't worry about drowsy but awake or if he falls asleep with the breast or the bottle. If you are feeding him at 2:00 a.m., just return him to his bed and get back to sleep yourself.)

If he does cry when you put him down, you don't have to leave a tiny baby alone in the dark. I couldn't have done that with my girls when they were this little. Sit by his side, pat him, and quietly 'sh-sh' him. It's very tempting to pick him up, but try to resist doing it repeatedly. Do go ahead and hold him, though, if he does begin to cry so intensely that he won't be able to wind himself down. Put him down again when he's calm – but don't wait until he's fully asleep.

Sleep Lady Tip

Avoid picking your baby up and putting him down repeatedly, as some baby books recommend. That often overstimulates babies and makes it even harder for them to go to sleep.

The brain takes longer to sort out daytime sleep, so napping will remain fairly disorganized this month – and probably until he's about four months. He will take three or four naps – don't worry about whether it's three or four, and don't worry about minor day-to-day variations (although you don't want total chaos). New parents often underestimate how frequently babies require sleep. If he stays awake more than two hours at a time, he will become overstimulated as well as overtired, and it will be harder for him to nap. That means that if he wakes up at 7:00 a.m., he should be napping by 9:00.

To help him get ready to nap, place him in a quiet environment a half hour or so before you want him to fall asleep (i.e., if he's going to nap at 9:00 a.m., start setting the stage at 8:30). That might mean nursing, or walking him a bit, or holding him while you sing him a song. If you feel ready, you can start working on putting him down drowsy but awake for his nap, although at this early age he may need to be a little higher on the 'drowsy' end of that scale.

By the end of this month, phase out motion sleep in cars, swings, and the like and get him napping in a cot or Moses basket. Many naps will still be short, just forty-five minutes or so, but gradually some of the naps should last an hour or more. If he usually wakes after only about thirty minutes, try to stretch out some of these catnaps by keeping him in his cot and soothing him back to sleep, comforting him the way you do at bedtime. It won't always work, but give it ten minutes or so and try again the next day. It's usually easier to work on this in the morning than in the afternoon.

Night feedings should taper off by the end of this month, certainly in the third month. If you find yourself nursing more frequently, particularly at night, ask yourself whether he is really hungry, when he last ate, and whether you should be offering comfort other than a breast.

Sleep Lady Tip

Even at this young age, some babies act on their growing recognition of their parents by trying to resist sleep. They want to stay awake and hang out with you, a pattern that may intensify as they go through peaks of separation anxiety in the coming months.

During this month, usually from six weeks on, babies begin to differentiate their cries, and that helps us figure out what's bothering them and how to fix it. There's a 'Change my nappy' cry. There's a 'Pick me up and hold me' cry. There's a 'Mum, I'm ready for bed now' cry, an 'I don't feel well' cry, a 'Give me back my dummy right now' cry, and, of course, a hunger cry. Don't treat all cries as hunger cries.

'With Holly, I always thought that crying meant hunger. So it was cry, feed, cry, feed. It was food first, then try something else,' said Marianne, that mother of three whom you will meet again in Chapter 13, 'Helping Twins and Siblings Sleep.' 'By the time I got to Ally, my third, it was try everything else before I tried food.' Instead of automatically nursing Dean and Ally for every cry, she'd walk them, rock them, pat them, and rub their backs, being careful not to do it so constantly that it would become a sleep crutch.

The Third Month (9–12 Weeks)

Babies this age on average need fifteen hours of sleep, ten at night and five spread out over three daytime naps. Many babies toward the end of this month can sleep six- to eight-hour stretches at night without feeding. They still need to eat about every three hours, but they don't need to eat as much at night. Bottlefed babies should eat four to five ounces per feeding every three to four hours.

During the third month, babies make a lot of progress, and you should get more rest. We can begin to work on improving both the quality and the quantity of her nighttime sleep, and toward the end of this month even begin to improve napping. The fussiness ebbs by the end of this month. They are awake more during the day, asleep more at night, and beginning to find their own natural sleep-wake rhythms. Your job will be to gently and subtly adjust and mold that rhythm into a flexible schedule. (She still isn't ready for the Sleep Lady Shuffle, and you can't push too hard yet for her to 'sleep through the night.' You will be able to help her sleep for longer stretches, and some babies will sleep most of the night by the end of this month.)

The Secret Language of Babies

Babies have a lot of different cries. I have been fascinated by Priscilla Dunstan's work on baby sounds, and many families have found it very helpful in understanding their babies' preverbal communication. Understanding what our little babies are trying to tell us, of course, makes it easier for us to meet their needs.

Dunstan, then a twenty-four-year-old first-time mum of a colicky baby boy in Australia, was an accomplished violinist and a trained opera singer with the equivalent of a photographic memory for sound. Her own quest to understand her fussy boy led to a nine-year journey of research, which produced the Dunstan Classification of Infant Cries. It's a bit daunting to capture baby sounds on paper, but I'll do my best, and you may want to watch her DVD, *The Dunstan Baby Language System* (www.dunstanbaby.com).

Dunstan believes that each cry contains a message, and she has identified five sounds that correlate with five biological infant needs:

1. *Neh* means hungry
2. *Owh* means tired
3. *Eh* means needs to burp
4. *Eairh* means lower wind pain (gas)
5. *Heh* means physical discomfort

The sounds are based on the baby's reflexes. For instance, a hungry baby reflexively begins to suck. That produces the sound 'Neh' – baby talk for 'Feed me!' If we understand these five sounds (which travel across cultures, races, and ethnic groups), referred to as the 'precry' stage, we can understand what a baby needs before the full-blown crying begins – what Dunstan calls the 'siren.' If you can meet the child's needs in this 'precry' stage, when the sounds are still soft, you can reduce stress for everyone in the family and help promote a securely attached child.

The Dunstan researchers also report that babies whose parents can understand their communication in this way sleep longer and better. They have also found that by boosting parental confidence and reducing some of the exhaustion, the Dunstan system may also help women reduce their risk of postnatal depression. Although not all parenting experts would agree, the Dunstan researchers do not believe that 'colic' is an unexplainable condition with its own cry; a baby whose needs are met won't have colic.

The 'Fussies'

At the end of the first month or start of the second, many babies enter that superfussy period. It isn't a whole lot of fun. Late afternoon or early evening is a hard time for parents, too. We're pretty worn out after taking care of a little baby all day; we're trying to get dinner on the table and summon up at least a shred of energy to converse with the spouse arriving home from work. Perhaps we are taking care of other small children who are tired and hungry themselves at this time of day, or older children who see absolutely no point in picking up their toys before watching TV. It helps to remember that the superfussies are a phase, not a life sentence. The fussiness peaks at about six weeks and wanes by about twelve weeks. Here are some tips to get you through this stage:

- Give the baby regular naps and avoid overstimulation.
- Cut back on socializing and having visitors in the early afternoon. Meet friends and relatives earlier in the day (or hire a babysitter or enlist a friend or relative for an hour or so once in a while so you can get out).
- Feed your baby in a quiet, dim room, without the distractions of televisions, telephones, or conversations.
- Do the best you can to keep older siblings away from the baby at this time of day.
- If possible, enlist Dad's help and convince him that instead of playing the action-packed games that fathers often favor, he should be 'soother in chief.' Fathers tend to arrive home just as the baby hits her fussy peak, between 6:00 and 7:00 p.m. It creates a discouraging and difficult dynamic.

I remember Bill was totally convinced that our first daughter detested him because he'd walk in the door, arms outstretched, and she'd greet him with a howl. Sometimes she'd fuss and scream for an hour in the early evening, and Bill learned how to be a very soothing dad, swaddling her, holding her, and walking her until she finally got calm. Good thing, too, because our second one fussed even more, doing an outstanding job of disproving the myth that it's easier with your second child!

Soothing Techniques

I often remind you to use your repertoire of soothing techniques, so you don't rely exclusively on nursing or feeding to calm your baby. We talk about soothing throughout the book, and many tools (like rocking your baby) are quite instinctual. But here's a quick checklist. Some, like swaddling, we use for only the first few months, but others, like gentle massage, are terrific through much of childhood.

Remember to respond to your newborn quickly, because once the baby gets hysterical, she's harder to soothe. Later on we try to strike a little more of that balance I discussed between immediately responding and letting them learn to self-soothe. But in the first few months, it's our job to create their calm.

If one technique doesn't work after about ten minutes, try another. If you get to the point where you are even more frustrated than your baby, let another adult take over. If you are alone and have reached the breaking point, let the baby cry for a few minutes in a safe place (i.e., his cot or bouncy chair) while you take a few minutes to calm yourself.

Here are some common strategies:
- Carrying your baby
- Swinging or rocking your baby
- Swaddling
- Repetitive soothing sounds or music
- Sucking a dummy
- Massaging the baby (I recommend some massage books in my resource list at the end of this book)

Sleep Lady Tip

Around the third month, babies start producing melatonin, a hormone that relaxes the muscles and promotes drowsiness. Linked to light and darkness, melatonin secretions rise in the evening. By regulating your baby's sleep, encouraging her to maximize her nighttime sleep, you are helping to establish good hormonal rhythms, which will in turn further improve her sleep.

Helpful changes are now occurring in her brain, and she's developing a better body clock. Some well-rested babies can now stay awake three hours at a stretch during the day. This isn't an iron-clad rule, so watch carefully and put her down if she starts looking or acting tired. Don't wait too long, because if you let her get overtired, she'll have more trouble sleeping and get fussier.

Make naps more structured. Toward the end of this month, at around twelve weeks, the morning nap should start to fall into place, lasting about one to one and a half hours and occurring around the same time each day. In a few weeks, you'll see the stubborn afternoon nap take on a more dependable shape as well. She will probably take a brief third and even fourth nap in the late afternoon, forty-five minutes to an hour depending on the quality and quantity of earlier naps. At this point, you should start putting her down drowsy but awake for the morning nap. (Afternoon naps are still harder.)

Babies are less portable now for day sleep; they need a quiet and familiar environment without a lot of light, noise, and distractions. They also need a deeper sleep, which their brains don't allow if they are in motion. She shouldn't be napping in car seats, strollers, and the like anymore; she needs to be home and in her cot or Moses basket. You can be a little more flexible if she falls asleep in a car, swing, or stroller during that third or fourth little nap.

You should have a bedtime routine – a very simple
one, bath, pajamas, maybe some infant massage or
baby yoga, a song or a simple picture book – that
you will build on as she gets older.

Bedtime should now look like bedtime, and it should be the same time every night, give or take fifteen minutes. Sure, she might just conk out on you at 8:00 one night when you had been planning to put her down at 9:00, but you don't want a completely scattered schedule: a 7:00 bedtime one night and 11:00 the next. You should start to see her natural bedtime window emerge toward the end of this month. Let that guide you.

You should have a bedtime routine – a very simple one, bath, pajamas, maybe some infant massage or baby yoga, a song or a simple picture book – that you will build on as she gets older. Nurse or bottlefeed her, swaddle her if she still likes it, and put her down drowsy but awake. If she knows how to put herself to sleep at bedtime, it will be easier for her to start learning to put herself back to sleep in the middle of the night without a round of 'comfort nursing.'

Your goal this month should be to lengthen nighttime sleep, working toward that six to eight hours of
uninterrupted sleep.

Babies still need six or eight feedings, but fewer will be during the night. At the beginning of the month, she'll probably still need a 10:00 p.m. or 11:00 p.m. bedtime feeding, but gradually you will move that earlier, to about 8:00 p.m. You'll know she's ready for the earlier bedtime either when she can sleep eight hours at a stretch overnight or when you see that she is fading earlier. Watch for sleepy cues, such as yawning, rubbing her eyes, or crankiness.

There is some natural variation to how long babies in this age range can sleep at night without a feeding – anything from six to ten hours is normal. Some babies will sleep all the way through the night, and others will semirouse themselves for one very brisk and businesslike nursing. They'll be only half awake, they'll eat, and they'll go right back to sleep.

Your goal this month should be to lengthen their nighttime sleep. I breastfed both of my children, but they both began sleeping through the night at this age. At eight weeks Carleigh slept from around 9:00 p.m. or 10:00 p.m. until 7:00 a.m., and Gretchen at ten weeks slept from 10:00 p.m. to 6:00 a.m.

If your baby is waking up for more frequent nighttime feedings, and you and your doctor have ruled out health and milk-supply problems, then you should begin gently helping her to change her pattern. Make sure your doctor agrees that your child is growing well enough and is healthy enough to have only one overnight feeding.

Whether you are breast- or bottlefeeding, make sure that she's eating well during the day, which means she'll have less incentive to eat at night. Give her full feedings, including both foremilk and hindmilk (see Chapter 5, 'The Right Start for Newborns and Infants') if you're nursing. Try not to let her graze or snack all day, because she'll get in the habit of eating all day and night, whether she needs to or not. Feed her in a quiet place with few distractions so she'll concentrate on her meal, not her environment. You may want to 'cluster feed,' which means you feed her frequently in the late afternoon and early evening. You have two choices as to how you reduce nighttime feedings.

Option 1 is a *dreamfeed*. Before you go to sleep, wake her for one final feeding. This 'dreamfeed' should ideally be between 10:00 and 11:00 p.m. (depending on when you fed her before bedtime). Keep the lights off, rouse her as little as possible, feed her, and put her back to bed quickly. Then do not feed her again during the night; instead, use other soothing techniques if she wakes up. Some babies, like my first child, respond well to a dreamfeed. Carleigh was happy to be woken gently, and she ate well and went back to sleep. If your child is like my second daughter, you may find that she doesn't eat much when you wake her, and then she gets up hungry a few hours later. In that case, you are probably better off trying the second method below. If you do dreamfeed, focus on feeding her quickly and getting her back to bed. Unlatch (or remove the bottle) as soon as she's done, and avoid any other interaction that will encourage her to stay up and play.

Option 2 is a *set-time feeding*. Set a time during the night to feed her, and then feed her only at that predetermined time. You can decide to feed the first time she wakes up, as long as it's been at least four hours after her bedtime feeding. Or you can choose a later time – for instance, her 'set time' can be the first time she wakes up after midnight (particularly if you know that's when she's been the hungriest or that she hasn't responded well to a dream-feed at an earlier time).

Some parents find that when they get on more consistent sched-ules, the babies just start skipping this final feeding on their own and sleeping longer, maybe eating a bit more during the day.

Whichever option you choose, stick to it; don't go back and forth. If she wakes up at other times, and she may the first few nights, use other calming and soothing techniques to help her get back to sleep. Sit by her and reassure her, but don't feed her until at least 6:00 a.m. If she's very upset, pick her up for some brief reassurance, but put her down when she's calm so she falls asleep in her bed, not your arms. Try not to pick her up and put her down over and over again. If you are clear and consistent, babies usually stop waking up for those other feedings within just a few nights.

Sleep Lady Tip

If you're worried your baby's going to feel little and lost in that great big cot, here's a trick to make a little nest within the cot. Roll up one or more baby blankets or towels to make a U and place them under the tightly fitted sheet, so they can't get loose and harm the baby. (One mum I know also fastened them with ponytail holders to make the rolls tighter.) Position the baby with her feet toward the bottom of the U. (Review the exact placement with your doctor so there's no suffocation or SIDS risk.)

If you have been cosleeping but want to switch her into her own bed, or if you have had her in a Moses basket but want to transfer her to a full cot, the end of the third month is the ideal time. Put her in the cot for daytime naps first, if she isn't there already. Give her about a week of napping in the cot to get used to it, then move her to the cot at night. Be consistent. If you want her in her cot, you have to keep her there all night, every night. Soothe her, stroke her, do what you need to comfort her, but don't just surrender and bring her back to your bed because you fear it's the only way you can get her to sleep. It's not.

The Fourth and Fifth Months

At four months babies should be able to sleep about eight hours at night without a feeding, and by five months they go for about ten or eleven hours. They sleep four to five hours during the day, spread out over three naps. One of our main goals at this stage is to help lengthen, organize, and improve the naps.

Babies still need to eat frequently, at least five times a day, every three to four hours. By five months, you may be able to work on stretching it closer to four hours. Occasionally, perhaps during a growth spurt, he may have to eat every two to three hours. Formula-fed babies will eat a bit less frequently, and keep adding about an ounce per feeding a month. By the end of the fifth month, the formula-fed baby will eat six to eight ounces at a time, at four or five feedings in twenty-four hours. Total consumption shouldn't exceed thirty-two ounces per day.

I get a lot of calls from parents of thirteen to sixteen week olds. Some mums go back to work around then, and they are frantic about juggling work and family when they are getting only a few hours of sleep – and frequently interrupted sleep at that. Also, many parents expect babies to start sleeping better after three months, only they think it just sort of happens magically and they get an unpleasant shock.

This is an excellent time, often the ideal time, to step in and coach a baby to sleep better. Bad sleep habits are not yet deeply ingrained, and the baby is experiencing physical and developmental changes, including an increased ability to soothe herself, that are very conducive to a more predictable schedule.

Developmental Changes

The fourth and fifth months are a time of transition. Colic and fussiness subside. Babies are more awake and more active. They experience an exciting burst of cognitive awareness, becoming more aware of sights and sounds and beginning to understand cause and effect and *object permanence*, realizing that people and things exist even when they are out of the baby's view. That's one reason they love hiding games and peekaboo, a great new element in the bedtime routine.

Along with this greater cognizance of new and old, here and there, familiar and unfamiliar, comes a bout of separation anxiety. When she wakes up at night, she may not be searching for a feeding anymore so much as a brief bit of reassurance that her parents are right where they are supposed to be.

Neurologically, the character of the baby's sleep is evolving, too. Over the fourth and fifth months, melatonin secretion rises and non-REM sleep increases, meaning she sleeps more deeply than she did as a newborn. But the non-REM also means that when she does have a partial arousal every three to four hours, it's more distinct, and she feels more awake. She may need a quick reassurance from you as she adjusts to this change, but she doesn't need a feeding.

Sleep Lady Tip

Babies this age are very sensitive to changes in routine. An unusually stimulating day, when you have a lot of visitors or are out and about in new places, can disrupt her night sleep. That will inevitably happen once in a while. Just take extra care the next day that she gets plenty of naps and has a little extra quiet time so you don't get into that vicious cycle of exhaustion leading to more sleeplessness leading to more exhaustion.

Some babies may cry out but quiet themselves by the time you reach the bedroom door, so you should tiptoe away before you wake her more. Others get more upset and disorganized and still need your help to calm down. Help her, but don't overdo it. Don't do so much patting or stroking or singing that she can't get to sleep without it. You want to comfort her, not create a new sleep crutch.

As your child's sleep becomes more organized, you can also start reading her tiredness clues. That means keeping one eye on the clock and the other eye on your baby. Is she active or is she yawning? Is she rubbing her eyes? Starting to nod off? These are all sleep signals. Pay attention, because it's a lot better for her to go to bed, whether it's naptime or bedtime, when she's getting tired than waiting until she's overtired. Cynthia's mum, Jayne, found that keeping a detailed sleep log helped her learn to recognize her four-month-old daughter's cues and rhythms, to see when her 'sleep window' was open. 'She'd yawn, rub her eyes, and start spacing out. I learned that by the second yawn, I'd better get her to bed for naptime.'

Bedtime

Because four and five month olds are more alert, they need an evening routine that helps them switch mental gears, unwind, and get ready for bed. Bedtime should be between 8:00 p.m. and 9:00 p.m., although you will shift that earlier to between 7:00 p.m. and

8:00 p.m. during the fifth or sixth month as daytime naps decrease and he sleeps longer at night uninterrupted. Remember to get him down drowsy but awake – it's increasingly important at this age. Some babies fuss and cry when you put them into the cot; some just nod off. If yours cries, sit by his cot, pat him, 'sh-sh' him, give him the reassurance he needs, but also give him some space to calm down and fall asleep on his own. Be his coach, not his crutch.

If he consistently falls asleep during that last prebedtime feeding, pay attention. He's telling you that he needs an earlier bedtime, so move it up fifteen or twenty minutes at a time until you find the right moment for him. That way he can finish nursing or taking his bottle and get into bed drowsy but awake.

Even if his bedtime is right, he may still occasionally fall asleep at the breast – or he may use the breast (or bottle) to put himself to sleep, thwarting your efforts to put him to bed drowsy. Remember, if his eyes are rolling back and he's suckling but not swallowing, unlatch him and put him down before he's completely conked out.

Sometimes the unlatching will wake him up and he will want to latch right back on, almost as if he's saying, 'Sorry! I didn't mean to fall asleep on the job. I'm still hungry!' In that case, go ahead and give him one more opportunity to finish. Help him stay awake by stroking his head or rubbing his palms, feet, or back. If he just reverts to suckling again and isn't taking in any more milk, assume he's done eating and is now trying to nurse himself to sleep. Unlatch him, burp him, swaddle him, and get him into the cot quickly.

At about five months, when Nina and Mitch also tackled Lydia's eating and napping patterns, they made a big effort to establish a calm and consistent evening routine. They kept the lights low and the television off. After a ten-minute bath, they moved into Lydia's bedroom and slathered a lot of nappy cream on her to prevent rashes. They dressed her in a 'sleep sack,' which kept her warm and cozy and freed them from worrying about dangerous or tangled bedding. They played a few quiet games, shunning any toys with 'crazy lights or noises' at bedtime. Nina then sat with her in a chair and read the same three little books that Lydia already recognized as part of her bedtime ritual. If Nina saw Lydia's sleep signals – yawning, eye rubbing, or diving toward Nina's chest — she sped up the bedtime process. She nursed Lydia but made sure to unlatch her and put her down drowsy but awake.

Around the fifth month, babies start to test how their actions can affect the world around them. They want to probe their powers, and your limits. You may see it at bedtime. One favorite experiment for these budding Einsteins seems to be 'If I cry, can I make Mummy come to my cot?' Respond and show her that yes, you'll come to check on her. But once you've reassured her, don't linger.

Feeding

You want to really focus on meeting the baby's nutritional needs during the day so he doesn't eat at night. He should be either sleeping through the night or eating only once at night. *Cluster feeding,* meaning more frequent feedings in the late afternoon or early evening, may help calm him, enhance his evening sleep, and also reassure you at night that he is getting enough food.

Sleep Lady Tip

With his new alertness and eagerness to take in his surroundings, your five month old may become more distractible while he eats. If so, try to feed him in a quiet, dimly lit place so that he can concentrate, with only a few breaks to look at Mum and smile.

The conventional wisdom on starting solids has shifted several times over the years, but these days most pediatricians introduce rice cereal or a similar food at six months. Some babies do well on solids earlier — discuss it with your doctor, but I think of this as a dietary issue, not a sleep solution. (If you try solids earlier and it doesn't go smoothly, just put it off for another month or so with your doctor's approval. It should be a pretty natural transition when the baby is ready.) Some parents introduce rice cereal early and give it at bedtime to make a baby sleep longer. After watching scores of families try this without significant success, I have my doubts. I think solids help those relatively few babies who still wake up repeatedly because they are truly hungry at night.

The more adept he is at putting himself to sleep, and back to sleep at night, the easier it is for him to give up nighttime feeding.

That problem is better addressed by making sure your baby eats more during the daytime. In those cases, a little cereal *during the day*, with your doctor's permission, might help shift the feeding clock. But if she is waking up because she has not yet developed good sleep habits, if she needs a bottle or breast to get through those partial arousals, or if she knows that at the first sound of her cry you will hustle her off into your bed, offering your child a few spoonfuls of cereal probably isn't going to solve the problem. You need to address the poor sleep habits themselves.

At four months, your baby should be able to sleep about eight hours at night without a feeding. At five months, he should be able to go for ten, often eleven, hours. The more adept he is at putting himself to sleep, and back to sleep at night, the easier it is for him to give up nighttime feeding. He may even do it without any help from you.

If he's getting up once to eat now, semirousing himself for one brisk and businesslike meal and then getting right back to sleep, I would leave it alone, as long as he is pretty good at getting himself to sleep and back to sleep. He'll probably outgrow that last feeding soon. If not, you'll learn how to gently end it at six or seven months. (Until he does outgrow it, you might want to have Mum nurse some nights and Dad give a bottle the other nights so you get a little more rest yourselves.)

Sleep Lady Tip

Until your baby outgrows middle-of-the-night feedings, you might want to have Mum nurse some nights and Dad give a bottle the other nights so you get a little more rest yourselves.

But if he's getting up frequently at night to eat, it's time to tackle it. With your doctor's approval, you want to get him down to one feeding at night, with the goal of stretching out the time he can go without the breast or bottle to eight and then ten hours.

Often it's the parent as much or more than the child who holds on to excess middle-of-the-night feedings, not quite convinced that the child won't starve. It's an understandable reaction because you've been so focused on feeding since his birth, and it's hard to feel certain that he just doesn't need all those feedings anymore.

A food and sleep log can help you see more clearly when he's hungry, when he's nursing for comfort, and how long he can go without food. Resist the urge to nurse at every cry – and pay attention to how your baby behaves. If he cries, you rush in, and he nurses for three minutes and then falls asleep, he clearly isn't hungry. He's using the breast as a sleep crutch, simply because he is used to it.

I'm going to give you two options for cutting back nighttime feedings, similar to the suggestions I made for three month olds. Make sure your doctor agrees that your child is growing well enough and is healthy enough to have only one overnight feeding.

Option 1 is a *dreamfeed* (which we learned about in the three-month section). That means you rouse him just enough to eat for one final feeding before your own bedtime, probably around 10:00 or 11:00 p.m., but then do not feed her again during the night; instead, use other soothing techniques if she wakes up. Some babies don't like being woken up to be fed at this time and don't feed well when they are sleepy, so you'll know pretty quickly whether dreamfeeding works with your child's temperament and body clock. If you do dreamfeed, focus on feeding her quickly and getting her back to bed. Unlatch (or remove the bottle) as soon as she's done, and avoid any other interaction that will encourage her to stay up and play or cling to you. At around five or six months, if the baby is healthy and growing well and you have your doctor's support, you'll start weaning off the dreamfeed if she hasn't started skipping it on her own. Slowly decrease the minutes you nurse, if you are breastfeeding, or start cutting back the ounces in a bottle. You can also decide in one fell swoop to just stop feeding at night. If she wakes during this transition, reassure her as you have at other wakenings.

Option 2 is a *set-time feeding*. Set a time during the night to feed her, and then feed her only at that predetermined time. You can decide to feed the first time she wakes up, as long as it's been at least four hours after her bedtime feeding. Or you can choose a later time – for instance, the first time she wakes up after midnight (particularly if you know that's when she's been the hungriest or that she hasn't responded well to a dreamfeed at an earlier time).

Either of these options is fine – *as long as you are consistent*. Choose one approach and stick to it. And feed her only once at night, and not again until at least 6:00 a.m. If you cave in, you are just giving her intermittent reinforcement, and those mixed messages only make it harder for her in the long run. If she wakes wanting food at a time that's not part of your feeding plan, find other ways of soothing her. Go briefly to her cot, reassure her, and comfort her with verbal and some physical reassurances. Comfort yourself too by reminding yourself that she is a healthy, well-nourished baby. If you are doing the Shuffle with a four or five month old, resume your bedtime Shuffle position if she wakes up at night

Some parents find that when they get on more consistent schedules, the babies just start skipping this final feeding on their own and sleeping longer, and maybe eating a bit more during the day. Usually, it only takes a few nights at this age for them to stop waking up.

Ari

'I'm a therapist, and I'd read all the books, and here I was exhausted, at my wit's end, nursing Ari three or more times a night – I was the boobie lady,' said Cheryl. When Ari was four months old, Cheryl and Gary decided to stop the nighttime nursing completely. Their pediatrician agreed Ari would be fine going ten hours without nursing.

In her professional capacity, Cheryl knew a great deal about child development and tears, but as a very hormonal, very emotional new mum (her own description), she couldn't deal with it, so her husband took over the night shift. Gary needed to spell out ahead of time precisely what to do and say when Ari woke up – a script of intervention. 'He needed to know what words to say, when to say 'hush, hush,' how long to sit in the rocking chair, how many minutes to pat Ari. Then he could carry it out,' Cheryl said. Perhaps because this couple had already started and stopped and started and stopped several other sleep systems, Ari did not respond as quickly as many four month olds. Still, in less than two weeks, he was on a very good eating and napping schedule and almost always sleeping through the night.

Lydia

To get five-month-old Lydia to sleep, Nina and Mitch took her into their bed, nursed every one and a half to two hours, rocked her, held her, and walked her – and often that worked only if Lydia could hear running water in the background! 'She was a motion junkie, a nursing junkie, and a white-noise junkie. I had to do this tummy-to-tummy rocking motion to get her to sleep in the bathroom with the water on,' said Nina, who on really tough nights had to tummy rock and nurse simultaneously.

Nina knew that Lydia was perfectly healthy and a good size for her

age and that she didn't need to eat that often. Knowing was on.
Doing something about it was much harder. When Nina asked the pedia-
tricians in her group practice, each gave her totally different advice, none of
it terribly useful.

One of the first things I had Nina do was to pay strict attention to
how Lydia behaved when she woke up at night. Nina immediately noticed
that the baby calmed down as soon as Nina picked her up. Lydia didn't
actually need to nurse; her mother's arm or shoulder were reassurance enough.
That knowledge made it easier for Nina and Mitch to proceed.

Nina remembered that Lydia had once gone six hours without nursing.
If she had done it once, her parents knew she could do it again, and they
finally got everyone in the pediatrics practice, including the nurse-on-demand
lactation consultant, to agree that six hours was a reasonable goal. They
knew that she almost always woke up at 2:00 a.m., which was six hours
after her bedtime. They decided to feed her at 2:00 a.m. or later and only
one time at night.

When Lydia cried – and she did wake up on and off and cry the first
few nights – Mitch went in to soothe her back to sleep. Once she woke
after 2:00 a.m. – her 'set time' – Nina nursed. But she put her back into
her cot instead of taking her into the family bed

Maude

Kathleen and Mickey had endured the poor sleep patterns of their first
child, Sean, until at nine months they used Dr Marc Weissbluth's cry-it-
out program. It worked, but the flood of tears made everyone tense and
miserable. With Maude, their second child, they wanted earlier and gentler
intervention. Kathleen was going back to work and didn't know how she
could function while caring for a four month old who 'did not sleep at all'
and a two and a half year old who got up at 5:00 a.m. (I also helped
the family with Sean's early rising, a common difficulty I discuss in my
chapters on older children.)

Although Kathleen and Mickey had tried to stop cosleeping with Maude
after the first few months, the baby seldom slept in her cot for more than
an hour or so. She would get up to nurse, and then mother and baby would
end up sleeping – or not sleeping – in the spare bed in the baby's room.
Kathleen had nursed Sean until nineteen months and was committed to

long-term nursing for Maude as well. She knew she had to stop all the nighttime nursing, but was afraid that would make her milk dry up completely. Her doctor convinced her that she could limit nursing without stopping it altogether, and guided her through a nursing and pumping schedule to help her body make the transition.

Kathleen and Mickey decided to use the set-time option. That would mean feeding Maude at midnight, and then not again until 6:00 a.m. As a two-time parent, Kathleen had learned that some tears 'aren't going to scar them for life. They aren't going to remember this when they are thirty and blame you.' Still, the first two nights weren't easy. Emotionally, Mickey and Kathleen both found it far easier to deal with Maude's initial forty-minute crying jag (knowing a parent was nearby) than they had with Sean's far more intense screaming (listening from afar). On the third night, Maude didn't cry — and she didn't wake up at midnight to be fed either; she slept all the way to dawn!

Kathleen and Mickey decided to pick up on her cue, and not feed her at night at all anymore. It wasn't always consistent after that. Some nights she slept, and some nights she woke up; sometimes she went right back to sleep, and sometimes she fussed a little, but nothing like that first difficult night. As she had hoped, Kathleen was able to nurse Maude for quite some time to come, only now she nursed in the morning and evening, pumped during the day — and slept at night.

A lot of babies at this age make it almost but not quite through until morning. They get up at about 5:00 a.m. to nurse, and then go back to sleep until 8:00 or so. If you find that her wake-up time is all over the place, her naptimes are haphazard, and on top of that her feeding times are starting to come right at naptime so she keeps falling asleep, then it may be time to phase out that 5:00 a.m. feeding (especially if you fed him earlier in the night). It's a hard time of day to cope, and you might have a few unpleasant days with some tears. But at this age, it's seldom more than a few days.

If you let these 5:00 a.m. mess calls continue, early rising becomes an extremely stubborn habit to change, and it can cause you grief for the next several years. If he protests when he doesn't get fed at 5:00, remember, you don't have to leave him alone to cry. You can stay with him and soothe him. Once the clock strikes 6:00, if he's still fussing, then do a dramatic wake-up (leave the room, count to ten, and come back in), get him up, change him, feed him, and start the day. (If he's fallen asleep, wait until he gets up on his own to feed him.)

Be consistent – that's incredibly important when dealing with early risers. Some babies will be up for good at 6:00; others will eat and fall asleep again. If yours gets up at 6:00, leave it alone for a bit while he adjusts to skipping that 5:00 a.m. feeding. Then, try keeping him in his cot until 6:15, then 6:30, and so on, in fifteen-minute intervals. Keep doing this until he gets to a point where he won't sleep later – or until you reach 7:00 or 7:30, which is a good time for a baby this age to start his day.

Napping

Gone are the days when a thirty-minute catnap would suffice. At four and five months, napping is all about length and predictability. Remember to watch both the clock and your baby's own behavior to know when it's time to put him down. You want to catch him when he's getting tired. Not after he's just fallen off the sleepiness cliff.

At this point, it's usually best if your baby naps in his cot. If you haven't got your child out of the car seat, swing, or stroller for naps, do so right now. He is just too old for it; the motion will hamper his ability to get the deeper, more restorative sleep he needs.

Sleep Lady Tip

Feeding him when he's up and alert, instead of ready to go to bed, helps weaken that food-sleep association and reinforces the message that he can get to sleep and stay asleep without a breast or bottle.

If you are committed to the family bed for the long haul, I would still recommend that he nap in his cot now. Some, although not all, mums who cosleep find they have to lie down with the child at naptime once or twice a day for three or four years. That can become quite limiting, especially if you plan to go back to work or have a second child. Plus, you can leave him alone in the cot safely. You must never let a baby nap alone in the family bed without close supervision. It's just not safe, particularly as they get older and more mobile.

Try not to nurse your child to sleep at any naps now. That's easier now that the feedings are further apart and you can plan the naps around them. For instance, a baby can wake up at 7:00 a.m., nurse, nap at 9:00, and not need another nursing until he wakes at 10:30.

Tracy and Drew, whose struggle with Lucas's reflux you can read about in Chapter 15, 'Medical Problems,' found that keeping a log greatly assisted them in detecting his emerging natural daytime sleep rhythms. Since his nap training was slow and difficult, the log also helped them discern the little bits of progress that made it easier to persevere. Tracy had nursed on demand but now structured Lucas's feedings, knowing he would nap longer if he wasn't eating all the time. 'I tried to be much more conscious about making sure that he was fed before going down for a nap, and to be very conscious of the gaps between feedings. When I was enforcing the nap rules, I didn't have to worry that he was awake because he was hungry; I knew when he ate.'

Tracy found it too hard to do full-fledged nap training twice a day plus deal with Lucas's evening problems, so they initially focused on nights and the afternoon nap. The morning nap they tried to stretch to forty-five minutes and left it at that. As he got more unbroken sleep at night and slept later in the morning, the sleep dominos all fell into place. He now slept until 7:00 or 7:30, which meant he was able to stay up a little later before the morning nap. Then, because the morning nap ran later, he wasn't so exhausted by the time his afternoon nap rolled around. That helped him sleep longer in the afternoon, further reinforcing the improving nighttime sleep, which then bolstered the next day's naps and so forth.

Ideally, four- and five-month-old babies should nap for ninety minutes or longer, morning and afternoon. A third late-afternoon nap can be shorter. He may well stir after ten minutes, and again after twenty to thirty minutes, predictable times for a partial awakening from a nap. Don't rush in and get him out of the cot at the first peep. See if he can get himself back to sleep, or if he's getting louder and fussier, try to help him get back to sleep. Go to him before he reaches that full-fledged screaming mode, which will wake him even more. Rub his back or 'sh-sh' him or use another comforting technique and see if that will coax him back to sleep.

You'll probably have to experiment a bit to see what type of comforting is effective at this time of day. Some babies will fall asleep again if you leave them alone, and get more awake if you try to soothe them. Others will want you in their room but won't want you to touch them. Be patient and give him at least twenty to thirty minutes to resettle himself. He may well reward you with another forty-five minutes' sleep.

Phase out your intervention at the partial awakening as he becomes more skilled at resettling himself. Don't let him get dependent on your patting or stroking him to sleep. Once his body clock adjusts to a longer nap, he should gradually learn how to get through that partial awakening on his own and not need your assistance.

Cheryl and Gary used to have the CD player going while four-month-old Ari napped. Naturally, the music stopped after forty-five minutes, just around the time his brain was doing its partial awakening anyway. That did it. 'I had the monitor on and I'd hear the music go off, and he would stir and I would buzz right into his room all happy and "rescue" him — I'd wake him up! I learned not to go in, and he'd just stir and go back to sleep. He'd sort of talk to himself — la, la, la, la — and fall asleep,' his mother said.

Nap training can be frustrating, but stick to it. Most families see progress in a week or two at this age, but you aren't alone (or incompetent) if it takes longer. If you put it off, if you don't help him learn to take adequately long naps at predictable times, it's going to be much harder to train him later.

Brittany

Lisa and Ted's first child was a poor sleeper until I worked with them when Teddy was about seven months old. Brittany, their second child, was a much easier sleeper. Lisa initially attributed this to Brittany's temperament, saying she was a cheerful, happy child. Actually, Brittany had her fussy moments, and she also had reflux, which often disrupts sleep. Her mum just knew how to deal with it better; she had learned from her experience with Teddy. Lisa followed the Sleep Lady's Eight Rules of Infant Slumber and gently taught Brittany to sleep without trauma to mother or child. 'With Teddy, I hadn't realized how important sleep was, or understood how much sleep a baby needed. I figured, when he's tired, he'll sleep!' she recalled. With Brittany, Lisa was much more careful to protect her child's sleep.

For the first ten weeks, Brittany slept in a Pack-'n-Play in her parents' room at night, where nursing was convenient. She either napped there or in a cradle in the family room. Lisa did not pay much heed to my rule about a quiet, sleep-friendly nap environment. With a three-and-a-half-year-old boy on the loose, she figured that was a lost cause. 'We couldn't tiptoe around with a boy in the house. I did the laundry, let the phone ring; visitors came over.' But Lisa let Brittany nap when she needed to nap, even if it meant disappointing a visitor who wanted to see her with her eyes open.

Despite her laissez-faire attitude about noise, Lisa imposed some gentle discipline and structure from the start. She did not nurse Brittany to sleep or routinely hold her to sleep at naptime. 'I did it once in a while. Who can resist holding a sweet sleeping baby?' Instead, she worked on 'drowsy but awake,' particularly at naptime.

She had carted Teddy around everywhere in a fairly haphazard way, but she didn't take Brittany out too much until she was old enough to have a nap schedule. Then they were able to get out and about in Brittany's awake time but avoid napping in car seats and strollers all the time. The unavoidable exception was the mornings they had to drop Teddy off at preschool, just as Brittany was supposed to nap. If she fell asleep in the car, Lisa transferred her out of the car seat and into her cot. She usually woke up briefly, long enough to figure out where she was, but then she generally fell asleep again. Lisa let her cry briefly or soothed her back to sleep.

Like most infants, Brittany experienced a fussy period, and the second month was the worst. Not only that, but Brittany fussed in the early evening – just as Lisa and Ted were trying to get big brother Teddy into bed! Lisa usually nursed Brittany then to help her calm down, but she didn't nurse her fully to sleep. Sometimes on very fussy evenings she would hold Brittany to sleep, but that was okay because she didn't do it all the time. It never became a sleep crutch because Lisa made sure to put her down drowsy but awake at other times. By the end of the second month, the fussies subsided. At eight weeks, Brittany was sleeping six hours before she woke to nurse. Then she would go back to sleep quite easily.

Lisa had learned with Teddy the importance of getting a child to bed tired, not overtired, so she watched for Brittany's sleep-window clues. Initially, it was quite simple. Newborn Brittany sensibly yawned when she was ready for a nap. Later on, she would still yawn as we all do, but it was no longer a reliable sign that she was ready for bed. Instead, Lisa noticed that Brittany sucked her thumb when she was tired or hungry, and seldom sucked when she wasn't. Because Lisa had her scheduled pretty well by then, a quick glance at the clock usually told Lisa whether the baby was hungry or tired. As Brittany was quite even-tempered after she got through that fussy stage, Lisa also knew that if she was cranky and teary, she probably needed to go to bed.

Once Brittany was ready for bed, she was really ready. Lisa had a good bedtime routine for Teddy, and she tried to follow a very similar one for Brittany – bath, nappy change and pajamas, book, prayer, lights out, and then a final song with a parent sitting near the cot in the dark. Then Lisa or Ted would leave, shutting the door behind them, and the baby would fall asleep. But sometimes Brittany was so sleepy that Lisa couldn't get past the nappy change! 'She'd start to cry as I was changing her. She wouldn't even let me sit down to read; she'd just lean toward her cot as we passed it. So we didn't always follow the whole bedtime routine. When she wanted to sleep, it was best to just put her to bed!' In cases like this I would suspect that this baby needed to go to bed a little earlier, that her parents were skating awfully close to missing the sleep window and facing the dreaded second wind. But with Brittany, her mother correctly intuited that it was just the way she was. Some kids go from zero to sixty. Brittany went from sixty to zero.

By the time Brittany was fourteen weeks old, she was sleeping from

6:45 p.m. until 5:30 a.m., when Lisa was so engorged that she woke her to nurse. Then she went back to bed until 7:45. Over the next month or so, Lisa stopped that early-morning feeding, and Brittany just slept. If she got up early and stirred out of habit, Lisa and Ted learned to just let her be. After a brief moment of fussing she would fall asleep again on her own. By five months, she was sleeping twelve hours a night, from 7:00 p.m. to 7:00 a.m. 'I used to think the difference was that Teddy was 'difficult' and Brittany was 'easy.' But now I sometimes do question whether part of Teddy's 'difficult' babyhood was just that he never got enough sleep!' Lisa said. 'I took all of Kim's great advice to heart, and I know it made a difference in Brittany. In me, too. I felt much more confident in scheduling sleep for my baby — and I know it was needed.'

7

Six to Eight Months

*A*t this age, babies need an average of eleven hours of uninterrupted *nighttime sleep and three and a half hours of daytime sleep spread over two to three naps.*

From six through to eight months, babies become more mobile. They roll over, sit up, maybe even stand while holding onto something. Many scoot or crawl, and the first teeth come in. Most babies sleep through the night fairly regularly, but if yours doesn't, it is still quite easy to get them on track. You may also find that at six or seven months, a baby who had been a good sleeper starts having difficulties. As she experiences her first wave of separation anxiety, she may resist being left in her cot at night or may start waking up more often to see you.

This chapter will help you promote nighttime security, develop a sleep-friendly schedule, and introduce appropriate wind-down evening activities. As your baby grows, bedtime can be fun as you begin to share quiet songs and games and create family rituals. But first you may have to break some patterns. If your baby is used to being rocked, walked, nursed, or stroked to get back to sleep in the middle of the night, you will need to help her discard those sleep crutches. If she's spent the first few months sleeping in unconventional places, like swings or car seats, you need to get her into the cot.

As you make changes you may have to tolerate some tears – but you don't have to let her cry endlessly or alone. Sit by her as she cries and stroke her head or pat her back a little; whisper soothing words. Her tears are her way of saying she is tired and frustrated, or wary of this change. But if you let her, she will learn to cope, adapt, and soothe herself to sleep – and it won't take as long as you fear.

Many, if not most, sleep problems at this age involve associations between sleeping and eating. You don't want her falling asleep at the breast, or with a bottle in her mouth, both because it interferes with sleep independence and because it's terrible for those little teeth that are going to come bursting out any day. You should also start setting recognizable mealtimes, so your baby is not eating all day, an incentive to get up to snack all night. Babies respond well to structured daytime meals. One mum told me that she felt like 'a dairy bar that was open 24/7.' But when she established 'regular business hours,' her child cut back on snacking, ate better meals, and slept longer.

> You don't want her falling asleep at the breast, or with
> a bottle in her mouth, both because it interferes with
> sleep independence and because it's terrible for those
> little teeth that are going to come bursting out any day.

You will meet several families in this chapter whose stories may sound like your own. Each followed my advice – but with enough freedom to match their family's needs and their infant's emerging personality. Some could tolerate tears at night; others couldn't bear more than a minute or two. They all found the right mix. So will you.

Developmental Changes

Separation Anxiety

Separation anxiety has its first peak at this age, and it increases when babies are overtired. At bedtime, he may fight sleep in order to be with you. He may also wake up more often wanting to see you. The gentle techniques I use throughout this book, including attachment to a lovey and helping your child learn to self-soothe, will ease his anxiety. Rarely if ever will you leave him alone to cry in the dark, and never for more than a few minutes. When he wakes up at night, you won't put a pillow over your head and hope the crying stops. You will respond immediately. He will learn that the people he loves are close at hand and watching over him.

A lovey helps the baby cope with nighttime
separation, making him feel safe and sound when
you are not with him.

Loveys

A *lovey,* a special stuffed animal or blanket, sometimes called a *transitional object,* can be a useful tool to ease separation anxiety and weaken other sleep-disrupting nighttime habits. If your child is not already attached to a lovey, help him forge that bond. A lovey helps the baby cope with nighttime separation, making him feel safe and sound when you are not with him.

If he has not yet shown a preference, pick a lovey for him, although he might select a different one when he gets a little older. Usually, a soft stuffed animal or baby blanket will do, but pay attention to his emerging preferences. For instance, if he's a hair twirler, look for a blanket with a fringe or a stuffed animal with a similar feature, like a Beanie Baby Jellyfish with tentacles. If he likes to rub and massage things, try a small thick blanket. Six-month-old Erin's parents, Corinna and Jeremy, just used a cloth nappy because she had already grown so accustomed to burrowing into it on their shoulders.

Sleep Lady Tip

Make your life easier by selecting a lovey that's easy to clean or wash (when in doubt, try putting it inside a tied-up pillow case and washing it in a gentle cycle). Some parents buy two loveys in case one gets lost or left at Grandma's house, but, be warned, babies are smarter than they appear! They discern slight differences in touch or scent and will not always accept a substitute.

The lovey should be small, soft, and safe – nothing that could choke or smother an infant and nothing that he could later use as a launching pad to climb out of the cot. Run any concerns by your health visitor.

Encourage the bond by wedging the lovey between you and your baby when you nurse or bottle feed him. Tuck it in his arms, or next to him for naps and bedtime and when he wakes up during the night. You may want to 'wear' the lovey for a few hours inside your own shirt, to impart more of that comforting and familiar scent of Mum. Play with the lovey, especially but not exclusively at bedtime. Incorporate it in peekaboo, or have the lovey blow kisses or wave bye-bye to baby.

Some children don't get attached at this age, particularly if they have another sleep crutch, such as nursing. If he doesn't bond, try again every now and then as he gets older. Anita, for instance, rejected the blankie her parents offered her as a baby but when she became a toddler, she adopted 'Lamby.' Teddy similarly spurned every plush toy he was offered but then cheerfully bonded to two plastic teethers when he was about thirteen months old, happily gripping one in each hand at bedtime.

New Mobility

Babies' increased mobility at this age can cause some new bedtime (or naptime) problems. Sometimes they roll themselves over on one side – but can't roll themselves back. Try not to interfere. Make sure she gets a lot of daytime tummy time, maybe on a fun patterned play mat, to practice these movements.

Sleep Lady Tip

If you are worried that your baby can roll onto her tummy but can't yet return herself to the safer back-sleeping position, talk to your doctor about whether you need to gently 'flip' her over or whether she has enough control over her neck and head movements to protect herself from SIDS while she develops her rolling skills.

Similarly, babies learn to sit up or stand by holding onto the cot before they learn to lie back down. Give them some time to practice during the day; they will figure it out. It may not be very graceful, but they'll manage, and the more you let them, the quicker they will learn on their own. Leaving her in place may mean she'll fall asleep sitting up and just plop over, but don't worry. She won't hurt herself, and once asleep she will wriggle herself into a comfortable position.

If you must intervene, do it *once* at what I call the 'magic moment.' In other words, if your baby is sitting up, help her lie down once at a moment when you think that she'll go down and stay down. If she pops right back up again, don't lay her down. That way you can avoid a prolonged sit-up/lie-down struggle – which the parent rarely wins.

Creating a Schedule

Sample Schedule

7:00–7:30 a.m.
Wake-up. Upon waking, nurse or bottlefeed and give solids.

9:00 or 9:30 a.m.
 Morning nap, one and a half to two hours. Upon waking,
 nurse or bottlefeed and give solids.

12:30 or 1:00 p.m.
 Afternoon nap, one and a half to two hours. Upon waking,
 nurse or bottlefeed.

3:30–4:00 p.m. (depending on previous naptime).
 Optional third nap, about forty-five minutes to an hour.

5:00 or 5:30 p.m.
 Nurse or bottlefeed and give solids.

6:00–6:30 p.m.
 Start bath and bedtime preparations, which may include an
 additional bottle or nursing.

7:00–7:30 p.m.
 Asleep.

When I ask new parents about their baby's schedule, some look
as perplexed as if I had posed a problem in quantum mechanics.
The prospect of developing a routine should not be so terrifying.
A good schedule can transform a tired and fussy baby into a rested
and contented one. I don't recommend completely rigid schedules,
but I do recommend devoting a few weeks to really focusing on
your child's sleep. That means building your other tasks, errands,
and activities around sleep, naps, and baby meals, not squeezing the
sleep, naps, and baby meals in haphazardly between all the other
things you have to do. Nap training, in particular, can be time-
consuming for a few weeks.
 Later on you'll have more flexibility – and when everyone is
rested, it will be easier to plan, and enjoy, a family outing or a
stroller walk with Grandma. But don't overdo the flexibility. Just as
we adults need basic structure in order to feel good and function
well, *babies need predictability, too.* Your baby will not be at her best

if her morning naps are at 8:30 one day and 11:30 the next, or if she goes to bed at 7:00 one night and at 11:30 on another. The trick is to get your child on the right schedule; try to stick to it pretty regularly, but know how to read her cues and modify the schedule when appropriate. Some days she'll sleep a little more, some a little less, just like you do (and you don't even have growth spurts).

Sleep Lady Tip

When travel, illness, or special events force you to deviate, get back on schedule as soon as possible. Schedule variations are much easier for a child who is well rested than for a tired baby whose life is always in chaos.

Corinna and Jeremy had a very erratic schedule for Erin until she was six months old. She catnapped thirty to forty minutes a few times a day, instead of taking two good solid naps, and her mum said she looked 'almost as sleepy after a nap as before one.' At night, they had to walk and walk her to get her to sleep – so much that her dad got tennis elbow from carting her around.

With my help, we set regular naptimes, regular mealtimes, and a regular bedtime. In the beginning, Corinna stuck close to home and worked her life around the schedule, but once it fell into place, she had a little more flexibility. Erin began eating and sleeping better, and Jeremy, who had a long commute and a late workday, adjusted his routine so that if he didn't get home in time to enjoy Erin in the evening, they got great daddy-daughter time in the morning.

Teddy was another baby transformed by remarkably few tweaks to his routine. He was waking up too early, napping too briefly, and nursing more frequently, not less, as he grew older, possibly in part because of some separation anxiety when he was about seven to eight months old. He was cranky and fell asleep as soon as he got into a car — all the classic signs, Ted and Lisa later realized, of an overtired child.

Lisa became more consistent about his schedule and lengthened the intervals between nursing. She also modified his naptimes by a half hour or forty-five minutes. She began putting him down at 9:00 a.m., instead of 9:45, for the morning nap and at 1:00 p.m., not 1:45, for the afternoon nap. 'Those forty-five minutes made the biggest difference in the world,' Lisa said. 'I had been trying to keep him up too long. I was missing his sleep window, and he would be so overtired by the time I tried to put him down that he couldn't sleep.'

He began eating better, sleeping better, and generally looking much more pleased with life. As his napping improved, he slept better at night, and his parents were able to teach him to sleep through until 6:30 or 7:00 a.m. instead of getting up for a sunrise snack every day.

There is no 'right' schedule for all babies, but the sample I gave you is a good framework. Some variation is inevitable; a baby who naps for ninety minutes starting at 9:00 a.m. is not going to be on the same clock as one who naps for two hours starting at 9:30. But the starting point, 7:00 or 7:30 a.m., and the end point, 7:00 or 7:30 p.m., should be about the same. If she's in child care or with a sitter part of the day, make your home schedule conform as much as possible to the child-care feeding and naptimes, as long as that routine is a sensible one. Consistency counts.

Okay. That's the scheduling ideal. Let's walk through it in more detail.

Wake-up. When you are ready to start your baby's day, turn on the lights, open the blinds, and say 'Good morning.' In the Sleep Lady lexicon, I call it *dramatic wake-up.* You want her to learn to distinguish between daytime awakenings and nighttime awakenings, between daytime feedings and evening ones.

Nurse or Bottlefeed. Nurse when she wakes up and play for awhile. Then get yourself some breakfast and feed her solids. (By six months, babies are starting solids.) This is her introduction to breakfast.

Morning Nap. About an hour and a half to two hours after she wakes up, it's time for bed again. Usually, the morning nap starts at around 9:00 or 9:30, a little sooner for early risers. Remember, that's when she should be asleep, not getting ready to sleep. The nap should last one and a half to two hours. A common error is starting the nap at 10:00 or 10:30. That's usually too late – and her fussing and grouching are her ways of telling you it's too late.

Look for sleepy cues to tell you when she's getting ready. She may rub her eyes, yawn, become less active, or get fussy. Some babies make special little 'put me to bed now' noises that an attentive parent can learn to interpret. If you don't detect any tired cues, try taking your baby into a quieter room. If she's in a kitchen, play-room, or some other place full of activity and stimulation, she may mask her sleepy signals. Try not to feed her right before you put her down.

Heidi recalled how eight-month-old Kevin would get all loose and limp when he got tired. She called him 'spaghetti boy.' 'If you hold him, he's like jelly,' she laughed. 'It's definitely a tired sign.'

Corinna and Jeremy's daughter, Erin, would rub her eyes and ears, and make a strange little noise that her mother learned meant 'Get me to bed right now or you'll regret it!'

Awake Time and Lunch. Plan to have two to three hours of awake time between the end of morning nap and the start of the afternoon one. This is a nice time to play, take a walk, or run some errands and have lunch.

If your agenda requires driving, try doing it at the beginning of this awake window, not the end. If she's more alert, there's less chance of her dozing off in the car and throwing off her nap schedule for the rest of the day, or of getting so used to napping in the car (not as restful as sleeping in a cot) that she won't nap in a cot. Some babies will want to have a bottle and eat lunch soon after the morning nap; some can wait. It's up to you, but don't wait so long that you run into the afternoon nap. You want to build that separation between nursing and going to sleep.

Afternoon Nap. No more than three hours should elapse between the end of the morning nap and the start of the afternoon one. Usually that means between 12:30 and 1:30. Watch both the clock and your baby; she'll signal when she needs to go down. Remember to leave her a little time to unwind, to get ready to sleep. Give her a few kisses, maybe a little rocking, and put her in the cot. Ideally, this nap should last one and a half to two hours.

Snack. When she wakes, she gets a snack – nursing or another bottle.

Optional Late-Afternoon Nap. Some babies take a brief third nap, forty-five minutes to an hour, in the late afternoon. If your baby is a poor napper and her two main daily naps are an hour or less apiece, then this little third nap is mandatory. Without it, she'll be running on vapors.

Don't worry if your baby skips this nap; most give it up themselves by nine months. And although I usually avoid motion sleep, it's okay if she dozes off for this little nap in the car on her way home. Eliminate the third nap if she sleeps so late, 5:00 or 5:30, that she has a hard time getting to sleep at bedtime. If she naps until 6:00, you'll have a hard time getting her to sleep at 7:00. She needs at least two hours between the end of this mininap and bedtime.

Dinner. Dinner, another nursing, and the third solids (if advised by your pediatrician) should be around 5:00. Again, there's a little variation depending on her afternoon nap, but don't let it get too late. Unless you have no choice for work or child-care reasons, don't postpone dinner until both parents are home. All that wonderful advice about how families should eat more meals together does not apply to infants! In fact, some couples find that if they get the baby fed and to bed early, they may actually have time to sit down at the dinner table themselves and have a real conversation.

Bedtime. Bedtime should be at 7:00 or 7:30. I define bedtime as when she's in her cot, not when you are running the bath, putting on pj's, or reading stories. Don't rush it. You need time to get her ready for bed, and she needs time to get herself ready to sleep. At this age, you should usually allow twenty to thirty minutes, plus whatever time you need for bathing and pajamas.

Sleep Lady Tip

Some mums find it easier to create that separation by no longer nursing in the baby's room. Or if you do want to stay in the baby's room, try nursing with a dim light on and turn it off when you want to signal that it's cot time. Some families also create some separation in the baby's mind by having Mum nurse but then hand off the baby to Dad, who gives some kisses and then puts her in her cot.

Enjoyable bedtime activities include gentle massage or baby yoga, ten minutes or so of quiet music, or looking at short, simple picture books. Peekaboo and other calm and gentle games are a big hit. She may enjoy funny little caresses, like having you kiss your finger and then touch it to her nose. Include the lovey in any bedtime games. Have the lovey caress the baby's nose, too, or have it play peekaboo.

If your baby is used to bedtime music, keep it soft and quiet. Use music to set the mood and cue the brain for sleep, but turn it off before she gets into her cot, or soon after if it's on a timer. You don't want her so accustomed to lullabies that she can't get to sleep or get herself back to sleep without them.

If you've been playing music until after she falls asleep, slowly ease it out. Put her in her cot with the music playing very softly. Try to turn it off before she's fully asleep, and if the CD ends, don't restart it. The same goes for toys with music and lights: Start bedtime with them on if that's what she is used to, but phase them out before she is fully asleep.

Bedtime Feeding. It's okay to nurse or give her a bottle right before bed as long as she doesn't depend on it to put herself to sleep and you aren't feeding her to sleep when she wakes up at night. If she does depend on nursing, and that's a very common pattern at this age, try to make the final nursing earlier in the bedtime routine, say, before a song or story. (More on nighttime nursers in a minute.) Try not to let her fall asleep sucking; put her down drowsy but awake.

The goal of getting her down drowsy but awake is crucial (see Chapter 2, 'Getting Started and Tips for Success'). If your baby has trouble with it, focus your energy first on getting it right at bedtime. It's not less important at 2:00 a.m., but it's a lot easier for us as parents to follow through when we are not half asleep ourselves and anxious about who else is being woken and when we'll all get back to sleep. Once you get it right at bedtime, it will be easier to carry this out at other times.

The Sleep Lady Shuffle

My Sleep Lady Shuffle is a gentle behavioral modification technique that lets you be a comforting presence as your child learns to put himself to sleep in his cot.

You are going to start out right by his side, and over a period of about two weeks you will gradually move further away until you will be able to leave the room. Often, nighttime wakenings will start to taper off because of the combination of a more structured, consistent daytime routine and this newly acquired ability to fall asleep. *When he wakes up at night during the Shuffle, as he will at the beginning, you will return to the position you were in at bedtime that night and soothe him. You might want to go by his cot briefly to calm and caress him before you return to that evening's position.* After we walk through the Shuffle, in my 'Problems and Solutions' section I'll talk about some specific reasons that babies at this age wake up at night and how to address them.

You should follow the Shuffle schedule, moving on to the next position even if your child has had a bad night or two, fussing or waking more frequently. Don't be surprised if there's a little regression or protest the first night of each new chair position. If your child gets sick during the Shuffle, you might want to pause and 'freeze' or maintain your position until he's feeling a little better.

You might even have to move a little bit closer during an illness to offer more comfort. But then resume your sleep coaching when he recovers.

Nights 1–3. Once bath, stories, bottle or nursing, and songs are over and your baby is in his cot drowsy but awake, sit in a chair right *next to his cot*. If he cries or fusses, you can stroke or pat him intermittently but don't do it constantly or you'll just create a new negative association. (You can do more touching on night 1, then taper off.) It's also important that the parent control the touch. Instead of having him hold your hand or finger, you should pat his. Make sure that you do not caress the child too steadily; do it on and off. You don't want to swap one negative association, like rocking, for another, like your constant touch or the sound of your voice. Don't depend too much on touch because on day 4, you will be further away and won't be touching as much. (The no-snuggles or no-picking-up-the-baby edict does not apply to a child who is sick, frightened, or startled by a loud noise, but make sure you don't do so much snuggling that he will expect it even when he is feeling better.)

Try not to pick him up – but if he's extremely upset, go ahead and pick him up, over the cot if possible. Hold him until he's calm, but keep it brief. Put him down again while he's still awake. You can sing during the get-ready-for-bed stage, but once it's time for sleep, you are better off making lulling 'sh-sh' or other soothing sounds. You might want to try closing your eyes. That makes it easier not to talk to him too much, and it also conveys a sleepy-time message. Don't stimulate him – bore him. Stay there until he falls asleep.

Nights 4–6. Move the chair *about halfway to the door*. (If the room is small or the cot is close to the door, then move all the way to the doorway, as in night 7.) Continue the soothing sounds, but stay in the chair as much as you can. Get up to pat or stroke him a little if necessary, or make the same soothing sounds as you have used the past three nights. Again, try not to pick him up unless he's hysterical, and if you do pick him up, follow the technique I described for the first three nights. Stay in the chair until he falls asleep. If you allow yourself to move to the cot side and pat him almost to sleep, you will defeat the whole purpose of moving your chair away. You will create a new sleep crutch.

Nights 7–9. Move the *chair to the doorway inside his room*. You should be dimly lit but still in his view. Continue the same soothing techniques from your chair, remembering to intervene as little as possible. Don't worry if he cries a little bit; keep quietly reassuring him. He'll know that you are there, and he will fall asleep.

Nights 10–12. Move *into the hall with the door open enough so that he can still see you*. You can keep making those 'sh-sh' sounds, not constantly but enough to let him know that Mum or Dad is close by and responsive. Stay until he falls asleep.

Children get ritualized easily. Make the changes every three days – or less. Dragging it out makes it harder, not easier, for your baby. Give it more than three days, and he'll expect you to stay exactly where you are – and get mad or upset when you try to double that distance.

Nights 13 and on. A significant number of babies start falling asleep and staying asleep by now. But many parents have one more step to take: giving him the opportunity to fall asleep without your presence. Leaving him to fall asleep without a parent in his room may seem like a huge leap for you, but it's not so big for him. All that chair moving has given him nearly two weeks of preparation. He has given up some negative associations, and he has learned that you are near.

Most parents stay in the hallway or in a very nearby room, where the child cannot see them but can hear them. You can make some reassuring 'sh-sh' sounds, not constantly but enough to let him know that Mum or Dad is close by and responsive. If he cries, try checking on him from his bedroom door – without going all the way into the room. Be calm and reassuring. Make some comforting sounds, conveying that you are not far away and that you know he can put himself to sleep.

I find that this final step, leaving him alone, is often harder for the parents than for the child. Try not to convey anxiety about possible tears to your baby. Give him credit for what the Shuffle has helped him achieve. Your baby really can soothe himself to sleep – if you give him the opportunity. Occasionally, a baby will cry a

Some Extra Reminders for the First Three Shuffle Nights

1. *Don't get into a power struggle about laying the baby down – you won't win!* If he is sitting or standing in the cot, pat the mattress and encourage him to lie down. Stay calm and say things like 'Sh-sh,' 'Night–night,' and 'It's okay, lie down.'

2. *You can stroke, pat, rub, sh-sh, or sing to your child intermittently through the rails of the cot.* But don't do it constantly until he falls asleep, or it will become his new sleep crutch. Stop when he is starting to fall asleep. (Some babies don't like to be touched as they fall asleep; follow your instincts and his cues.)

3. *The parent controls the touch.* Don't let the baby fall asleep grasping your finger or hand, for example, because he will wake up when you move, and it will start all over again. Pat or stroke a different part of his body or the top of his hand.

4. *If the baby becomes hysterical (most don't), pick him up to calm him.* Stay in his room; don't walk around the house. Don't let him fall asleep in your arms. When he's calm, kiss him, put him back in the cot and sit near him in the chair. Make soothing sounds and pat or stroke him. If you pick him up and he's immediately calm, then you've been 'had.' Instead of you training him to sleep, he trained you to pick him up! Wait a little longer next time. Trust your instincts and your knowledge of your child. You will know within a night or two whether picking him up helps or further stimulates him.

5. *Stay by his cot until he is sound asleep at bedtime and during all night wakenings during the first three days of the Shuffle.* If you rush out of the room the second he closes his eyes, he will wake up and be upset, and you'll have to start all over.

6. *Return to your Shuffle position, and follow these rules each time the baby wakes during the first three nights* (as long as you and your pediatrician have decided to end night feeding): Go to the cot, give him a kiss, encourage him to lie down if necessary, and sit in the chair. Do this at each awakening until 6:00 a.m.

little for a few nights, but don't rush in and rescue him prematurely. Let him calm down and nod off. If you check on him from the doorway, try to be fairly unobtrusive about it and don't check too frequently. You want to calm him, not stimulate him into getting more awake each time you approach. It should get easier on you quickly.

Problems and Solutions

Many babies have *negative associations,* or *sleep crutches,* that they need to get themselves to sleep or back to sleep. They may want to be fed, held, rocked, and so forth. Work on eliminating these associations at bedtime and when your baby wakes up during the Shuffle. These directions emphasize the first three nights, when you will sit right beside your child and comfort him. *From night 4 on, if your child has not yet discarded the crutch, go to his cot side and comfort him very briefly, and then return to your bedtime Shuffle position for that night.* If your child wakes up once in a while after the Shuffle, I usually recommend that you make a quick, reassuring visit to his cot side, make sure he's okay, and then return to the hallway or your bedroom, whichever makes you feel more comfortable. Don't forget to use the lovey.

If despite following the advice in this section your child is still waking up at night, take another look at his routine. Are you putting him to bed a little too drowsy? If so, he may have learned to put himself to sleep at bedtime when you've done much of the sleep preparation work for him, but he can't get himself back to sleep at night without your assistance. Try putting him down at bedtime when he's a tad less drowsy and a bit more awake so he can perfect those self-soothing skills. You might also try moving bedtime earlier by fifteen minutes or a half hour and maybe create a little more separation between that last nursing or bottlefeeding and bed. Try leaving a soft light on while you nurse, which will help him break that suckle-sleep association.

Time Checks

Sometimes we need to modify the Shuffle because a child is over-stimulated by the parent's presence by his cot or bed. He wants to engage and engage, and no matter how much you soothe and 'sh-sh,' he'll still keep trying to engage you. In this situation, you may want to try working with 'time checks,' a variant of what some call 'Ferberizing.' At bedtime, do your nighttime routine, getting your child calm and soothed before placing him down. Then kiss him and tell him you will check on him before leaving the room.

There is no magic rule about how often you should check on him, and you may have to experiment a bit. If you do it too quickly, he may treat it like a game and get even more stimulated. If you are away too long, he may get worked up and upset.

Start with every seven minutes, and gradually increase it, but trust your own instincts and make necessary adjustments. When you check on him, go directly to his cot and give him a quick reassuring pat. But don't linger: You will defeat the whole purpose if you stand there for a half hour patting him to sleep.

Eliminating Nighttime Feeding

One of my hardest tasks is convincing mothers that most healthy six- to eight-month-old babies on a normal growth curve don't need to eat at night. Even a smart, thoughtful mother who knows this in her head may still have a fear in her gut of letting her child go hungry. 'My baby was in the ninety-eighth percentile for weight, and I still worried about starving her,' one mum I worked with told me.

The overwhelming odds are that the main reason your baby still gets up in search of breast or bottle is that you allow it! Don't be hard on yourself if your baby developed this habit. You have loads of company. It is a time-tested way of getting you and your baby back to sleep quickly, but now you can try some alternatives.

Families I've worked with have tried several techniques for

eliminating nighttime feedings. Choose what feels right for you. Even if you start with the gentler steps, please read this entire section because you'll find some tips on soothing your baby or adjusting mealtimes that may be helpful. Also, please check with your pediatrician and make sure that your child does not have a medical or growth issue that does require more frequent feedings. Some babies who haven't yet outgrown their reflux, for instance, might still need more frequent small meals, but even with these babies, try to do as much of the feeding as possible during the day, or else you'll be living with the sleep-disrupting side effects of reflux long after her tummy problems are over.

Whatever approach you take, it will be easier if you try to reset her hunger clock so that she takes in more calories by day and is not looking around for more at night. I know some babies, even this young, who do a remarkable job of resisting food all day so they can feast all night. Here are steps that might help:

- Review your daytime feeding schedule, and keep a written log of her diet. Talk to your doctor about whether she's getting the right mix of milk and solids.
- Try to nurse or bottlefeed her in a quiet, dim place without television, phone calls, or other distractions. That may help her feel more like it's a night feeding. This advice holds true during growth spurts, too. She may need an occasional night feeding midspurt, but by concentrating on enhancing daytime feeding, you'll minimize the nighttime ones.
- Overnight, try cutting down on nursing time. If she usually feeds for twenty minutes, give her fifteen. Keep cutting back every few days until she's ready to give it up. Make sure you are unlatching her when she finishes eating heartily; don't let her just gently suckle and doze. Get her back to bed while she's drowsy but awake.
- Same with a bottle. Let her eat, but don't let her play with it. With a nighttime bottle, you can also try to switch to a smaller bottle, put less formula in the bottle, or gradually dilute the formula so that when it gets very watery she might decide it's not worth getting up for. But when you cut the nursing time

all the way back to five minutes, or the bottle to just three ounces, it's time to stop. Anything smaller is just a tease.

If you want to cut back nighttime feedings but you, or your pediatrician, think your baby still needs to eat once during the night, you have two choices:

Option 1 is a *dreamfeed*. Wake her for one final feeding before your own bedtime, probably around 11:00 p.m. Do not feed her again during the night. Use other soothing techniques if she wakes up. Some babies don't like being woken up to be fed at this time, and don't feed well when they are sleepy, so you'll know pretty quickly whether dreamfeeding works with your child's temperament and body clock. If you do dreamfeed, focus on feeding her quickly and getting her back to bed. Unlatch (or remove the bottle) as soon as she's done, and avoid any other interaction that will encourage her to stay up and play or cling to you.

Option 2 is a *set-time feeding*. Set a time during the night to feed her, and then feed her only at that predetermined time. You can decide to feed the first time she wakes up, as long as it's been at least four hours after her bedtime feeding. Or you can choose a later time – for instance, the first time she wakes up after midnight (particularly if you know that's when she's been the hungriest or that she hasn't responded well to an earlier dreamfeed).

Either of these options is fine – *as long as you are consistent.* Choose one approach and stick to it. And feed her only once at night, and not again until at least 6:00 a.m. If you cave in, you are just giving her intermittent reinforcement, and those mixed messages only make it harder for her in the long run. If she wakes at a time that's not part of your feeding plan, find other ways of soothing her. Go briefly to her cot, reassure her, and then return to your Shuffle position and keep comforting her with verbal and some physical reassurances. Comfort yourself too by reminding yourself that she is a healthy, well-nourished baby.

Some parents find that when they get on more consistent schedules, the babies just start skipping this one feeding on their own and sleeping longer, maybe eating a bit more during the day.

Now let's talk about how to cut out all night feedings when you and your pediatrician agree that your baby is ready to sleep eleven hours. Here are three ways to phase out the feeding as you begin the Sleep Lady Shuffle:

Option 1 is a dreamfeed, as outlined above before your bedtime. Only do this for three nights and then stop.

Option 2: Follow the advice I gave above for *'set-time' feeding*. Do this for three nights only.

Both of these approaches give her body three days to adjust to taking in fewer calories at night. If she wakes at times other than the set-time feeding (which she will), sit by her cot and comfort her.

Sleep Lady Tip

If she wakes before her set-time feeding and stays awake fussing until the set time, do not then feed her. You don't want to train her to cry! Get her back to sleep for at least a little while before you feed her. For example, if she wakes up at 11:00 and fusses until midnight, don't pick her up and feed her just because the clock strikes 12:00. That will just teach her to fuss or cry for an hour until you give in, and that's not the best way to minimize tears. So get her to sleep, if it's only for thirty minutes, until she wakes up again. So if she wakes up at 11:00, fusses until 12:00, finally falls asleep at 12:10, and wakes up at 12:45, you can feed her. She learned to get to sleep without that food. While she's fussing, try not to pick her up, but if she gets hysterical, go ahead and hold her and re-assure her briefly. Some babies adjust in three or four days. Some take a little longer, but if you are consistent, the tears will ebb quickly, and she'll wake less frequently.

Don't feed her until after 6:00 a.m., when you can both start your day. Don't forget to do 'dramatic wake-up.'

Usually, parents will move their seat away from the cot on the fourth night of the Shuffle, but we're going to modify it for this night weaning. *So on the fourth night, stay next to the cot. Do not feed her overnight at all.* Each time she wakes up, go sit by her cot and soothe her, both by making gentle and calming sounds and by patting or stroking her. Sometimes it works better if the father does the comforting at night, since the baby knows he can't nurse – and he can't cave in and decide to nurse.

A third option, although less popular, is a bit more gradual. Feed the baby as frequently as she is used to – but feed her less. If you breastfeed for fifteen minutes, shave off a few minutes each night. If you bottlefeed, put an ounce or so less in the bottle. Each night, cut back a little more and make sure you unlatch her as soon as time is up. Some parents find this approach gentler and easier; others find it a nuisance to watch a clock and keep track of nursing times and unlatch or measure liquid ounces in the middle of the night when they are very sleepy. You know what will work for you.

Don't drag this out. Pick a target date for the phaseout to be done, usually within a week. Fine if it goes faster, but don't prolong it.

Be consistent. Choose one approach and stick to it!

At seven months, Anita was still getting up to eat several times a night, migrating among her cot, car seat, and parents' bed. She had never slept through a single night of her life. Penny and Jim tried limiting the feedings to once a night – a set time at 4:00 a.m. But it didn't help. Anita didn't understand why she could get fed at 4:00 a.m. but not at midnight or 2:00 a.m. 'Looking back, I realized it was confusing her,' Penny said. It was classic intermittent reinforcement – rewarding Anita with food just often enough to motivate her to keep waking in search of it. Penny and Jim realized they weren't going to make any progress unless they made a change.

With my help and her pediatrician's support, Penny overcame her lingering doubts about whether Anita still needed to eat at night and became confident that she could wean Anita at night without having to stop nursing altogether. Penny still nursed at bedtime, but she nursed at the beginning of the bedtime routine, not the end, to weaken the nursing-sleep association in Anita's mind.

When Anita woke up at night, Penny or Jim – they decided that they would not leave it all to Jim – would soothe her but would not feed her. I gave them the choice of staying in her room until she fell asleep again or going in and touching base and then leaving. Penny chose the second approach, but only up to her comfort point. 'I was able to go in, spend a few moments with her, and then leave. If she was crying a lot and it was becoming more intense, I could go back in and soothe her again. If she was crying a little but it seemed like she was about to fall asleep quickly on her own, I didn't go back. It wasn't based on strict time limits and rules; it was based on how I felt and how I thought Anita felt.'

On those nights when Penny did return to Anita's room, she was careful not to pick Anita up. That could have just teased Anita into thinking she was going to be nursed, creating more frustration when those hopes were thwarted. It could also have led to a new negative association, with Anita waking up at night and expecting to be picked up and rocked and snuggled back to sleep.

Change came quickly. Anita decided that if she wasn't going to get fed, she wasn't going to bother waking up. By the fourth night, Penny had to go in for only one brief check. By the fifth night, Penny heard Anita get up briefly and stir, and then drop right back to sleep on her own. From then on Anita slept all night and was happier, and more well rested during the day. She even began eating better during the day, further reducing the incentive to get up at night. 'I was amazed,' said Penny. 'That's all it took!'

Phasing Out Walking and Rocking to Sleep

Many of us walk or rock our newborns to sleep – or start this habit when we find that nursing doesn't get them to sleep anymore. If your child is six months or older, it's time to phase it out. You'll know it's a problem if your child needs to be walked for more than a few minutes at bedtime, if she wakes up again as soon as you stop walking, or if she needs to be walked each time she wakes up at night. The same goes for rocking.

Focus on bedtime, when you are most awake and better equipped to follow through consistently. Begin by doing all the walking or rocking in her bedroom, not all over the house. This helps create a positive association between the bedroom and sleep.

Scale back the amount of time you walk — even if she isn't entirely asleep when you stop. In other words, if you usually walk thirty minutes, try walking twenty minutes for two or three days, then scale back to fifteen minutes for two or three days, then ten.

Put her down when she's drowsy but awake — think about that 7 or 8 on the drowsiness scale.

This is the point when parents usually look at me with alarm and say, 'But if I put her down, she'll cry.' Yes, she might. Sit by her cot and soothe her. Don't engage too much — just whisper some gentle reassurances and stroke her a bit now and then. If you do pick her up, do so briefly to calm her and then put her back down. Continue your reassurances, and maybe try rocking her body a little bit with your hand while she's lying down. Some babies this age still find comfort in being swaddled with their arms free when you put them back down. It makes them feel like you are still holding them.

Erin needed to be walked — and walked and walked — at bedtime and for her nap. At first her mum, Corinna, didn't mind all that much — newborns are so snuggly and all the pacing was good post-pregnancy exercise. But Erin got heavier and heavier, and walking got harder and harder. Jeremy devoted a special pair of deck shoes to baby walking. Corinna developed pain in her arms. 'I lost all my baby weight fast, but my arm was about to break!' Corinna said.

They didn't follow the phase-it-out approach. They just stopped the walking. But to prepare Erin, they first made some schedule adjustments. Her bedtime had been around 9:00 or 9:30. When they moved it up to 7:00 or 7:30, she wasn't so overtired and therefore didn't need her sleep crutch as much. They also got her up at a more consistent hour in the morning, moved her nursing and solids closer together, and rescheduled her naps so she wasn't going as long without some rest.

When they were ready to make the change, instead of making a long march around the house, they just included a brief and calming stroll around her room as part of her bedtime routine. They put her down awake, sat next to the cot, and soothed her as they did the Sleep Lady Shuffle. There were some tears, but not nearly as many as they had feared. 'I thought it was going to take two hours that first night. I made Jeremy come home from work early, and we were going to order a pizza,' Corinna said. 'But it took a half hour, and it got easier each night after that.'

Erin was a little unusual in that she didn't demand to be walked if she woke up at night – and she didn't wake up every night. Often babies who want to be walked to sleep at bedtime will insist on the same nocturnal promenade in the middle of the night. If your baby gets up crying, go to her immediately and reassure her. Stroke her a bit and whisper 'sh-sh' or 'night-night' or a similar soothing sound. But avoid lifting her out of her cot, and definitely don't cave in and start walking.

If, despite your reassuring presence, she gets really hysterical – if she reaches the point where she is crying so fervently that she can't remember what she is crying about – go ahead and pick her up. Help her calm down – but keep her in her room. Build pleasant associations between her room and sleep. Don't pace the halls; don't hand her any new crutches to replace the walking. Hold her gently for a little while until she is calm. Put her down calm and drowsy but awake. Let her do that final piece of falling asleep on her own. You can sit beside her as she does.

Donna rocked her eight-month-old daughter, Elsa, to sleep in her arms. Elsa then woke up to nurse three times a night, and still got up between nursings, wanting to be rocked back to sleep. She was also a poor napper and needed a dummy at bedtime.

Donna began by focusing on putting Elsa to bed while she was drowsy but still awake and soothing her while she fell asleep without her dummy. She initially scaled back nursing to every five hours, and around the fourth or fifth night she stopped nursing at night. The pediatrician said this was fine; Elsa was petite but healthy. Donna still nursed Elsa at bedtime, but instead of rocking her after she ate, she would burp her, kiss her, and put her into the cot, sitting next to her and soothing her.

By the end of the first week, Elsa was waking up only once at night instead of four, five, or six times, and she went back to sleep easily without nursing, rocking, or using her dummy.

Sleep Lady Tip

This is critical for easing a baby off a walking or rocking sleep crutch. If he fusses and you pick him up and he calms down immediately – or worse if he falls asleep right in your arms – you've been 'had'. You are supposed to be training him to sleep. Instead, he trained you to pick him up. Wait a little longer next time. Trust your instincts and your knowledge of your child. You will know within a night or two whether picking him up helps him calm down, further stimulates him, or just shows that he's already got your number.

Dummy (Pacifier) Withdrawal

You don't have to take away the dummy at this age. It's your choice, and what you choose may depend on how often he's waking up and demanding that you find his dummy and plug it in again for him. Here are some options:

- Let him keep the dummy
- Let him have it only at naptime and bedtime
- Let him keep the dummy only at naptime (which can be harder than bedtime for a baby to calm himself)

If you are keeping the dummy for at least some portion of his sleep time, you may try to help your baby find it himself. If you've noticed that your baby is able to grip and maneuver the dummy on her own – most babies develop the pincer grip between six to eight months – you may want to leave several strewn around the cot so he can find one himself, instead of demanding that you come in over and over again to retrieve and replug it. You may have to put it in his hands a few times until he catches on.

If you are weaning the baby from the dummy – well, *weaning* isn't really the right word. It's not gradual. It's either in the baby's mouth or not. You'll have to do some extra soothing if you take away the dummy. See if he'll start bonding to a lovey. Pick a night when you are ready to cope with a little unpleasantness and put him to bed without his dummy. Make sure you have an especially nice and calming bedtime routine, and try to get him to bed drowsy but awake. Stroke or soothe him instead of giving him the dummy, using techniques similar to those I advise for parents who are breaking the nighttime nursing or walking habits. Do the same thing each time he wakes at night. If you cave in once after he's cried for an hour, you aren't teaching him to sleep without the dummy. You are teaching him to cry for an hour in order to get a dummy.

I worked with a set of twins who were definitely caught in the dummy trap. The parents spent so much time traipsing in to replug one dummy or the other that they finally just took the twins out of their cots and put them in Pack 'n Plays at each side of the parents' bed. But it wasn't really all that much better – they didn't have to keep running all night into the other room, but they were still constantly swinging their arms and replugging 'nuks.' We stopped this by adjusting their schedule, moving the babies back to their cots, and improving the bedtime routine to help them settle down. We used the Sleep Lady Shuffle to improve their ability to sleep without their dummies.

Unconventional Beds

Some babies learn to sleep in unconventional places – swings, car seats, and the like. Maybe your baby had reflux, and you placed her upright in her car seat to digest when she was very little, and she got used to dozing off there. Maybe the soothing movement of the swing just helped relax her to sleep. But she can't sleep there forever.

I worked with one little girl, nearly eight months old, who had spent every single night of her life and all her naps in a moving swing. If she woke up at night, her mother nursed her and then put her back in the swing. This child was actually quite advanced developmentally, crawling at five months and standing at six months. But she didn't have a clue as to how to sleep lying down. It took her three weeks to learn.

Her parents did the Sleep Lady Shuffle. They would lay her down in her cot, and she would promptly sit up and fall asleep sitting. Then she'd fall over, which naturally would wake her up – mad. She'd sit up again, fall asleep again, topple over again, and wake up. One of her parents sat nearby, soothing her, but avoided picking her up unless she was really frustrated. They would go through this ritual several times at bedtime, and several times when she woke up in the middle of the night. Eventually, she would get so tired that she would lie down and go to sleep, although she wasn't particularly happy about it. But within a few days, she was waking up less frequently, and less furiously. It was taking her parents only five to ten minutes to get her back to sleep.

Initially, her mum kept the swing for naps, although she turned the swing off when the baby fell asleep, phasing out that feeling of being rocked. By the end of the first week, she had made enough progress that her mum put her in the cot for naps as well. It took another two weeks for all the problems to resolve, but her parents noticed that when she began napping in the cot, instead of the moving swing, she seemed to be much better rested.

Early Birds

Early risings sometimes have a very simple solution. If too much light is coming into the baby's room, buy room-darkening blinds (also good for napping). If an external noise – dustmen, songbirds, or a dad with a long commute who has turned on the shower – is waking her, you might want to try a white noise machine or a fan. Unfortunately, it's not always so simple.

If your child is awake at 6:00 or 6:30 a.m., cheerful, refreshed, and ready to start his day – even if you aren't – you'll probably have to live with it. That's a common and biologically appropriate wake-up time for a baby or small child. Remember to adapt the meal and nap schedule to suit his early hours. The first nap should be one and a half to two hours after he wakes up.

If baby is now sleeping through the night and napping well but still waking before 6:00 a.m., you might try making his bedtime later, shifting it in fifteen-minute intervals to see if that will coax him into sleeping later, but be careful. He may still wake up at 6:00 but be more tired and cranky because he's no longer getting enough sleep at the front end. Pay attention to his sleep window, his sleepy signals and behavior. Don't force him to stay up when he really needs to go to sleep, or he won't be able to fall asleep when you want him to. If you do make a trial run on the later bedtime, try letting that third little afternoon nap run a little later so he isn't too overtired when you put him down. You may also use the techniques I outline below for problematic early risers, but they may or may not work for a child whose early wake-up time is appropriate for his own internal clock.

Babies who wake up before 6:00 a.m., or who wake up cheerful at 6:00 or 6:30 but are a total grump by 7:00, are a different story. You need to intervene and coach him to sleep later. The longer you endure early risings, the harder it is to change the pattern, so I strongly suggest you address it now, even if it takes a few weeks to see results. Once they're older, it can take months.

Make sure your early riser is getting enough daytime sleep because nap deprivation can cause poor night sleep and early awakenings. You can try adjusting an early bird's morning nap, moving it later in half-hour increments. Make sure he doesn't start his morning nap before 8:00 a.m., and then gradually push it back to 9:00 a.m. This might help shift his whole body clock and coax him into sleeping later. But be careful. Watch his sleep windows and use your intuition, because you don't want to postpone his nap so long that he is too wired to fall asleep. If you think he is waking up very early because he is hungry, try waking him for a final feeding about 11:00 p.m. as an interim step, and also work on making sure he takes more food during the day.

When you hear your early bird stir, go to him very quickly. Try to soothe him, and offer him a lovey. Try to get him and his lovey back to sleep without taking him out of his cot. Even if he doesn't doze off again, do not turn on the lights or let him out of his cot until 6:00 a.m. – even if he wails with impatience. When I say 6:00, I mean 6:00. I don't mean 5:45 or 5:50. Or even 5:59. Letting him get up earlier, while it is still dark, sends a confusing message, and is another example of intermittent reinforcement. He cannot understand why he can get up in the dark at 5:45 a.m. but not at 2:15 a.m. Also, many parents I've worked with have learned the hard way that if they let him get up at 5:45 a.m., he'll gradually wake up earlier and earlier.

> Letting him get up earlier, while it is still dark, sends a confusing message, and is another example of intermittent reinforcement.

At this age, I usually recommend that the parent stay in the room while the child gets back to sleep in the early morning. But keep your interaction minimal. Try sitting in a chair with your eyes closed. Say that Mummy (or Daddy) is still sleeping and act like baby should be sleeping as well. When the clock finally strikes 6:00 – and it can seem like it takes forever – leave the room for a minute or two. He may cry, but it's only one minute. You'll be right back.

Sleep Lady Tip

If you feel your presence in his room is encouraging your baby to stay awake, you can try leaving his room and see if he falls asleep again on his own. Stay out until 6:00 a.m., or check on him period-ically until 6:00 a.m..

Whether you've been out for a minute or much of the last hour, when you reenter the room, do a *dramatic wake-up.* Open the blinds, turn on the lights, sing a cheery morning song – a reverse lullaby. Think of it as a morning routine, just like you have an evening one. The idea is to help the baby distinguish between day and night, to know when it is really time to get up and start his day. Your message must be clear: 'I'm getting you out of the cot because it's morning time – not because you were crying.'

Early Risers

If your little one wakes up before 6:00 a.m., he's probably overtired. Overtired children don't sleep as well, or sleep as long, as well-rested ones. He may be:

- Going to bed too late
- Not napping enough
- Staying up too long between the end of his afternoon nap and going to bed (try not to let that interval exceed four hours)
- Going to bed when he's past that 'drowsy but awake' mark. If he's too drowsy, he won't know how to get himself back to sleep when he's more alert – including at 5:00 a.m.

Napping

Napping is hard for babies. Nap training is hard for parents. Nighttime problems are usually solved reasonably quickly. Fixing day sleep requires more patience and more perseverance. It is time-consuming and usually involves tears.

Babies, like adults, simply have trouble sleeping when it is not dark. Our brains are programmed to be awake during daylight and asleep at night. In addition, babies aren't yet very good at helping themselves switch gears from active to restful. And even at this young age, they can resist sleep. They fight it off because they would much rather stay up to play, explore, and be with you. That doesn't mean they are having separation anxiety problems; it just means they are forming nice, healthy attachments.

Sleep Lady Tip

Don't go directly from a stimulating activity, like dancing her around to your favorite radio station, straight into the cot.

NAP READINESS. Remember that babies from six to eight months need two naps a day, about one and a half to two hours apiece. The short third nap in late afternoon is optional as long as they are getting two decent naps earlier in the day, but it's required if their earlier naps are skimpy. Start by reviewing your child's schedule. Pay close attention to her daytime sleep windows. You may be putting her down a bit too late, when she's already revved up with a second wind.

You can tackle naps at the same time you start the Sleep Lady Shuffle at night. Start with the nighttime Shuffle, and the next day at naptime put your chair in the same place and follow the same steps and the same soothing techniques. Move your chair every three days, even if she didn't nap well that day.

However, some families choose to concentrate on night sleep and not tackle naps at the same time. In that case, use whatever techniques you can to make sure your child gets good daytime sleep (more on that in a moment). Despite my insistence on consistency, you don't have to be in the same position at naps as you are for bedtime and night wakenings. It's okay if you start nap training days, weeks, or even months after the bedtime Shuffle.

CREATE A GOOD NAP ENVIRONMENT, both in terms of reducing stimulation levels and physical surroundings. Give her wind-down time, maybe an abbreviated version of her bedtime routine. Read a book, or listen to quiet music. Nursing or bottlefeeding sometimes helps to create this transition time, but try not to let her fall asleep while eating. Remember to put her down drowsy but awake – although she can be a little bit drowsier than at nighttime.

A DARK, QUIET ROOM. Some babies need near total darkness to nap, even if they want a little more light at night. If you live in an especially noisy home, you might want to try a fan or place a white-noise machine on low volume across the room from the cot. If you are concerned that she will get so dependent on the machine that she won't be able to sleep without it, use it only for naps and slowly reduce the volume as her sleep improves.

FOLLOW THE SAME BASIC RULES AS BEDTIME. If she stands up in the cot, put her down once; if she stands up again, ignore it. Don't feel obligated to feed her before every nap, particularly if you are working on breaking a food-sleep association. If you've been rocking or swinging her to bed, concentrate on phasing it out at naptime. Cut the rocking or swinging time in half at the beginning, and work on getting her down drowsy but awake.

THE LONGEST HOUR. Even if you do everything right to set the stage for naptime, brace yourself. You may have to devote the next full hour (twice a day if you are training for morning and afternoon naps) to getting her to sleep.

CHECKS. As you work through the Shuffle at naptime, do what you must to console her – and yourself. Sometimes a parent's presence, however, will make her stay awake instead of falling asleep. If she's either trying persistently to engage you or getting madder and madder that you are there but won't do what she wants, then try leaving the room. Come back to check on her frequently, every five to fifteen minutes, whatever feels right to you. And even though I constantly tell you to be consistent, it is okay to do timed checks at naptime but follow the Shuffle at night. They will be separate enough in the baby's mind.

Corinna stopped walking Erin to sleep at naptime and just put her down in her cot. Corinna sat right outside the room with a magazine and said, 'It's okay, Mummy's right here.' She entered the room briefly about every fifteen minutes for additional reassurance. They reached the point where she could put Erin down, then move away from the hallway and do things around the house. She would still check on her every fifteen minutes. It never took a whole hour for

Erin to fall asleep, and over a period of a few weeks, she fell asleep faster and faster.

Give it a full hour. Then, if your baby still hasn't fallen asleep, leave the room for at least one complete minute – that's sixty seconds, not ten seconds – even if she complains. No matter how little tolerance you have for tears, you can manage sixty seconds. Come back in and, with a little drama and flourish, take her out of her cot and act like naptime is over, much like you do at morning wake-up time. You want to convey the idea that when she gets up it's because you've decided it's time, not because she has been crying.

If she doesn't sleep a wink during the morning hour, try to get her down for her afternoon nap earlier than usual because she's going to be overtired. Pay close attention to her sleepy clues. Catch her when she's ripe for a nap, maybe in as little as forty-five minutes.

IF YOU HAVE AN OLDER CHILD TO TAKE CARE OF, you may have to leave the baby's room and make frequent checks. I had to do this when my second child was an infant and my first was three and at home in the afternoon needing Mummy. For me it was quite difficult because I felt pulled between my two children, and Gretchen, the baby, was crying more than I really wanted.

Marianne, who'd had three kids in three years, was convinced that each baby was a more capable napper than the one before simply because she didn't have as much time to rock, sing, and soothe the youngest at naptime. She had to leave the littlest one, Ally, in her cot at naptime and go to deal with whatever toddler antics needed her attention.

Donna couldn't sit next to Elsa's cot for an hour twice a day for the Shuffle because she had four-year-old Kit to attend to – and some of Elsa's natural nap windows coincided with the time she had to take Kit to preschool. Donna did the best she could, which meant working around the preschool schedule and leaving Elsa in her room when Kit was home. She checked on Elsa frequently (more like the Ferber method). It wasn't easy on any of them, and it took forty-five minutes of coaxing to produce forty-five minutes of napping. But forty-five minutes of sleep was still better than Elsa's earlier little dozing sessions, and gradually the naps lengthened as Donna stayed as consistent as she could be under the circumstances. With two parents around to share child-care responsibilities, Elsa napped better on weekends, and those longer and easier weekend naps probably helped her overall progress.

CATNAPS. Ideally, your baby will sleep for an hour and a half or more, but often babies sleep less than forty-five minutes. I call these *disaster naps,* because they are less than a full sleep cycle. All those little naps do is give her just enough oomph to resist sleep, but she'll be cranky and tired again in no time.

You have a few options to try to prolong those naps. Remember that if she's getting up after twenty or thirty minutes, she might not really be fully awake; she may be experiencing a partial awakening. Instead of taking her out of her cot as though her nap was over, go to her quickly and try to soothe her back to sleep for another half hour or hour. If this works, gradually give her more opportunities to resettle herself without so much assistance from you. As she develops this skill, you won't have to jump in so quickly when you hear her stir. A little 'sh-sh' from the hallway might do the trick. Gradually, with your help and consistency, she will start sleeping for longer periods of time on her own.

If you can't get her back to sleep after trying for an hour and she has slept only twenty or thirty minutes total, you should modify her schedule for a while until napping improves. If she takes a brief morning nap, make her afternoon nap earlier. She's not going to manage to stay awake for three hours until the second nap if she's running on vapors, not without driving both you and herself crazy.

Use both the clock and your child's cues to make adjustments before she falls apart. She may need her 'afternoon' nap at 11:30 or noon, and then need a third nap later in the afternoon. Don't let her take the third nap too late, or else it will throw dinnertime and her evening routine so far off that you'll be back where you started. Wake her by 4:30 p.m. Be flexible at this stage. If you try and fail to get her to nap at 9:00 or 9:30 a.m. but at 10:00 or 10:30 she seems sleepy, try again.

Parents often ask me if it's okay if a child takes two or three forty-five-minute naps. At this age, probably not. One clue is her behavior. Does she seem rested or tired? Happy or cranky? Is she waking up a lot at night? Too little day sleep often leads to fitful and disrupted night sleep.

IF YOUR CHILD SKIPPED A NAP, or dozed only briefly either in the morning or in the afternoon, you need to *implement an emergency backup plan* to make sure she sleeps one way or another for a decent interval in the afternoon. You don't want a baby so completely miserable and sleep deprived that you undo all the progress you've made at bedtime – even if it means temporarily ignoring all my rules about no motion sleeping. Put her in a car, the stroller, or her swing – whatever works to get her a nap.

But if you use a backup technique, be careful which one you choose. Don't backslide into one of the habits you have just broken. For instance, if you have been working on ending cosleeping at night, don't put her in your bed for this nap emergency. Try a car ride instead. If you have been phasing out rocking and walking at night, don't walk or rock at naptime. Find another nap tool, and rely on it for the short term.

Nap-Coaching Tips

It's easier to get a baby to take the morning nap than the afternoon nap. Don't miss that opportunity.

Afternoon nap training is tougher. Don't get discouraged; it's normal.

Keep a sleep log during nap training. Watch her sleep windows.

If it's 2:00 or 3:00 p.m. and the baby has not napped well enough, you may need to resort to your 'backup' plan, such as a nap in the stroller or car, to avoid an exhausted baby and a bedtime disaster.

You will be tied to the house during nap coaching. If you feel like all you are doing all day is trying to get your baby to nap, then you are doing it right! The payoff: You'll have more freedom (and a happier, rested baby) once you have a predictable napping schedule.

If you have a babysitter or child-care setting that can do the nap training, thank your lucky stars. If your caregiver is reluctant to do the training, see if you can win her over with a simple explanation of the sleep science. If not, explain that your child needs a full 'sleep tank,' and if that means the sitter has to use a sleep crutch like rocking to get the child to nap, or to resume a brief or interrupted nap, that's okay.

If motion sleep is part of the short-term fix, try to minimize it. If you use a swing to get her to sleep, turn off the motor once she's out and let her nap with it off. Ditto for the car. Drive around to lull her into sleep if you must, but then pull over or come back home so she can sleep without the car's motion. Transfer her to a cot if it won't wake her, or sit out there with her, in the car or right nearby if the weather permits, and let her sleep. Read a book or snooze yourself – tend your garden if the weather's nice. I'm not too comfortable with letting a baby sleep in a car unattended, even in 'safe' neighborhoods.

Unfortunately, after everything you went through to get her to nap, you can't let her nap too late or your evening will be even rougher than your day. Wake her by 4:30, 5:00 at the absolute latest, and keep bedtime at its normal hour.

PARENTAL STRAINS. Just about every parent I've worked with has found nap training tedious, but emotional reactions vary. Some parents tolerate daytime tears, finding it easier emotionally to have a child cry when it's not dark.

> *Penny found Anita's crying easier to take at naptime than at night. 'I wasn't so exhausted; I wasn't trying to sleep myself,' she said. 'And I knew Anita was exhausted; I knew she really needed this nap. That allowed me to put up with some crying. She cried for forty-five minutes once, but that was the worst. Usually it was twenty to thirty minutes, and even that stopped in a week and a half.' Anita began sleeping for a solid hour, and then gradually extended her nap to an hour and a half.*

Other mums report exactly the opposite reaction, that they can't take being alone in a house with a screaming child when the other parent is off at work and unable to provide on-site support and encouragement. Caregivers at home, whether a babysitter or a grandma, often find it hard to deal with the nap routine or the tears. My advice then is don't push it. If it's too hard on you, if it's too hard on your child-care provider, if it's creating more tension instead of less, then don't worry about it right now – as long as your child's nighttime sleep is improving.

Use backup measures, temporary fixes, or improvised solutions to get your child some daytime sleep for the short term. Nurse her, pat her, swing her, do what you have to do. *But don't give up on naps completely or convince yourself that she doesn't need them.* She absolutely does need them, and she will need them for another three to four years.

But don't feel guilty if you can't follow all my advice right now. Give yourself (or your babysitter) permission to let the training slide for now, and just do what you have to do to get your child some daytime sleep, preferably at predictable times. As nighttime sleep improves, the daytime sleep might fall into place on its own. If not, take a deep breath and try the training again in another month or two. Keep reminding yourself that good daytime sleep promotes better nighttime sleep; it helps you get through it.

You may go through a stage when some of your nap tricks no longer work. Don't panic. It just means that changes in her bedtime and overnight sleep are helping her discard her sleep crutches. It may mean she's on the brink of learning to nap better, with a little more coaching from you. It's your signal to start nap coaching.

Cosleeping

If you started out cosleeping but have found that it is not right for you, or if you start the night with the baby in her cot but end up bringing her into your bed even if it's not what you intended, please turn to Chapter 12, 'Whose Bed Is It Anyway?' I'll also review safety rules and give you advice for how to improve sleep if you wish to continue sharing the family bed but are finding that no one is sleeping very well in it.

Adam

From early infancy, Adam needed to be walked, rocked, bounced, held, and nursed – and even that wasn't enough. A full-term, seemingly healthy baby, Adam in fact had a number of developmental delays and digestive diffi-culties that were not immediately apparent or swiftly diagnosed. Neither his hearing nor his vision developed properly at first, so for the first few months he heard and saw less than other babies. He also had a severe, but somewhat atypical, form of reflux that was hard to diagnose. Instead of spitting up, he would pant and gasp as acid reflux hit a spot in the back of his throat, closing his trachea. Sleep was almost impossible. 'I knew from the time he was five days old something was wrong,' Margaret remembered. 'By the time he was ten days old I was keeping a log. I had to hold him constantly, eighteen to twenty hours a day. He never slept more than twenty minutes at a time.'

By the time six months had passed, Adam's reflux was under control and his hearing and eyesight had caught up. But the early difficulties had created poor sleeping habits, depriving him of the chance to learn to self-soothe. Margaret and Robert went through one or two hours of bedtime contortions every night, finally getting him down at 8:30 or 9:00. He would sleep reasonably well for three hours or so and then wake up repeatedly for the rest of the night. He spent a lot of time in their bed, nursing and dozing, but seldom getting much deep sleep.

Daytime wasn't much better. Naps seldom lasted more than twenty minutes. An overnight sleep study in a clinic shed some light on his idiosyncratic sleep patterns. Even when he seemed to be awake and thrashing, he was in fact neurologically asleep. From that, his parents learned that sometimes they were actually stimulating him into being more awake when they thought they were lulling him to sleep. But even armed with more knowledge about Adam, nights didn't get any easier.

The family sought me out when Adam was seven and a half months old. Within three weeks, we had him going to sleep in his cot in a matter of minutes with minimal tears. It wasn't perfect. He still woke up once or twice many nights, but now the awakenings were brief and far less upsetting and disruptive. Everyone was getting more rest and feeling much happier.

Robert took the lead in the Sleep Lady Shuffle, with a few minor adjustments to suit Adam's needs. We developed an extremely detailed and structured nighttime routine. We wanted Robert to give Adam enough of the physical contact he craved so he could feel secure, but not so much that it prevented him from changing sleep patterns. From a chair near the bed, Robert patted Adam's back intermittently for thirty seconds, with his hand through the cot slats. He said, 'Sh-sh. Go to sleep,' the same sounds he would make consistently each night. Then Robert paused, and patted Adam again for another thirty seconds. When Adam tried to stand up, Robert removed his hand and did not interfere with Adam's movements. He said, 'Sh-sh. Go to sleep,' again, followed by another thirty seconds of patting. The first two nights, he did this for an hour and a half before Adam fell asleep. When he woke up during the night, Robert did exactly the same thing, making sure that Adam got an utterly consistent message.

By the third night, Robert followed the same routine, but it took only forty-five minutes. On the fourth night, Robert patted Adam for ten-second intervals and made sure he paused for at least twenty seconds in between. He did this pat-stop, pat-stop routine for a total of only five minutes. After that, he continued to make his reassuring 'sh-sh' sounds, but he had moved further away from Adam now, and did no more patting. Adam fell asleep in a half hour (as did Robert in his chair!). The fifth night Robert did one sequence of 'sh-sh' and ten seconds of patting when he initially went in. Then he waited a full minute. Then he did another ten-second sequence and waited a full minute. He followed this cycle five times, and then sat quietly in the chair in Adam's room, occasionally still murmuring a reassuring 'sh-sh.' Adam fell asleep in thirty minutes.

On nights 6 and 7 Robert and Margaret could see the difference. Robert put Adam down and said, 'Sh-sh. Go to bed,' once. Then he just sat in the room, a few feet from the cot. Adam cried but fell asleep within an hour on night 6 – and in twenty minutes on night 7.

On the next two nights, Robert was able to move the chair further from the cot, reaching the door on the ninth night. He stayed there, at the door, for another four or five days (a little longer than I usually recommend), and finally was able to leave the room. Adam cried, but his mother described it as a normal wind-down crying: quiet whimpering with a few bursts of harder tears, but decreasing in intensity. None of that ear-piercing shrieking they had earlier endured. And it was only for a few minutes, not the hours they had experienced in the past.

Encouraged, Margaret and Robert decided that they were ready to stop going in to him when he woke in the middle of the night, to see if he could get himself back to sleep on his own. This was a change for a couple who had earlier rushed to respond to his every tear. They braced themselves – but he cried softly for only five or six minutes and then drifted back to sleep. They decided it was less disruptive for his sleep and theirs if, instead of getting out of bed and interacting with him and risking waking everybody up even more, they just let him cry those few minutes and put himself back to sleep. He still woke up, but his whimpers never lasted very long.

They followed this practice into toddlerhood. Adam never became a perfect sleeper, and he still has some hypersensitivity issues they may want to explore before he starts school. But the best measure of how much their life improved was their decision to have a second child. They had a little girl – and she is a much better sleeper!

8

Nine to Twelve Months

*B*abies at this age on average need eleven hours of sleep at night and three during the day. At nine months, babies should nap for about an hour and a half in the morning and about one and a half to two hours in the afternoon. Most have given up that brief, third late-afternoon nap. By twelve months, the morning nap is about an hour, and the afternoon nap is about an hour and a half.

Many of the problems and solutions encountered in babies from nine to twelve months old are quite similar to those found in babies from six through to eight months old, but there are a few sleep-related developmental differences. These babies are more mobile, crawling and pulling themselves up in their cots, and can pop up each time you put them down at bedtime. Some walk by their first birthday, a major developmental milestone that can temporarily disrupt sleep. Increased activity can tire them out, so you have to pay very close attention to their sleep window, when they are most ready and able to fall asleep. Some can fight sleep, and conceal that window. If you wean during this period, that can also alter the rhythms of bedtime.

The families in this chapter had experiences that are quite typical for this age. Many expected their babies to resist sleep changes far more fiercely than they did, and they anticipated having a lot more difficulty in coping with tears. All of them found the baby responded better than they expected. The parents found that the tears were not as intense as they had feared, and they didn't feel so bad about letting him shed them as long as they were by his side.

> 'The key to success with sleep training was realizing that crying wasn't abandonment; it wasn't torture,' Megan said. 'We learned that sleep was so important to his growth and development that not teaching him to sleep was hurting him. We thought we would be bad parents if we let him cry. But we learned that ten minutes of crying didn't hurt him. We realized he was okay, and that made us feel so much better. You've got to just tell yourself over and over again – what you are doing is right.'

Developmental Changes

Separation Anxiety

Babies have peaks of separation anxiety at about nine months, when they are crawling and sitting, and at twelve months, when they are standing, walking, and climbing. Those physical leaps often make them wake up more at night, at least temporarily, and the accompanying cognitive leaps make them more aware of strangers, places, and change.

Right around the first birthday, babies experiencing these anxiety peaks often start to test their parents to see what the response will be. One common test is to start bawling when the parent, particularly the mum, leaves the room at night. They are saying, 'What are you going to do if I cry? Can I make you come back and stay with me?' This can make bedtime a more wrenching time for both the child and the parent, even with babies who had been going to bed easily at a slightly younger age.

> Amy had slept quite well from around five months until around ten months. Then a bad stomach virus and a wave of separation anxiety combined to wreak havoc with her shut-eye. 'Whatever it

was, it came with a vengeance,' her mother, Linda, remembered with a grimace. Amy started waking up at night, once, then twice. Then she started fighting going to bed at all – she wanted Mum and Dad.

'We tried walking, talking, rocking. Eventually the screaming would get so bad that one of us would take her down to the basement and lie on the couch with her, and the other would stay upstairs and try to get some sleep.' Their home and work lives got more and more stressful. They followed my program, which made Amy feel more secure and sleep better at night.

Loveys

If your child has not already grown attached to a lovey, encourage one now. The lovey makes the baby feel safe and secure, particularly at bedtime or when he wakes up at night. Put a few stuffed animals or blankets in his cot, and see if one has special appeal. Or try to choose one matched to his own habits and preferences.

One mum noticed that her son kneaded her fingers as she nursed him to sleep. She got him a little stuffed cow, and with a little steering from her, he gradually shifted his kneading habit from her finger to the cow's horns. After that, he was able to use his little cow to soothe himself at night.

To encourage the bond with the lovey, hold it between you and the baby when you are nursing or bottlefeeding him, and include the lovey in bedtime games like peekaboo. You may want to wear it inside your own shirt for a few hours to impart that *eau de Mum*. If he doesn't bond despite your efforts, try a lovey again in a month or two – or maybe he'll choose one from among the presents he is sure to collect on his first birthday.

New Mobility

Most babies can now pull themselves up and stand – which creates some new twists at bedtime or naptime when you put them down in the cot and they can pop back up again. I usually tell parents not to intervene, or to put the baby down once, but only once. While you are sitting next to the cot, pat the mattress and encourage your baby to lie down. If you sit, he will be more likely to sit down to be on your level. Babies do tend to learn how to get up before they can get back down, so let her practice during the day. Let her stand up and try to get down holding on to the coffee table – after you babyproof the corners and put some pillows around if needed. Games like ring-around-the-rosy are also good for developing up-and-down motions. But do the practicing games out of the cot, during awake time, not at naps or bedtime.

Eating and Sleeping

Introduce a cup before the first birthday, even if you are still nursing, and even if you plan on nursing for some time to come. As babies get older, they can get emotionally attached to the bottle or breast. It basically becomes a lovey, and that can contribute to an ingrained habit of waking up at night in search of it. Nurse or bottlefeed at set times, and use the cup at set times, giving him water, milk, soy milk, formula, diluted juice, whatever your doctor recommends.

Mums often find that they and the baby both like nursing in the morning and evening and using the cup during the day, especially with solids at mealtimes. Don't let him fall asleep on the breast or with the bottle, and don't let him be dependent on nursing to fall asleep or stay asleep, or you'll be up nursing him back to sleep all night for months to come. To ease the switch from bottle to cup, make sure you keep encouraging the attachment to a lovey (other than the cup itself).

Some mothers wean their babies in the nine- to twelve-month range, and some babies basically wean themselves no matter what their mothers intended. If your baby is looking around a lot while nursing (or taking a bottle), mouthing the nipple without sucking, trying to slide off your lap before you finish feeding him, or impatiently looking like he's got better things to do, that's the signal.

When It's Time to Wean

Weaning from the breast should be an easy, natural transition. Some mums wean after just a few months, particularly if they are going back to work. Others breastfeed for a year or longer. If you wean before the first birthday, you'll wean to a bottle. If you wean around the first birthday, I recommend going from breastfeeding to a cup. Weaning seldom disrupts sleep, but sleep that is already disrupted can make weaning harder if the baby is already overtired and unhappy. Weaning is also more difficult if she has not learned how to fall asleep without a breast or bottle in her mouth. There's no 'right' way to wean, but the most common advice is to drop one daytime feeding one week, drop a second one the second week, and so on (some mums go slower, which is fine – do what works for you). Many mothers continue nursing the first thing in the morning and once at bedtime well beyond the first birthday. That's only a problem when the baby can't go to sleep, or back to sleep, without being breastfed. (The same applies to bedtime bottlefeeding.) In that case, you are facing a sleep issue, not a weaning issue.

Many mums report that the easiest feeding to drop is a midday one. It's easier on their bodies and on their babies. If you are switching to the bottle, have someone else offer the bottle to the baby. If the baby is using a cup, start giving him a cup of milk with whatever meal corresponds most closely to the nursing time. After a week, or whatever feels right to you, do the same for another feeding.

The final two breastfeedings are usually the wake-up one and the bedtime one. Some families keep those two feedings for quite a while; it's your choice. When you decide to give up the morning feeding, have Dad if possible get the baby up in the morning and offer a breakfast bottle and solids (if your baby is eating solids). Mum shouldn't join the breakfast scene until the baby is settled.

If you are stopping that last prebedtime feeding, use the bottle or a sippy cup, then go into the baby's normal bedtime routine. Make sure you allow a little extra time for her routine so she has plenty of time if she needs some extra soothing. It might help to have Dad do the last step of the bedtime routine for a couple of nights, or if she's not yet on a cup, have Dad give her the final bedtime bottle. Remember that you don't want her drinking milk at bedtime indefinitely, as it's bad for her teeth. Talk to your pediatrician about when to switch to water at night (and not juice!).

If your breasts get engorged, try placing ice packs on them. Watch out for clogged ducts and mastitis, and report problems to your doctor quickly to get relief and avoid more serious difficulties.

Sleep Lady Tip

If you have to wean suddenly because of a medical condition or other emergency, use a pump, if possible, but slowly decrease the amount and frequency you pump over about fourteen days. Some lactation consultants suggest drinking sage tea or putting sage leaves in a salad, as the herb can reduce milk supply.

Whether you do it now or in a few more months, weaning should be a natural, easy transition. But nothing is easy and natural when you are dealing with a sleep-deprived, overtired baby, particularly one who hasn't learned how to fall asleep without a breast or bottle in his mouth.

Creating a Schedule

Sample Schedule

7:00–7:30 a.m.
   Wake-up. Nurse/bottle/cup and breakfast.

9:00–9:30 a.m.
   Start the morning nap. If your child is sleeping eleven to twelve hours uninterrupted at night he might be able to

stay awake until 10:00 a.m. (or three hours after waking up). Some children need a small morning snack after the nap.

12:00–12:30 p.m.
Lunch with nurse/bottle/cup.

1:00–2:00 p.m.
Start the afternoon nap. Snack upon awakening.

5:00–6:00 p.m.
Dinner with nurse/bottle/cup.

7:00–7:30 p.m.
Bedtime with nurse/bottle.

Although I don't believe in completely rigid schedules, young children do need consistency and predictability. During the first weeks of sleep scheduling, you are better erring on the side of too much rigidity than too little. This section gives you detailed advice on how to set up a schedule for this age group. (If you want to read even more about scheduling and the relationship between food and sleep, review the scheduling section in the previous chapter.)

Schedules obviously vary somewhat from one child to the next. A baby who wakes up at 6:30 a.m. will have a slightly different timetable than one who gets up at 7:30. But this is a good model, so try not to deviate too much. Especially don't let the baby stay up too late at night, no matter how much fun he seems to be having.

Remember Dr Weissbluth's mantra: Sleep begets sleep. A well-rested child sleeps better than an overtired one. Babies who don't get enough sleep during their naps, or who don't go to bed on time in the evening, tend to wake up more frequently in the middle of the night, and to wake up earlier in the morning.

'One of the first things Kim did was talk to us about schedules – map out the intervals, when Amy should be awake, when she should

be napping. That was news to us! She had always been a catnapper. Talking about an actual schedule was a big thing,' said her mother, Linda.

The big scheduling differences between younger and older infants center on eating. Check with your doctor, but healthy children from nine to twelve months on a normal growth curve can almost always go eleven to twelve hours at night without a feeding. If your child is still waking to eat frequently, you probably have to either adjust his body clock or change his habits.

Separating food time from sleep time, and creating recognizable meal and snack times instead of nonstop nibbling, helps create a sleep-friendly structure. Feed her at recognizable mealtimes: break- fast, lunch, and dinner. Many babies also have morning and after- noon snacks, but you want to get away from the idea of constant feeding and grazing all day (and all night). If your baby goes to bed or takes a nap right after a meal, make sure there is some time between nursing or bottle feeding and going into the cot. You want to break that suckle-snooze association and teach her that milk is part of mealtime, not part of sleep time.

Wake-up. A good time to wake-up is 7:00 to 7:30 a.m., although some children do get up earlier for the first few years. Even if your child tends to sleep later, it's generally a good idea to start waking him by 7:30 to regulate his sleep rhythms and avoid pushing naps and bedtimes too late. (If he sleeps later but takes good naps and sleeps well at night, don't worry about it;

give him plenty of time to adjust when he gets older and has to wake up for preschool.)

Just like you have bedtime rituals, create morning ones. Throw open the blinds and greet the new day with special games or songs. Sleep experts call this a *dramatic wake-up* and it helps your baby better define in his own mind the difference between waking time and sleeping time. This can be a good opportunity for some of those active, stimulating games, like flying baby, that dads like to play but that aren't a great idea in the last five minutes before bed. It's also nice for parents who get home from work late to start their day having fun with the baby.

Morning Nap. Give him some wind-down time to prepare for his nap. It doesn't need to be as long as the bedtime ritual but he does need time to transition from all that revved-up morning activity to morning sleep. Try to get him down by 9:00 or 9:30 – a little earlier if he's an earlier riser, a little later if he sleeps an uninterrupted eleven or twelve hours at night. But don't let him stay up for more than a three-hour stretch. Watch for his sleep windows. Many babies yawn, suck their thumb, or rub their eyes. Others have more idiosyncratic signals like twirling their hair or just getting a zonked-out glassy-eyed look.

'Amy rubs her eyes, that's a sleep clue. But she's a sleep fighter; she is good at masking her cues. We had to learn to pay very careful attention to her cues because she would push and push and fight as hard as she could, so we thought that she wasn't tired, that she just didn't need a lot of sleep. In fact, she needed two or three hours more than we had been giving her. She was sleep deprived,' Linda said.

The morning nap should be about one and a half hours for a nine month old and an hour for a twelve month old. If your child sleeps longer but still naps well in the afternoon and makes it to bedtime, don't worry about it. If, however, he takes a long morning nap and then has trouble sleeping in the afternoon and is a wreck before bedtime, knock off fifteen to thirty minutes from the morning nap. The afternoon nap is generally a longer and more important one, and it's the one he's going to keep after he gives up the morning nap a few months from now.

The interval between the morning nap and lunch is often a good time to run some errands or go outside and play. He has just slept and is less likely to doze off in the car or stroller and throw off his afternoon nap schedule. Some kids need a small snack right after the morning nap. Others wait until lunchtime.

Lunch. Lunch is around noon or 12:30. At this age it's usually solids, with nursing or a bottle or, even better, a cup. Try to have some playtime after lunch or take a walk. Don't have lunch so late that you go directly to the afternoon nap; you are trying to weaken associations between food, particularly the bottle, and sleep.

Afternoon Nap. The afternoon nap usually starts between 1:00 and 2:00 – or around three hours after the morning nap ends. Remember to keep an eye out for that sleep window, and give him some wind-down time to transition to sleep after a period of active play and exploration. This nap should last one and a half to two hours for a nine month old and one and a half hours for a twelve month old. He'll probably want a snack when he gets up.

Dinner. Keep dinnertime early, between 5:00 and 6:00, even if both parents aren't home or aren't ready for dinner yet. Your life will be saner, and he will sleep better if you keep him on an early schedule. I find that babies have an eating 'window' (much like a sleep window), and if you miss it, they eat poorly. Either they wake up hungry in the middle of the night, or we wake up worried that they didn't eat enough.

Bedtime. Bedtime should be at 7:00 or 7:30, and by *bedtime* I mean in the cot, not in the bathtub or on your lap reading stories. Babies this age can fight sleep much more vehemently than younger infants. I worked with one who would shake his head vigorously to stay awake at the tender age of nine months.

Allow plenty of time for him to unwind, and develop ways of cueing his brain that it's time to sleep. You should start brushing his teeth at this age, even if there aren't many teeth. Some parents like to get the toothbrushing out of the way before they begin the rest of the bath and bedtime routine. If the baby hates having his teeth brushed, you don't want to get him all cuddly, cozy, and ready to sleep only to have him kick up a great big stimulating fuss over his dental hygiene.

Make sure the bedtime routine is in the bedroom, not wandering all over the house, and keep the games and stories pretty much the same every night. Some babies, especially when they get a little older, will insist on exactly the same routine every night, down to the last detail, and heaven forbid that you try to vary the story. Allow about fifteen to twenty minutes. Babies are getting a little more interested in picture books and simple rhymes and songs now, and they like Peekaboo and other simple games. Remember to include the lovey in the games.

Christina and Andy had a pretty good bedtime routine for Sally even before I met them. We tweaked it a little, mostly eliminating a feeding too close to her bedtime. She would have dinner, a bath, then a story, and go to bed. That was at nine or ten months, and it worked so well for her that at nineteen months, her routine had hardly changed – a little extra playtime with Dad, and two stories instead of one. 'Andy has tried to put her down without those stories, but she won't go,' Christina said, laughing. 'Rituals! I swear by them.'

Keep any bedtime music soft and quiet. Use music to set the mood and cue the brain for sleep, but turn it off before she gets into her cot, or soon after. You don't want her so accustomed to lullabies that she can't sleep without them. If you've been playing music until after she falls asleep, slowly ease it out. Lower the volume and try to turn it off before she's fully asleep. Similarly phase out bedtime use of toys with noise and lights.

If you walk or rock your baby, keep it brief and stay in her room. Put her down drowsy but still awake so she can learn to do that final part of falling asleep on her own. The goal of getting her down drowsy but awake is crucial. If your baby has trouble with it, focus your energy first on getting it right at bedtime. It's not less important at 2:00 a.m., but it's a lot easier for parents to follow through when we are not half asleep ourselves. Once you get it right at bedtime, it will be easier for you to carry this out consistently at other times.

Bedtime Feeding. It's okay to nurse (or give your baby a bottle) right before bed as long as she doesn't rely on it to get herself to sleep and you aren't nursing her back to sleep when she wakes up at night. If she does depend on the breast or bottle, and many babies do, try to put the final nursing earlier in the bedtime routine, say, before a song or story. Try not to let her fall asleep at the breast. Remember, drowsy but awake!

Some mums find it easier to create that separation by no longer nursing in the baby's room. See if it's a good tool for you. If you want to remain in her room, try keeping the light on while you nurse and turning it off when you want to signal to her that it's cot time.

Megan and John had no schedule whatsoever for Bruce – unless you call haphazard twenty-minute naps and a 10:00 p.m. bedtime a schedule. But Megan and John wouldn't have solved the other problems without fixing the schedule.

Bruce had had severe colic for his first four months, and an extremely kind grandmother used to come over and help every day, comforting the baby and giving Megan and John a bit of a break. Once he was over the colic and feeling better, she'd still come over to play with him almost every night. What baby will willingly crawl off to bed when his grandma is around to cater to his every whim? He used to rub his eyes and yawn a bit around 8:00, but nobody paid much attention, even though his sleep window was gaping open. After all, he was wide awake and having so much fun. 'He was enjoying himself so much, acting like a crazy man the entire evening,' Megan said. Later they realized that Bruce was clearly telling them he needed to go to bed at 8:00, but when nobody responded, he got a rush of cortisol, a second wind, to stay up until 10:00. No wonder it was so hard to get him to sleep when Grandma finally went home.

Along with sleep coaching, they put him on a more consistent nap schedule and told Grandma that although they and Bruce loved her dearly, she had be out the door at 7:00 p.m. when he was in his bath – or stay all night and deal with the consequences.

The Sleep Lady Shuffle

Many families I work with, including those in this chapter, use the Sleep Lady Shuffle to help the baby shed these negative associations. I introduced the concept in Chapter 1, 'The Sleep Lady System,' but we'll review it here, paying particular attention to the needs of this age group. When your child wakes up at night during the Shuffle, go to her cot to comfort her briefly and then resume the position you had been in at bedtime that evening until she falls back to sleep. We want to respond consistently to all wakenings. Use the tips I offer in the 'Problems and Solutions' section to address your child's sleep crutches or habits that make it hard for her to fall to sleep again on her own during the night.

You should follow the Shuffle schedule, moving on to the next position even if your child has had a bad night or two, fussing or waking more frequently. *Don't be surprised if there's a little regression or protest the first night of each new chair position.* If your child gets sick during the Shuffle, you might want to pause and 'freeze' or maintain your position until she's feeling a little better. You might even have to move a little bit closer during an illness to offer more comfort. But then resume your sleep shaping when she recovers.

Nights 1–3. Once bath, stories, and songs are over, sit in a chair *next to your baby's cot*. If she cries or fusses, you can stroke or pat her intermittently (especially the first night), but don't do it constantly or you'll create a new negative association. You can sing during the get-ready-for-bed stage, but once it's time for her to sleep, stick to calming 'sh-sh' or other soothing sounds. You might want to close your eyes. That makes it easier not to talk to her too much, and it also conveys a sleepy-time message. Remember, if she stands up in the cot, put her down only once. Then pat the mattress and encourage her to lie down. This works better if you are sitting by the cot, at her level, instead of standing over it.

It's also important that the parent control the touch. Instead of having her hold your hand or finger, you should pat hers. Make sure that you do not caress the child too steadily; do it on and off. You don't want to swap one negative association, like rocking, for another, like your constant touch or the sound of your voice.

Don't be too quick to pick her up during any stage of the Shuffle – but if she's really upset and you do need to pick her up, go ahead and do so, over the cot if possible. Hold her until she's calm, but keep it brief. Put her down again while she's still awake. Tell her that it's okay, and stay in the chair until she falls asleep.

Nights 4–6. *Move the chair about halfway to the door.* (If the room is very small, or the cot is close to the door, then move all the way to the doorway, as in night 7.) Continue the soothing sounds, but stay in the chair as much as you can. Get up to pat or stroke her a little if necessary, or make some of the same soothing sounds as you have used the past three nights.

Nights 7–9. *Move the chair to the doorway,* still inside the room. You should be dimly lit but still in her view. Continue the same soothing techniques, intervening as little as possible. Stay in the chair as much as you can. Don't worry if she cries a little bit; keep quietly reassuring her. She'll know that you are there, and she will fall asleep.

Nights 10–12. Move further away, usually to *the hallway,* but still *within her direct line of vision.* Make your 'sh-sh' sounds, not constantly but enough to remind her that you are close by and responsive. Stay there until she falls asleep.

A few things to remember. Children get ritualized easily. Make the changes every three days – or less. *Dragging it out makes it harder, not easier, for your baby.* Give it more than three days, and she'll expect you to stay exactly where you are, and get mad or upset when you double that distance.

Nights 13 and on. It's time to leave your baby to fall asleep on her own – if she's not sleeping already. Don't panic – it's probably harder for you than for her. She's had two weeks to prepare for this. She has surrendered some of her sleep crutches and is more secure in her sleep skills. She recognizes your support and responsiveness.

You now need to move away from your baby's room. How far away you go is up to you. You should be out of her sight, but it's fine if you want to *stay within earshot, down the hall or in a nearby room.* If she's whimpering or crying a bit, try calming her from the bedroom doorway. See if you can soothe her with your voice from the doorway. But if you find you must go to her cot do so briefly. Then return to the hallway out of view, but close enough that she can hear your soft, soothing sounds. Listen to your intuition and check on her again from the doorway in a few minutes if you think she truly needs you. But try not to intervene too much or backtrack on all the great work you – and your baby – have done. Very rarely do babies cry for more than a few minutes after experiencing the Shuffle. Keep in mind that she has gained confidence that you are nearby and responsive. She's ready to master this skill. See 'Some Extra Reminders for the First Three Shuffle Nights' on page 141.

Amy's parents put her on a more regular nap schedule, lengthened what was basically a good bedtime preparation routine, and began the Shuffle. She cried at first, and she cried a lot the night they moved the chair to the doorway. But Linda and Miguel had been dealing with hysterical crying for the past two months, and at least now they could see that she was adjusting to the new bedtime arrangements. Within about ten days, they were out of her bedroom and able to give her verbal encouragement and instructions from their own room across the hall. 'We'd say, 'Lie down, lie down,' and she would lie down and go to sleep,' Linda said.

Through the measured paces of the Sleep Lady Shuffle, Amy had regained trust that her parents were nearby, that they would check on her and be there if she needed them. But she also figured out that they weren't going to take her out of the cot, even if she screamed, and that she had to go to sleep.

When Amy got a little older, fifteen months or so, she would sometimes take charge of her own bedtime when she got tired early. 'She'd pull herself out of my lap and point to her cot!' On the other hand, if Miguel's or Linda's parental antennae picked up a little anxiety one night, they could bend the rules a bit. They didn't pick her up, and they didn't return to the earlier chaos and the basement couch. But one parent would occasionally sit on the floor in her doorway at bedtime and give her the little extra reassurance she needed. This let them keep those normal peaks of separation anxiety

*in check, without disrupting her whole sleep routine. It's a good
example of how parents can be flexible and respond to their child's
needs, once their baby has mastered the fundamentals of independent
sleep.*

Problems and Solutions

Babies who have trouble getting to sleep and staying asleep often
have *negative associations,* or sleep crutches. These aren't actually
bad behaviors per se; they only become negative when they block
sleep independence. For instance, children should be hugged and
snuggled. But if they are hugged and snuggled until they fall asleep,
and each time they wake up at night, they will never learn how
to fall asleep on their own or get themselves back to sleep at
night.

Similar negative associations involve a dummy that has to be
replaced constantly; walking, rocking, serenading, or swinging a baby;
or nursing or feeding a baby even when he is seeking food purely
for comfort, not out of hunger. Our job as parents is to help the
baby erase these sleep-harming associations and create positive new
ones that will help him get the sleep required by his growing body
and that miraculously expanding mind.

Troubleshooting

If despite following the advice in this section your child is still
waking up at night, take another look at his routine. Are you putting
him to bed a little too drowsy? If so, he may have learned to put
himself to sleep at bedtime when you've done much of the sleep
preparation work for him, but he can't get himself back to sleep at
night without your assistance. Try putting him down at bedtime
when he's a tad less drowsy and a bit more awake so he can refine
those self-soothing skills. You might also try moving bedtime earlier
by fifteen minutes or a half hour, and maybe create a little more
separation between that last nursing or bottlefeeding and bed. Try
leaving a soft light on while you nurse, which will help him break
that suckle-sleep association.

Time Checks

Sometimes we need to modify the Shuffle because a child is over-stimulated by the parent's presence by his cot or bed. He wants to engage and engage, and no matter how much you soothe and 'sh-sh,' he'll still keep trying to engage you. In this situation, you may want to try working with 'time checks,' a variant of what some call 'Ferberizing.' At bedtime, do your nighttime routine, getting your child calm and soothed before placing him down. Then kiss him and tell him you will check on him before leaving the room.

There is no magic rule about how often you should check on him, and you may have to experiment a bit. If you do it too quickly, he may treat it like a game and get even more stimulated. If you are away too long, he may get worked up and upset.

Start with every seven minutes, and gradually increase it, but trust your own instincts and make necessary adjustments. When you check on him, go directly to his cot and give him a quick reassuring pat. But don't linger: You will defeat the whole purpose if you stand there for a half hour patting him to sleep.

Eliminating Nighttime Feeding

Many parents who are still feeding nine- to twelve-month-old babies all night look at me with a great deal of skepticism when I tell them this, but healthy babies this age who are on a good growth curve don't have to eat at night. Not even once. Not even a little bit. They can go eleven to twelve hours or so without a feeding.

Check with your doctor, but if your baby is still waking to eat at night, you're dealing with a habit, not a nutritional need. Either your child's hunger clock needs a little readjusting, so he eats more during the day and doesn't have a growling tummy at night, or he is using nighttime nursing or bottlefeeding as a sleep crutch.

At this age, I usually recommend that you simply stop the night feedings. Instead, comfort the child, sitting by his bed and patting him intermittently, murmuring 'sh-sh' or making other reassuring sounds. A parent recently told me she was worried about going 'cold turkey.' I reminded her that she wasn't leaving her baby alone to cry; Mum or Dad would be right at her side to soothe her. Instead of 'cold turkey,' I encouraged her to think of it as 'warm and fuzzy turkey.'

Sleep Lady Tip

If the baby wakes before her 'set-time' feeding and stays awake and fussy, don't feed her as soon as the clock strikes her 'set time.' If you do that, you risk training her to cry and cry. Instead, get her back to sleep for at least a little while before you feed her. For example, if she wakes up at 11:00 and fusses until midnight, don't pick her up and feed her at the stroke of 12:00. Get her to sleep, even if it's just for thirty minutes until she wakes up again. So if she wakes up at 11:00, fusses until 12:00, finally falls asleep at 12:10, and wakes up at 12:45, you can feed her. She learned to get to sleep without that food. While she's fussing, try not to pick her up, but if she gets hysterical, hold her briefly. Some babies adjust in three or four days; others take a little longer. Your consistency will help her adapt more quickly.

Still, if that's too abrupt for you, here are two ways to phase out the feeding as you begin the Sleep Lady Shuffle:

Option 1 is a *dreamfeed* for two or three nights. Wake him for one last feeding at about 10:00 or 11:00, about three hours after he goes to bed but before you turn in for the night.

Option 2: Follow the advice I gave in the previous chapter for one *'set-time' feeding*. Do this for three nights.

With either option, don't feed her again until 6:00 a.m., when you can do a 'dramatic wake-up' and start your day. If she wakes up at other times, and she probably will for a few nights, sit by her cot and comfort her. By morning, she will be hungry, which in turn will help her eat more during the day, meaning she'll be more satisfied before night.

Usually parents will move their seat away from the cot on the fourth night of the Shuffle, but we're going to modify it for this night weaning. *So on the fourth night, regardless of whether you choose option 1 or 2, stay next to the cot. Do not feed her overnight at all.* Each time she wakes up, go sit by her cot and soothe her, both by making gentle and calming sounds and by patting or stroking her. Sometimes it works better if the father does the comforting at night, since the baby knows he can't nurse her – and he can't cave in and decide to nurse. Move your chair in three-day increments after that.

I know a lot of us have anxiety about not feeding our children at night; we are afraid that we are hurting them, that we are leaving them with severe pangs of hunger that they can't articulate. We aren't. They will be fine. If you are consistent – meaning you don't cave in and feed him some of the time at night – he'll probably give up those nighttime feedings in just three to four days. If you are inconsistent, it's just going to be more difficult, more prolonged, and more confusing for him.

If your baby takes more than three to four days, don't worry – there is nothing wrong with him; just stay calm and consistent, and he'll adjust and be fine. (If this is a particularly anxiety-provoking topic for you, go back and review the section in Chapter 7, 'Six to Eight Months,' where I go into more detail about how to increase food intake during the day.)

Greta and Matt used the Ferber technique successfully with Jordan, their first son, but with Frederick, their second, it was a disaster. 'He cried for forty-five minutes, and I couldn't stand it. Plus the crying seemed to stimulate him, to keep him up more,' Greta said. But at eleven months, Frederick was 'nursing a hundred times a night,' or at least once an hour. He would end up in his parents' bed, often dozing on top of his mum, who did not find this a restful arrangement.

Greta and Matt combined the Sleep Lady Shuffle with a complete halt to overnight nursing. Greta continued to breastfeed during the day, but not so frequently. Less nursing meant that he ate more solids, which in turn meant he wanted to nurse less. Giving up the constant nursing, Greta could concentrate on developing alternative soothing skills and give Frederick more of a chance to develop his own self-soothing skills. At bedtime, Greta also had to train herself to make sure he didn't fall asleep on the breast, so she could put him down drowsy but awake.

Greta and Matt moved through the Shuffle fairly quickly, sometimes moving every two days instead of three, because Frederick was so easily ritualized. In other words, after two nights, he expected his mother or father to be sitting in a specific place and got upset when they changed the chair's position. If we had let it go to a third night, it would have been even harder for him to adjust to the changed chair position. They also recognized immediately that they should keep the touching and patting to a minimum, because it seemed to make him more alert, not more sleepy. 'It didn't help to have my hand on him. It worked better if I stood nearby and occasionally said something or touched him,' Greta said.

Bedtimes improved really quickly, but night wakenings took a little longer. When Frederick woke up, Matt went very quickly into his room to soothe him. After eleven days, he began sleeping through the night, although it did take a good deal longer to get him to sleep later in the morning.

Daytime weaning came easily for Christina and Sally, but at ten months Christina was still having trouble cutting out her daughter's two last breastfeedings. At bedtime, Christina nursed Sally to sleep in a rocking chair, staying there until she was sleeping soundly enough to be gently transferred into the cot. At 4:00 a.m., Sally woke up and Christina and Andy took her into their bed to be nursed again.

Contemplating doing anything that would upset Sally was very difficult for Christina. She had about zero tolerance for tears, and she interpreted every cry as a sign of hunger. 'She was my little baby, and I couldn't let her cry,' Christina recollected. 'I nursed her too much; every little cry, I thought she was hungry. I never let the poor child cry. I didn't realize that crying was part of her way of communicating.'

Christina was apprehensive about the Sleep Lady Shuffle and the prospect of tears but had become convinced that she owed it to herself and to Sally to help her daughter learn to sleep. She and Andy considered which parent should sit in the chair, and Christina decided that as hard as it would be for her to listen to Sally's tears up close, it would be absolutely unbearable for her to listen to them from further away. 'I knew if I was watching her, I would know she was okay.'

Sally was a classic example of an easily ritualized baby who just swapped one sleep crutch for another. She gave up her nighttime nursing – but within two nights was demanding bedtime patting instead. It was very hard for Christina to keep the touching inter-mittent, to let Sally go to sleep without Mum's hand resting on her through the cot. Christina also had to resist – and she didn't at first – putting Sally down over and over again when she stood up. Sally would keep doing it, because she knew Mum would rub and pat her as she got her to lie back down, and Mum would keep doing it because Sally would cry if Mum stopped.

Sally cried a fair amount the first three nights, even with her mum being much too involved. The first night was a tough forty-five minutes, the second was thirty, the third twenty. (This is why it helps to keep a log, because twenty minutes seems really rotten until you look at your log and see that night 3 was less than half the tears of night 1.) On the fourth night, it was time for Christina to move the chair to the door – and things began to fall into place. It took the rest of the week, but the wakenings grew shorter and less frequent. Within a week, she was sleeping through the night. Her mum said, 'She became an awesome nighttime sleeper.'

Phasing Out Walking and Rocking to Sleep

When nursing no longer does the trick, or when we cut out night-time nursing because we know it interferes with sleep, some of us end up walking or rocking our babies to sleep instead. A few minutes of walking or rocking at bedtime is fine, but if he demands prolonged rocking or a five-mile hike, or if he needs to be walked and rocked repeatedly during the night, it's time to stop.

As with so many sleep problems, the easiest time for you to insti-tute changes is at bedtime, when you are more awake and more likely to be consistent. Begin by doing all the walking or rocking in the bedroom, not all over the house, to create a positive association between the room and sleep.

Scale back the amount of time you walk or rock every few days. Stop walking when he's reached a 7 or 8 on the 10-point drowsy scale, and put him down in his cot. We want him to be aware that he is going into the cot. We don't want to somehow secretly slide him in or trick him, because when he has a partial awakening he'll get mad if he thinks he went to bed in your arms but now he finds himself stuck in the cot. The safest bet is to read him a book and do a little rocking as you slowly make your way to turn off his light. Blow kisses to the moon, give him a kiss and a hug, and put him into the cot.

Sit by the cot and soothe him. If he gets really hysterical, pick him up briefly and put him down as soon as he's calm. If he calms down in two seconds once you've picked him up, you know you've been had! He didn't need to be picked up as badly as you thought he did. Offer swift comfort when he wakes up, but don't start the walking and the rocking again. Resume your Shuffle position and be consistent.

I worked with one little girl who slept poorly during the day and more poorly at night. Her mum nursed her much too often, but by this age, nursing no longer guaranteed that she would fall asleep. Instead, her parents spent an unbelievable amount of time bouncing her to sleep in their arms. They bounced at bedtime, they bounced at naptime, and they bounced each time she woke up at night. An extremely alert baby who hated missing out on any of the action, she even learned to jerk herself awake when she started falling asleep midbounce.

We addressed it by cutting bouncing time in half for two days, and then cutting it back drastically. They would bounce and give her kisses as they turned off her bedroom light, and then they would bounce her over to and into the cot. That was it. She wasn't too happy at first, but her parents were comforting yet consistent. Luckily, she was a resourceful little thing and soon learned to hum herself to sleep!

Dummy (Pacifier) Withdrawal

Dummies have their place, but by this age their place is not in the cot, unless your baby is one of the rare ones who uses it to go to sleep at bedtime but doesn't seek or demand it when she gets up in the middle of the night – in which case you wouldn't be reading this section!

If you are, as one mum put it, 'rebinking' all night, you can either take away the dummy or, if that seems too harsh or difficult, let her keep it but help her learn to put it back in her mouth by herself. You've probably noticed that she can put Cheerios, banana pieces, and teethers in her mouth; there's no reason she can't handle the dummy. To make it easier, leave several in her cot so one is always within easy reach.

If your child has not yet learned how to 'rebink' herself, when you retrieve the dummy, put it in her hand, not her mouth. For a few nights, you might have to guide her hand to her mouth, but at this age they learn pretty quickly. Some children this age want one dummy in each hand.

If you do let her keep the dummy, she may well attach to it as she would to a lovey, and you may eventually have to confront dummy withdrawal more directly. But some parents prefer to wait until their children are a little older to cross that hurdle. I would encourage you at this point to limit the dummy to cot and car so that your child will experiment with other forms of self-soothing. Some parents take the dummy away at night, but leave it at naptime when it is harder for babies to settle themselves.

If you decide to go without the dummy, or if you try to let her take care of her own dummy but she resists and still wakes up in search of it repeatedly, pick a night when you are ready to cope with a little unpleasantness. Make sure you have an especially nice and calming bedtime routine, and try to get her to bed drowsy but awake.

Don't give her the dummy. Stroke or soothe her, just as you would a child you were weaning. Instead of giving her the dummy, use techniques similar to those I advise for parents breaking night-time nursing or walking habits. Do this each time she wakes up at night. Consistency counts. Keep in mind, if you cave in after she's cried for an hour, you aren't teaching her to sleep without the dummy. You are teaching her to cry for an hour in order to get a dummy.

Unconventional Beds

In the early months, many babies sleep anywhere except their cot – car seats, bouncy chairs, cradles, Moses, and wicker baskets that have been passed down for generations. But they can't fit in a basket or bouncy seat forever, and by the time your baby is nearing the end of the first year, he should be in his cot (unless you are committed to long-term cosleeping). If your child is still spending his nights in a less conventional setting, change it now. Use my Sleep Lady Shuffle to get him into a cot, and keep him in the cot, consistently, when he wakes up at night. Use that lovey to ease the transition.

Bruce, the baby who had those evening playdates with Grandma, was walked, rocked, held, and put to bed in an unusual manner. His parents had held him almost 24/7 in the first four months – partly because he was colicky, partly because they thought it would make him grow up to be an affectionate person, and partly because they just couldn't resist holding their beautiful first child in their arms. 'We were so amazed by him, we just held him and stared at him,' Megan recalled.

Eventually, she and John decided they needed to put Bruce down – but by then he had his own thoughts on the matter. Sure, he was fine in his cot – playing with an excessively interactive mobile that did a better job of waking him up than calming him down. But sleep in the cot? Forget it. Bruce slept in a bouncy chair – and they placed the bouncy chair in their bed. Even so, he was up several times every single night, and they would either bounce him back to sleep in his chair or take him out and walk him and then try to 'secretly sneak him back into the bouncy chair before he knew it.'

As his first birthday approached, they decided something had to give. They did the Sleep Lady Shuffle, and although it wasn't an overnight fix, the worst they ever faced was a half hour of crying. Within two weeks, it was bye-bye bouncy chair; he was cheerfully going to sleep in his cot and staying there all night long.

Early Birds

If your child is awake and raring to go at 6:00 or 6:30, you'll probably have to accept that, even if your own preference is to sleep another hour or so. Many babies do wake up early, and feel fine that way. Remember to adapt the meal and nap schedule to suit his early hours.

The first nap should be one and a half to two hours after wake-up. (For a baby who sleeps eleven hours uninterrupted at night, the nap can be three hours after wake-up if he doesn't seem too tired or cranky before he hits the three-hour mark.) You might also try shifting bedtime later in fifteen-minute intervals to see if that will coax him into sleeping later, but be careful. He may still wake up at 6:00, but be more tired because he's no longer getting enough sleep at the front end.

Pay attention to his sleep window and his behavior. Don't force him to stay up when he really needs to go to sleep, or he won't be able to fall asleep when you want him to. Room-darkening blinds may help, and white-noise machines can be useful if there's a lot of early-morning noise – birds singing, dustbins crashing. You may also try the techniques I outline below for problematic early risers, but they may or may not work for a child whose biological clock is set just fine for him, but not for you.

That laissez-faire approach doesn't hold for a baby who wakes up *before* 6:00 a.m., or who wakes up cheerful at 6:00 or 6:30 but is falling apart by 7:00. You need to step in and teach him to sleep later. As Greta and Matt can attest, the longer you endure early risings, the harder it is to change the pattern. Address it now, even if it takes several weeks to see results. If you wait until he's a toddler or preschooler, it can take even longer. Make sure your early riser is getting enough daytime sleep, because nap deprivation can cause poor night sleep and early awakenings. You may have to change his nap schedule, too, to make his morning nap a little later. Try moving it back a half hour or so, but don't let him get so overtired that he is too wired to nap.

Early Risers

If your little one wakes up before 6:00 a.m., he's probably overtired. Overtired children don't sleep as well, or sleep as long, as well-rested ones. He may be:

- Going to bed too late
- Not napping enough
- Staying up too long between the end of his afternoon nap and going to bed (try not to let it exceed four hours)
- Going to bed when he's past that 'drowsy but awake' mark. If he's too drowsy, he won't know how to get himself back to sleep when he's more alert – including at 5:00 a.m.

When your early bird stirs, go to his room immediately. You want to try to get him back to sleep ASAP, not let him scream himself awake. Give him his lovey and try to soothe him back to sleep without picking him up. Even if he doesn't doze off again – and not all babies will at first – do not turn on the lights or get him out of his cot until 6:00 a.m. no matter how much he protests. Getting him up earlier sends a confusing message and is another example of intermittent reinforcement.

At this age, I usually recommend that the parent stay in the room for this early-morning routine. If, however, you feel your presence is encouraging him to be more awake, as often occurs with older children, you can try leaving his room after a bit of reassurance and see if he falls asleep again on his own. Check on him every ten to fifteen minutes. If you stay in the room, keep the interaction minimal. Try sitting in a chair with your eyes closed. When the clock finally strikes 6:00 and he's not falling asleep – and it can seem like it takes a very long time to reach 6:00 – leave the room for a minute or two. He may cry, but try not to let it bother you, as you will be right back in a minute.

When you come back in, make a big deal out of 'good morning' time. Do your dramatic wake-up. The morning routine is the flip side of the bedtime-routine coin. Your goal is to help him distinguish between day and night, to know when it really is time to get up. Your message must be clear: 'I'm getting you out of the cot because it's morning time – not because you were crying.'

While Frederick's nights were increasingly easy, early morning was not fun. He woke up at 5:00 a.m. with a high-pitched scream. 'It was the toughest time to deal with, because you knew you were less likely to go back to sleep,' said Greta, voicing a sentiment I hear often from parents.

Either Greta or Matt would go to him and tell him to lie back down. Sometimes he would fall asleep right away. Sometimes he'd cry the whole hour. 'It was very unpredictable,' Greta recalled. But they didn't pick him up. Then at 6:00 a.m., they'd leave the room for two minutes. When they came back, they would say, 'Good morning!' and act like the previous hour of protest had never occurred.

It took longer to change this early-waking pattern than it had to get rid of that constant nighttime nursing, but eventually Frederick began sleeping until 6:00. His parents would love to have him sleep another hour, but they keep reminding themselves that he's getting eleven hours of solid sleep – and they relish that extra fifteen or thirty minutes he occasionally grants them.

Napping

Parents often wonder why overtired children don't nap easily. You know the answer by now: Overtired children are too tired to nap. Their high cortisol levels make them feel alert, even wired, despite being sleep deprived. This applies to babies who go to bed too late at night, babies who wake up too early in the morning, babies who nap in moving cars and strollers, babies who skip naps, babies who take short catnaps instead of longer restorative naps – and babies who do all of the above. You need to review your child's schedule and get him on a nap schedule consistent with his natural sleep windows. I confess, nap training is my least-favorite part of sleep training, but it's an essential one.

Children this age still need two naps – one in the morning, and a longer one in the afternoon. The transition to one nap usually doesn't come until around fifteen to eighteen months. Don't attempt it too early.

If you let your baby sleep too long in the morning, he will have trouble sleeping in the afternoon, and there is no way a nine to twelve month old can make it all the way from morning nap to evening bedtime without making everyone in the family pay the price. *Limit the morning nap to one and a half hours for the nine month old, one hour for the twelve month old.* And not before 8 a.m. Get that afternoon nap started about three hours after the morning one ends. An occasional exception is okay. If he's been sick, or slept poorly one night, or had an unusually active morning exercising brand-new crawling or walking skills, he might need a longer nap once in a while, but don't make it a habit.

By nine months, most babies give up that third late-afternoon mininap. If he's still taking that third nap but it doesn't interfere with bedtime, don't worry about it; he'll give it up soon. Similarly, if he's not napping particularly well earlier in the day, let him keep the mininap while you work on lengthening and improving his two main naps. However, if he is taking the mininap and then having trouble getting to sleep at a reasonable bedtime, you are going to have to force the issue and not let him take that late-afternoon snooze.

Nap training isn't fun, and it often involves tears. Some of us as parents can cope with a crying baby in daylight more easily than we can at night. We are more rested and we just don't feel as bad leaving them alone when it's not dark. But some of us have a terrible time doing nap training ourselves at home when our spouse or partner isn't there for moral support.

I always tell families to try the nap training – and try it for more than a day or two. But if a little voice inside your head is saying that you really can't do this, listen to it. Give yourself permission to stop the training. That doesn't mean you should abandon your efforts to get your child to nap, or that you should convince yourself that your child doesn't need to nap. He does need to nap, even if he is trying his level nine-month-old best to convince you otherwise.

Ilan, my coauthor's son, stopped napping at ten months. He wouldn't nap for her, he wouldn't nap for his father, and he wouldn't nap for his loving babysitter who had got dozens of babies to nap in her long child-care career. He'd occasionally doze off in the car, picking his big brother, Zach, up from school, or even slump over in his high chair late in the day. His parents finally concluded he was one of those rare babies who just didn't need to nap. They were wrong. I didn't work with Ilan's family until he was almost two, but then we did get him to resume napping for two, two and a half, or sometimes three hours on weekdays. (Weekends, when he was excited that Zach was home, remained a problem.)

The moral of the story is that if you can't stomach the tears, you don't have to. But I want to be very clear here: *You don't have to nap train him if it's too much for you now. But you do have to make sure he naps, one way or another.* Put your energy into improving his night-time sleep, and use whatever tricks you know to get him to sleep during the day, even if that means bending my rules and relying in part on some motion sleep.

You may find that when nighttime sleep improves, daytime sleep will follow. Or you may find that you have to return to nap training again a few weeks or months from now. But once you see that these techniques really do improve nighttime sleep and make your child happier, it may be easier for you to stick to nap training the second time around.

Here's nap training in a nutshell (if you want more details on napping and using the Shuffle during the day, go back and read the 'Napping' section in Chapter 7, 'Six to Eight Months'). Put your child in a cot drowsy but awake and give him an entire hour to fall asleep for the morning nap. Do the same – for an hour – for the after-noon nap.

If you want to stay with him and do the Shuffle, even if it takes the whole hour, that's fine. If, however, you sense that your pres-ence keeps him awake, don't stay in the room. Leave the room and go back and comfort him every ten minutes or so. You can also sit right outside his doorway, where he knows you are nearby, and use the hour to read, knit, stretch, do leg lifts, or catch up on e-mail. Not all babies will take that full hour, or they may only take the full hour for the first few days.

If he doesn't sleep at all during the morning hour, try to get him down for his afternoon nap earlier than usual because he'll be overtired. Watch his sleepy clues, and catch him when he's ripe for a nap. That could be in as little as forty-five minutes after you let him get up from the morning nap (or morning nonnap).

Give him that entire hour to fall asleep in the afternoon, but when the hour is up and he's still awake, enter his room and do a dramatic wake-up. If he nods off but only catnaps, waking up after only twenty or thirty minutes, resettle him and start your sixty-minute count again.

Nap-Coaching Tips

It's easier to get a baby to take the morning nap than the afternoon nap. Don't miss that opportunity.

Afternoon nap training is tougher. Don't get discouraged; it's normal.

Keep a sleep log during nap training.

If it's 2:00 or 3:00 p.m. and the baby has not napped well enough, you may need to resort to your 'backup plan,' such as a nap in the stroller or car, to avoid an exhausted baby and bedtime disaster.

You will be tied to the house during nap coaching. If you feel like all you are doing all day is trying to get your baby to nap, then you are doing it right! The payoff: You'll have more freedom (and a happier, rested baby) once you have a predictable napping schedule.

If you have a nanny, babysitter, or child-care setting that can do the nap training, thank your lucky stars. If your caregiver is reluctant to do the training, see if you can win her over with a simple explanation of the sleep science. If not, explain that your child needs a full 'sleep tank,' and if that means the sitter has to use a sleep crutch like rocking to get the child to nap, or to resume a brief or interrupted nap, that's okay.

Have a backup plan for the afternoon. Do whatever it takes to get him to sleep, including a car ride if necessary, because letting him get even more overtired will just add to your vicious no-sleep cycle.

A common error is to offer the child a brief 'comfort nursing' right before naptime. What often happens is that the baby dozes off after about fifteen minutes while nursing – sort of a little 'power nap' on the breast. It gives him just enough sleep to fight off a genuine nap. Mums should either eliminate prenap nursing or schedule it earlier in the day.

Irene got Brad off the nighttime bottle and out of her bed extremely quickly, but nap training took two stressful months. 'The nanny was reluctant to do it, so I did it when I was home but I wasn't home every day, so it took a long time and was very difficult,' she said. Still, her perseverance paid off, and Brad finally abandoned those unhelpful twenty-minute catnaps and started taking two solid naps every day. When he got older, his transition to one nap went quite smoothly, and at eighteen months he was napping – for Irene or the nanny – two to three hours every afternoon.

While Bruce's nighttime sleep improved quickly, naps were tough. Some days, Megan bundled him into the car and drove until he fell asleep, which usually didn't take long. She didn't want to risk waking him up by trying to carry him back into the house through the cold winter air, but didn't want to keep driving either, knowing that he would not sleep as deeply in motion. So she'd take along a bunch of blankets . . . and her laptop. When he fell asleep, she'd drive home, park in her driveway, drape herself in blankets, and get some work done for a job at a local magazine.

Cosleeping

If you are bedsharing, please see Chapter 12, 'Whose Bed Is It Anyway?' If you want to continue cosleeping, I can help you improve the quality of your family's sleep. Pay a lot of attention to helping your child learn to nap on his own, which will be a big help now and as he develops more sleep skills in the future. If you have been cosleeping but want to stop, I'll give you suggestions on how to follow through. If stopping is on your agenda, age nine to twelve months is a good time to do it, before the heightened separation anxiety that occurs around the first birthday.

Jason

You met Tess briefly in the opening chapter, where she was struggling with her mother's chemotherapy and her son's sleeplessness. Jason was ten months old at the time and usually slept with Tess, while her husband, Ron, unable to sleep with a baby in the bed, exiled himself to the guest room for eight months. Jason nursed and nuzzled all night long. 'It was an all-you-can-

eat buffet, all night long,' Tess said, laughing. 'And I was his walking, talking comfort item.'

Tess knew she was going to have to make some changes, but she wanted them to be ever so gentle, and I didn't want to push Tess beyond her emotional limits. So we tried just getting rid of the 2:30 a.m. feeding, we tried having her place a pillow between her and the baby and turning him away from her, we tried having her wear extra layers of clothing at night. 'I'd be up from 2:00 a.m. to 5:00 to skip that 2:30 feeding, rocking him, blind with exhaustion. I knew deep down that it wasn't going to work, but Kim let me go through all of that because I needed to. It was about exorcising my demons. Then, with my mother sick, I was on the verge of collapse.'

Tess had her own emotional baggage. As a child, she had experienced sleep terrors and sleepwalking, and slept with her parents until she was eight. 'I have my own memories of being in my room and going into my parents' room. I think I would have dropped dead if they had said, 'No, you can't come in.' I was the third child by fifteen years, so I got away with a lot.' She had also endured two devastating miscarriages before Jason, so all the normal anxieties of motherhood were magnified in her mind. And of course she was dealing with a seriously ill mother with whom she was very close. On the other hand, she knew her tear aversion was a little over the top. 'I'm a lawyer. I'm a prosecutor. I can be coldhearted. But I can't stand to let my baby cry. I was insane!'

Finally ready for more direct action, she got Jason a lovey, a 'taggy' blanket. She kept one at her home and one at her mother's New York home. 'He loves tags; every toy we got him, he just went for the tag.' They coslept on the floor in his room for nearly two weeks, more than the two or three days I usually recommend, but there was so much situational stress here, we needed extra emotional padding.

When the time came to put Jason into his cot, she handed him to his father and checked into a hotel, where she spent the night explaining to a friend on the telephone that she was afraid letting her baby cry might make him feel abandoned and turn him into a serial killer someday. Meanwhile, Ron, not exactly a tear warrior himself, invited one of his friends over to the house for moral support.

The baby cried for an hour, and Ron stayed in the room but did not pick him up. Yet despite that difficult bedtime, Jason woke up only once

overnight when he cried for twenty minutes. The next night was easier —
twenty minutes of crying at bedtime, and he needed only brief checks and
reassurances from his dad.

The third night, Tess checked out of her hotel and took her turn. Jason
cried less than night 1 but more than night 2, and although Tess still found
tears distressing, she had seen the evidence with her own lawyerly eyes that
he was not hurt, that he was 'his usual happy self,' and that he was already
sleeping better. She sat near him, saying 'sh-sh' and murmuring soothing
things to him, but kept her distress in check and let him cry.

Over the next week or so, it kept getting easier. Jason would go to bed
without much fuss and wake up only once or twice, crying but not needing
to nurse, falling asleep again within twenty minutes. The first few nights
Tess sat by his bed, but then discovered he fell asleep more easily if she
just went in to make sure he had his dummy and blanket and left again.
Usually he'd fall asleep right away. On the rare nights when the tears
ramped up, those moments when he cried to the point where he probably
forgot what he was crying about, one of his parents would soothe him and
he'd go back to sleep.

'It was only ten days of trauma — although it felt like a year. And then
it was such an amazing turnaround. In three days he went from nursing
all the time to not nursing the entire night, from sleeping with me to sleeping
in his cot. It took ten days to consolidate, but the change in the first three
days was amazing,' Tess said. 'I let the sleep issues get completely out of
control because I was so unwilling to let him cry, I waited much too long
to deal with what was a real problem. Now I look back and don't know
what I was thinking.'

9

Thirteen to Eighteen Months

*A*t this age toddlers need an average of eleven and a quarter hours of *uninterrupted sleep at night and two and a quarter to two and a half hours during the day. Children at the younger end of this age bracket take two naps, in the morning and afternoon, but by eighteen months most consolidate to one midday or afternoon nap.*

Early toddlers are prone to behavioral sleep problems. Their increased mobility (including walking), a peak in separation anxiety around the first birthday, and emotional attachment to such objects as bottles and dummies can all complicate bedtime and contribute to nighttime awakenings.

At around fifteen to eighteen months, toddlers transition from two naps to one. That's a tricky stage because there is usually a point when one nap is not enough and two naps are too many. The result is an overtired child who doesn't sleep well at night. This chapter will give you techniques to help speed up and smooth out that transition, but you will probably still face a bit of crankiness for about three weeks as her body adapts.

As if that wasn't enough, temper tantrums often emerge at this age, and toddlers start testing their parents. Bedtime is a common battleground for toddlers flexing emerging willpower muscles. A soothing bedtime routine is extremely important for children this age, and adhering consistently to routines and setting clear rules is essential – because the next stage is only tougher.

Developmental Changes

Separation Anxiety

Separation anxiety hits a peak right around the first birthday. Saying 'night-night' to parents can be tough. That nice, long transition to bedtime, good focused time with one or both parents, helps ease the fears. Although one year olds can't say much, they understand an awful lot, so give plenty of verbal assurances that you are nearby.

Even after some parents complete the Shuffle successfully, they like to stay in the room as the baby falls asleep to help with the separation. That's okay as long as you don't fall back into all your pre-Shuffle habits, and she doesn't wake up at night needing you to go sit there again and again. If you choose not to stay in the room, it may help if you reassure the toddler that you'll be nearby – and then keep your word. Instead of going downstairs to clean the kitchen, which can seem very far away from the cot, stay in a nearby room so she feels your closeness as she nods off.

Loveys

Loveys, usually a special stuffed animal or security blanket, are very useful as children cope with separation anxiety. Many families have told me their babies resisted all attempts to have them bond with a special toy the first year, but quickly attached to an object around the age of one. They may choose one of their own at this age, maybe from among that batch of first birthday presents. They may also abandon the lovey they favored in infancy and choose a new one.

> 'Alex had a whole cot full of animals, and we had been trying to get him to attach to one since he was six months old. He ignored them, wouldn't even touch them. But when he got older, he got interested. While we were concentrating on his sleep, we chose one, a Good Night

Moon bunny, and tried to use it consistently. When he got a little older, he started asking for a different animal each night,' his mother, Adele, said. It wasn't a typical pattern, but it was a successful one. He was able to happily snuggle up with whichever one he selected as his evening's companion.

At thirteen months, Teddy suddenly got attached to two plastic teethers. He wasn't teething — he just wanted to grip one in each hand when he went to sleep. The problem was they were so small that they'd fall through the cot slats, and he'd wake up and scream if he couldn't find them. 'It wasn't easy to keep crawling under the cot to get them,' Lisa recalled. She began a concerted effort to transfer his affections from the teethers to a Barney. It took a while, but Barney eventually trumped the plastic rings and was much less likely to end up on the floor.

To encourage the bond, incorporate the lovey in bedtime and naptime rituals. For instance, if you play peekaboo before bed, the lovey should play peekaboo, too. If you stroll around the room saying good night to favorite objects, the lovey should say good night, too. Tuck the lovey in the cot with her at bedtime and naptime. At some point, your baby might mimic bedtime activities for the lovey, giving her lamb or teddy bear a good-night kiss and tucking it in.

Even if the lovey bond hasn't stuck before, I strongly recommend making another effort now. Toddlers often get emotionally attached to the breast or their bottle, sippy cup, or dummy, and they may wake up often at night wanting a bottle or cup, not because they are really hungry or thirsty but because it helps them feel secure. Easing the attachment to the breast, bottle, and so on goes hand in hand with strengthening the attachment to the lovey — you'll have trouble fostering the lovey bond if you don't reduce the previous attachment simultaneously.

Some parents worry if a toddler starts lugging the lovey around with him all the time. That may be a minor inconvenience, because you have to remember to take the lovey with you, but I don't regard it as a problem. Dummies are a little different, and I don't recommend having toddlers walk around with them all day. It may interfere with communication and speech development. Consider getting rid of the dummy, or restricting it to bedtime and naps.

Eating and Sleeping

As parents, we have to adjust to the idea that milk isn't the heart of our children's diet anymore. By the first birthday, they get most of their nutrition and their calories from table foods or solids. Pediatricians usually recommend they take two to three glasses of milk (approximately 600ml/20oz) – the advice varies a bit, so consult your doctor. If you toddler eats a lot of dairy products like yogurt, she's getting her calcium and vitamin D, and doesn't need to drink as many glasses of milk.

Remember, she's not an infant anymore, so pouring milk into her right before bedtime will not prolong her sleep. To the contrary, it might just fuel her habit of associating milk with sleep, and wanting to drink all night. It may also invite her to wake up and let you know loudly that she has a soaking wet nappy. Introduce a cup now if you haven't already, even if you plan to continue nursing. Offer the sippy cup – of water, milk, formula, diluted juice, whatever your doctor recommends – at each meal.

Sleep Lady Tip

There's no 'right' way to wean, but the most common advice is to drop one daytime feeding one week, drop a second one the second week, and so on.

Using a Cup

If you wean, and many mothers do around the first birthday, I recommend going from breastfeeding to a cup, not to a bottle. Weaning should be an easy, natural transition. It seldom disrupts sleep, but sleep that is already disrupted can make weaning harder for an overtired, unhappy baby. Weaning is more difficult if she has not learned how to fall asleep without a breast or bottle in her mouth. (For more on weaning, see Chapter 8, 'Nine to Twelve Months.')

Sleep Lady Tip

To transition from bottle to cup, start with the first morning bottle. Fill it with only 90–120ml/3–4oz, and then move quickly to breakfast. After a few days, offer a sippy cup of milk. Then start reducing the amount of milk in the bottles that you offer before (or after) lunch and dinner. Give him a cup with his meal instead. You may find that if you give him the bottle after his meal, he won't really want it much anymore, because he won't be hungry.

Many mothers continue nursing the first thing in the morning and once at bedtime well beyond the first birthday. That's only a problem when the baby can't go to sleep, or back to sleep, without being breastfed. (The same applies to bedtime bottlefeeding.) In that case, you are facing a sleep issue, not a weaning issue, and I'll talk more about how to change those patterns later.

If your child is using a bottle rather than a sippy cup, make the switch now, particularly if the bottle is a sleep crutch. Check with your pediatrician; if there are any growth concerns and the doctor recommends sticking to the bottle for a while, you can still address the sleep associations. Give the bottle when your child is awake, after a nap, for instance, instead of right before naptime or bedtime.

If your child becomes fussy during the day and asks for a bottle, look at the clock and your sleep log. Is he really hungry, or does he want the bottle for comfort or out of habit? Can you comfort or distract him in some other way? Maybe he's overstimulated and needs a few quiet hugs from you, or a few minutes on your lap with a book. Maybe he's tired and it's time for his nap. Perhaps he is signaling that he needs to go to bed a little earlier than usual.

Don't assume that the bottle is the only thing that will make him feel calm and happy.

When you are ready to wean him from the bedtime bottle, follow a similar strategy. Reduce the amount every two or three days, from 220ml/8oz, down to 180ml/6oz, to 120ml/4oz, to 60ml/2oz. Then offer him a sippy cup of water instead. Sometimes a baby protests when he hits that 120ml/4oz mark because it is no longer enough fluid for him to suck himself to sleep. Find other ways of comforting him, and stick to your plan.

Some families deal with the bottle-cup issue before they start sleep shaping, but it's often best to do them simultaneously. You can modify the Sleep Lady Shuffle slightly. For instance, you might want to add one night at the cot side (so you would be right next to the cot for four days, not the three I usually recommend). Night 1 you might cut the bottle to 180ml/6oz, night 2 to 120ml/4oz, night 3 to 60ml/2oz, and on the fourth night, take the bottle away but stay by the cot to give him a little extra help adjusting. On the fifth night, start the next phase of the Shuffle, moving away from the cot. There are other ways to modify this, and you may want to tweak the system a bit to fit your family, but keep in mind that if the bottle is the child's sleep crutch, you will have to help him give it up so he can learn how to soothe himself to sleep. We'll also talk more about night weaning later in this chapter.

Creating a Schedule

Sample Schedule

(Shift earlier if your child wakes between 6:00 and 7:00 a.m.)

7:00–7:30 a.m.
   Wake-up and breakfast.

9:00–9:30 a.m.
   Start of one-hour morning nap if she's still taking one.
   She'll probably want a snack right before or after the nap.

11:30 a.m.–12:30 p.m.
   Lunch (depending on morning-nap timing).

12:30–1:30 p.m.
   Start of afternoon nap. About an hour and a half if it's a
   second nap, about two to two and a half hours if it's the
   only nap of the day. Snack after nap.

5:00–5:30 p.m.
   Dinner.

6:00–6:30 p.m.
   Start bath/bedtime routine.

7:00–8:00 p.m.
   Asleep.

Children need regular naptimes, regular bedtimes, and three
recognizable mealtimes. Their bodies need the routine to regulate day and night hormone cycles, and to keep them in sync
with their internal clocks. Their little hearts and minds need
certainty and predictability to feel secure. But I also believe in
some flexibility.

The sample schedule is a good starting point, but you can adjust it. For instance, if your child is an early riser, move the morning nap earlier. You may also have to play with the schedule a bit to accommodate the needs of your other children. Sleep times are averages. Some kids sleep more, some sleep less, but the variations are a lot less than many parents think. If your child is napping and sleeping poorly, chances are you are underestimating how much sleep she needs.

Even when you do achieve a workable schedule, natural variations inevitably occur. Some days she will eat or sleep a little more, and some days she will eat or sleep a little less. Growth spurts, runny noses, new teeth, or just a bad mood – toddlers have their off days just like we do – can all create minor variations in her daily routine. But don't let the schedule get totally out of whack. As you learn to read her sleep cues and she becomes better rested, you will be able to tinker with the schedule more easily. Watch her daytime behavior. If she's easy and content, she's probably on a pretty good schedule. If she's fussy and demanding, she may need longer naps, an earlier bedtime, a later wake-up time – or all of the above.

If you have to skip a nap because of a doctor's appointment or some other essential interruption, most toddlers fare better missing the morning nap than the afternoon one. You can temporarily move the afternoon nap up a bit to compensate for a missed morning one.

Barring unusual dietary or health concerns, thirteen to eighteen month olds should have three recognizable mealtimes a day. Most snack twice a day, either before or after the morning nap (usually before, but it depends on your child's precise schedule) and upon awakening from the afternoon nap. Check with your doctor, but healthy children in this age group on a normal growth curve can almost always go eleven to twelve hours at night without food. If your child is still waking to eat frequently, you have to adjust her body clock, change her sleep habits, or both. I'll give you some tips on how to do that later in this chapter.

Sleep Lady Tip

Don't give a bottle at bedtime in the hope that it will make her sleep longer – those days are long over.

Wake-up. A good wake-up time is anywhere from 6:00 to 7:30. Remember that one of the basic rules of sleep hygiene is to wake-up and go to bed at about the same time every day. If your baby wakes up before 6:00, the 'Early Birds' section below will help you teach him to sleep later.

Some toddlers sleep past 7:30. If it works for you and your family – and by *works* I mean that she is getting good naps and at least eleven to eleven and a half hours of uninterrupted sleep at night – that's fine; leave it alone. When she gets closer to starting preschool, make sure you leave plenty of time for her to gradually adjust to an earlier wake-up. But an 8:30 or 9:00 a.m. wake-up throws off many toddlers. They nap too late or inconsistently, and they go to bed too late and don't sleep well at night. You can either just start waking her at 7:30 – gently at first – or you can adjust more gradually. Get her up about ten minutes earlier than usual, hold it there for two or three days, then another ten minutes earlier, and so on.

Morning rituals, the counterpoints of your evening ones, are still a good idea to reinforce her understanding of wake-up time versus sleep time. Throw open the blinds, switch on the lights, sing some cheery good-morning songs, and start your day. It's your choice whether you feed her immediately or have some playtime. Parents who come home late from work (usually, but not always, fathers) often make mornings their special game time.

Morning Nap. While she's still on a two-nap-a-day schedule, her morning nap should begin around 9:00 or 9:30. If she's sleeping well at night, the morning nap should be two to three hours after she woke up. Watch the sleep windows to determine exactly what time is right for her. Remember to provide that wind-down time to get ready for sleep, maybe a book or two or an abbreviated version of her bedtime routine.

She will probably sleep about an hour, maybe an hour and a half. I discourage longer morning naps because the afternoon nap is usually the more important one, the one that she will hold on to for another two or three years. If she sleeps two or three hours in the morning, consider waking her after ninety minutes or else she is going to have a tough time going down for her afternoon nap. After the morning nap is a nice time to visit the playground, go for a walk, or do some shopping. She will be refreshed and less likely to doze off in the car or stroller and throw off her afternoon nap schedule.

Lunch and the Afternoon Nap. A lot of parents don't realize that toddlers get hungry more quickly than we do. Lunch is often at 11:30, almost always by noon or 12:30. You've usually got some playtime after lunch and before nap. Usually you will aim for two to three hours between the end of the morning nap and the start of the afternoon one. Again, watch her sleep signals to get her down at the right time.

The afternoon nap usually lasts about one and a half hours. Once she consolidates to one nap, aim to get her down sometime between 12:30 and 1:30, and she'll probably sleep two to two and a half hours. A pretty typical afternoon nap runs from about 1:00 to 3:30, but it can vary thirty minutes in either direction. When she gets up, it's time for another snack and some playtime before dinner.

Dinner. An early dinnertime, 5:00 or 5:30, is usually wise, even if that means she doesn't eat with her parents. She can always have fruit or a bit of dessert with you while you eat dinner. The early schedule helps both her eating and her sleeping. I find that children have eating windows, too, and if you feed them too late, they don't eat very well. The last thing you want is a poor dinner eater who then wakes up demanding a midnight snack. (You'll get enough of that in adolescence!)

Bedtime. Aim to have her asleep – asleep, not getting ready for bed – between 7:00 and 8:00. Watch her cues and trust your own intuition. You might move bedtime a little later, 8:00 or 8:30, after she has begun sleeping consistently through the night and at naptime and has caught up on all her missed sleep. Remember, she still needs, on average, eleven hours and fifteen minutes of sleep at night.

Toddlers need a lot of transition time to prepare for sleep, in terms of both brain hormones and emotional readiness to separate from their parents until morning. Bedtime routines must be structured and predictable, and they absolutely cannot be rushed. Leave enough time – maybe it will be half an hour for your child, maybe an hour (including bath time) – and make it a fun and loving time, a time she eagerly anticipates.

Keep the bedtime routine in her bedroom, not all over the house, so she incorporates the message that it is time to slow down and get ready to sleep. It's okay to start downstairs with some prebedtime evening rituals, but as soon as the bath is done, stay in the bedroom. Get any unpleasant aspect of bedtime over at the beginning, so you can spend the rest of it calming down in enjoyable ways.

As I mentioned, she won't need a feeding prior to bedtime, but some toddlers still like to nurse briefly or have a cup of water before bed. If she's taking a bottle at bedtime, switch to a cup and think about water instead of milk. You can do this gradually if you like, moving from an 220ml/8oz bottle to a 120ml/4oz bottle and then to a cup. Some people use milk or formula and dilute it for a few nights before switching to water.

If you walk or rock your baby before sleep, keep it brief and keep it in her bedroom. If she still listens to music at bedtime, start phasing it out before she actually gets into her cot. Put her down drowsy but still awake.

Relatively minor changes in the bedtime routine can sometimes make a big difference for a toddler. Adele and Geoff used to read Alex a book in their bed, but they moved his story time to his own room, which helped him transition to his cot. They also got much more attuned to his sleep windows. 'I got more hyper about paying attention. He pulls at his eyelids – which I hate. And he pulls his hair. Sometimes he just gets really wound up or can just be staring and walking around and out of it. I began to recognize that any of those signs meant he needed to go to sleep,' his mum said.

Now that your baby is standing and probably walking, be prepared for some cot gymnastics. Many babies stand in their cot; you put them down, and they bounce right back up. For a one year old, this is literally stand-up comedy. But no matter how hilarious she thinks it is, try not to join in the merriment or she'll play jack-in-the-box all night. Pat the mattress, put her down once, and then pat her. If she gets up again, keep patting the mattress as a signal to her, but don't keep lying her down. This works better if you're sitting rather than standing over the cot. She'll get down when she's ready, and she'll be ready faster if you don't help her turn it into a game.

Ellen and George adopted James from Korea when he was six months old. He bonded quickly with his new parents but remained shy, somewhat fearful, and apprehensive about change. He was also a terrible sleeper, waking frequently and needing a lot of help to get back to sleep. Severe chronic ear infections made the whole situation worse, because he woke up often, in pain and in need of comfort.

Before working with me, they had rocked, walked, or patted him until he fell asleep, and then tried to gingerly slip him into the cot without waking him. I think that usually backfires — if a toddler goes to sleep in one place, he's going to open one eye at some point and then bolt wide awake when he finds he ended up somewhere else. In addition, James had coslept with his foster parents in Korea. When he got to the United States, Ellen and George didn't take him into their bed, but they didn't teach him to fall asleep on his own, either. At bedtime and when he woke up at night, they had to walk, pat, or rock him, over and over again. 'He was totally reliant on me to get him to sleep,' Ellen recalled.

At eighteen months, Ellen and George worked with me to change his schedule. They shifted the 9:30 bedtime to 7:30, but made only very minor changes to what was already a specific and stable bedtime routine. 'We bathed him every night, instead of every other night, and then we put on his pajamas, gave him a cup of water, and read three books — the same three books every night in the same sequence,' said Ellen. 'We put on the music box for two minutes; we hugged him and put him in the cot.'

The Sleep Lady Shuffle

Many families I work with use my Sleep Lady Shuffle to change sleep habits, to gently and gradually have the parent fade away from the bedside. Let's see how it applies to a child at this age. *Night wakenings usually taper off during the Shuffle, but when she does wake up, pat or comfort her briefly by her cot and then resume the position you were in at bedtime that evening.* The goal is a consistent response to all wakenings.

You should follow the Shuffle schedule, moving on to the next position even if your child has had a bad night or two, fussing or waking more frequently. Don't be surprised if there's a little regression or protest the first night of each new chair position. If your child gets sick during the Shuffle, you might want to pause and 'freeze' or maintain your position until she's feeling a little better. You might even have to move a little bit closer during an illness to offer more comfort. But then resume your sleep shaping when she recovers.

Nights 1–3. Once bath, stories, and songs are over, *sit in a chair next to your baby's cot.* If she cries or fusses, you can stroke or pat her intermittently, but don't do it constantly or you'll just create a new negative association. You can touch more on the first night. You can sing during the get-ready-for-bed stage, but once it's time for her to sleep, stick to calming 'sh-sh' or 'night-night' sounds. You might want to try closing your eyes. That makes it easier not to talk to her too much, and it also conveys a sleepy-time message. Stay there until she falls asleep. If she gets up, remember not to keep putting her back down.

Make sure that you, the parent, control the touch. Instead of having her hold your hand or finger, you should pat her. Make sure that you do not caress her too steadily; do it on and off. Count to yourself if it helps – count to ten touching, then count to sixty not touching, then touch for another ten counts. You don't want to swap one negative association, like rocking, for another, like your constant touch or the sound of your voice.

Try not to pick her up – but if she's really upset, keep it brief and put her down as soon as she seems calmer. Don't let her fall asleep in your arms. Tell her that it's okay, and stay in the chair until she falls asleep. *Do this for each wakening.* Make sure you read 'Some Extra Reminders for the First Three Shuffle Nights' in Chapter 7, 'Six to Eight Months.'

Nights 4–6. Move the *chair about halfway to the door.* (If the room is small or the cot is close to the door, then move to the doorway, as in night 7.) Continue the soothing sounds, but stay in the chair as much as you can. Get up to pat or stroke her a little if necessary, or make some of the same soothing sounds that you have used the past three nights. If you allow yourself to move to the cot side and pat her almost to sleep, you will defeat the whole purpose of moving your chair away. You will create a new sleep crutch.

Nights 7–9. Move the *chair to the doorway inside her room.* You should be dimly lit but still in her view. Continue the same soothing techniques, remembering to intervene as little as possible. Don't worry if she cries a little bit; keep quietly reassuring her. She'll know you are there, and she will fall asleep.

Nights 10–12. Move into the *hall with the door open enough so that she can still see you.* You can keep making those 'sh-sh' sounds, not constantly but enough to let her know that Mum or Dad is close by and responsive. Stay until she falls asleep.

Children get ritualized easily. Make the changes every three days – or less. Dragging it out makes it harder, not easier, for your baby. Give it more than three days, and she'll expect you to stay exactly where you are – and get mad or upset when you try to double that distance.

Nights 13 and on. Most parents stay in *the hallway or in a very nearby room, where the child cannot see them but can easily hear them.* You can make some reassuring 'sh-sh' sounds, not constantly but enough to let him know that Mum or Dad is close by and responsive. If she cries, try checking on her from her bedroom door – without going all the way into the room. Be calm and reassuring. Make some comforting sounds, conveying that you are not far away and that you know she can put herself to sleep.

I find that this final step is often harder for the parents than for the child. Try not to convey anxiety about possible tears to your toddler. Give her credit for what the Shuffle has helped her achieve. Your toddler really can soothe herself to sleep – if you give her the opportunity. Occasionally a toddler will cry a little for a few nights, but don't rush in and rescue her prematurely. Let her calm down and nod off. If you check on her from the doorway, try to be fairly unobtrusive about it and don't check too frequently. You want to calm her, not stimulate her into getting more awake each time you approach. It should get easier on you quickly.

Most parents have to take one more step and move farther away, doing what I call a 'job check,' telling the child where they will be, what they will be doing, and promising to be back very soon: 'Mummy is going to get her pajamas. I'll be back in five minutes' or 'Daddy is going to brush his teeth, and then I'm going to come back and blow you another kiss.' These checks work best with older toddlers who have more developed language skills.

Some families stay in this position for a while; the toddler still needs those ten or fifteen minutes of reassurance. Others get to the point where they can put the child to bed, say good night, and leave. Sometimes they need to come back for one last 'curtain call' before she goes to sleep, but the goal is to reduce the number of checks. Use your instincts about what will work best for your child. You might have to let her regress a little once in a while. For instance, if you are leaving her to fall asleep on her own, and she does it successfully, she may still have a spell now and then when she needs a little more reassurance and you have to stick closer by her for a few nights. I don't mean going back to the start of the Shuffle, but you might have to hang out in the hallway one or two nights, or revert to making checks briefly before you can leave her on her own again.

A few points to stress: Children get ritualized easily, so make your changes every three days, not every four, six, or eight days. *Dragging it out makes it harder, not easier, for your baby.* She'll get accustomed to you sitting in a certain place, and get mad or scared when you try to double the distance.

Time Checks

Sometimes we need to modify the Shuffle because a child is over-stimulated by the parent's presence by his cot or bed. He wants to engage and engage, and no matter how much you soothe and 'sh-sh,' he'll still keep trying to engage you. In this situation, you may want to try working with 'time checks,' a variant of what some call 'Ferberizing.' At bedtime, do your nighttime routine, getting your child calm and soothed before placing him down. Then kiss him and tell him you will check on him before leaving the room.

There is no magic rule about how often you should check on him, and you may have to experiment a bit. If you do it too quickly, he may treat it like a game and get even more stimulated. If you are away too long, he may get worked up and upset.

Start with every seven minutes, and gradually increase it, but trust your own instincts and make necessary adjustments. When you check on him, go directly to his cot and give him a quick reassuring pat. But don't linger: You will defeat the whole purpose if you stand there for a half hour patting him to sleep.

Diane and Peter had a rough first night with Chloe, then thirteen months, doing the Sleep Lady Shuffle, but then so many of their nights were rough nights with their first-born child. Chloe would fall asleep drinking a bottle in her mum's lap, and often woke up unhappy when Diane tried to place her in the cot. Chloe had been weaned, but she had an attachment to her bottle, and woke up several times a night demanding it.

Like many babies I work with, Chloe had had severe reflux, and she threw up a lot. There was no way her parents were going to do a cry-it-out program, knowing that if she cried hysterically, she'd start vomiting again. Diane said that people sometimes told her not to worry if the baby threw up one more time at bedtime, to just let her cry. But they didn't understand that if your baby is already throwing up a zillion times a day, 'you can't stand having her throw up one more time.' Plus, neither parent nor child gets to sleep any faster when a baby throws up in her cot. Projectile vomiting is not exactly a spalike experience. Sheets and pajamas have to be changed, and the baby needs to be washed or bathed again.

Chloe did cry a lot the night she began the Shuffle, but with a parent seated by her cot, she stayed just this side of hysterical and didn't throw up. (I had recommended that Diane do the last nighttime feeding a little earlier, before bedtime, which I think reduces the chance of tears leading to vomiting at bedtime.) She stood in her cot sobbing with her arms outstretched, and then she'd get tired and 'flop down.' Then she got up and sobbed some more.

The second night was much easier. Chloe cried for fifteen minutes, less intensely, although she was up a few times during the night. By the fourth night, she was standing in the cot, pacing and talking, but the hysterics were over. By night 6, she went to bed with far fewer complaints, and she slept right through until morning.

Nap training took longer, partly because she decided to break with the usual pattern and tried to give up her afternoon nap, not her morning one. That doesn't work too well because a thirteen month old just can't go that long between naptime and bedtime.

The Sleep Lady Shuffle also helped James. Ellen and George took it slowly, knowing that he did have a lot of separation issues and that his adoption a year earlier had already turned his whole world upside down.

By the second week they were leaving his room after twenty minutes, and making frequent checks on him. Ellen found that he sometimes did better when they left the room because he became irate when they were present but not picking him up. And when they were in the room, he didn't always want to be touched; he just wanted a parent's silent presence. 'He needed to know I was around, but it was insulting to him if I touched him but wouldn't take him out of the cot,' she said. That's not at all uncommon; some babies don't like physical contact while they are trying to fall asleep.

James's problems didn't go away overnight, but Ellen and George did begin to detect an improvement after only four nights, not enough to make it easy on them – Ellen sometimes bawled harder than James – but enough for them to know they had embarked on the right path.

Starting on night 16, he slept through for five nights in a row. At *about day 20 or 21, he was ready to let his parents leave the room and fall asleep on his own. That's when she dubbed him the 'Olympic sleeper,' and once his problems were solved, they stayed solved. Not even the birth of a little sister threw him off. Two years later, he had a brief period during which he needed a little extra reassurance at bedtime, when he went through one of those normal periods when preschoolers get the 'scaries.' But he got over it quickly and returned to his well-established sleep-champ patterns.*

You might remember Ellen from the first chapter in this book. She was the mum who wrote out the cue cards to use in the middle of the night. Sleep training was really hard on her. It's hard on a lot of parents – and think of the extra anxiety an adoptive parent feels. The cue cards reminded her not just of what she had to do – but why she had to do it. 'It was my first really tough parenting task, but I saw it was bigger than sleeping. It felt like a life lesson,' she said. 'It was about teaching him to self-soothe; it was the first baby steps of understanding limit setting. I could see all the parenting issues coming down the road. This is where my husband and I had to step up to the plate and take hold of this problem for him." I admired their perseverance as they tackled bedtime, naptime, and those three or four middle-of-the-night awakenings simultaneously and with impressive consistency.

Problems and Solutions

Babies who have trouble getting to sleep and staying asleep have what sleep experts call *negative associations,* or *sleep crutches.* These behaviors aren't bad in and of themselves; they become bad only when they interfere with sleep – yours or your baby's. For instance, children should be hugged and snuggled, but if they are hugged and snuggled until they fall asleep and each and every time they wake up at night, they will never learn how to fall asleep without being hugged and snuggled. And no matter how much we love hugging and snuggling our children, 3:00 a.m. is not necessarily the preferred time. Dummies, swings, walking, rocking, or midnight nursing can also become sleep crutches. Our task is to help our children free themselves from these crutches.

Night wakenings usually taper off during the Sleep Lady Shuffle, but they don't always stop immediately. I've stressed the first three nights, when you will be tackling these problems initially, and you will return to sit by your child's cot side to comfort him. *Starting on night 4, just quickly go to his cot for reassurance, and then resume whatever position you were in that evening for the bedtime Shuffle so you give a consistent message for all awakenings.* If your child still wakes up sometimes after the Shuffle is completed, it's generally best to comfort him from the doorway, or give him a quick reassuring pat in his cot and then comfort him from the doorway.

If these techniques don't eliminate those final night awakenings, you might be putting your child to bed when he's too drowsy. Remember, you want a 7 or 8 on that drowsy-but-awake scale. Maybe you are at a 9.

It's easier for a toddler to put himself to sleep at bedtime than in the middle of the night – particularly if he was 90 percent asleep before his head hit the pillow. Try putting him down when he's a bit more alert, even if it means backing up and doing a few more days of the Shuffle. You may find that an earlier bedtime also helps him conquer the night awakenings. Try moving bedtime a half hour earlier. If you are still nursing at bedtime, try doing that feeding a little earlier in the evening to further weaken the link between suckling and sleeping. Sometimes it helps to keep a low light on while you nurse to help her break that suckle-sleep association.

Eliminating Nighttime Feeding

Healthy toddlers should be able to go from dinner until breakfast without a feeding, eleven or twelve hours. Check with your doctor, but if your baby is still waking up to eat at night, it's probably a habit, not a nutritional need. Either you need to adjust her hunger clock so she eats more during the day, or she is using the bottle or breast as a sleep crutch. Or maybe both. If she's still nursing, shorten feeding sessions so that she is actively nursing, not just sucking or dozing with the nipple in her mouth. Adjust your nursing schedule so she's not falling asleep on the breast. If she is using a bottle, consider switching to a cup.

Sleep Lady Tip

If you don't feed your toddler at night, she'll wake up hungrier in the morning. If she's hungry in the morning, she'll eat more during the day. If she eats more during the day, she won't wake up as hungry in the night. It's the opposite of a vicious circle.

With infants, I often recommend gradually eliminating night-time feedings, but after the first birthday, it's usually best to just stop it cold. When she wakes up wanting to nurse or take a bottle, sit by her side and find other ways to calm and comfort her. Pat her or her mattress a bit, whisper 'sh-sh,' tell her it's night-night time. Don't cave in and feed her, or the inconsistency, the intermittent reinforcement, is going to make the change more prolonged and difficult for her.

If you can't bear stopping cold, try a 'set-time' feeding for three nights (outlined in Chapter 7, 'Six to Eight Months Old'). On the fourth night don't feed her at all and instead stay by her bedside an additional night and soothe her. Overnight weaning from either breast or bottle usually takes just a few days at this age.

Phasing Out Walking and Rocking to Sleep

If you are still walking or rocking your child to sleep, and having to walk or rock him back to sleep over and over again all night long, stop it. There are easier ways to get weight-bearing exercise that don't involve serious sleep disruption! A few minutes of walking or rocking before bedtime is fine, as long as you can then put him down without him squawking and he doesn't wake up at night demanding another stroll. But if walking or rocking has become a sleep crutch, just get rid of it. It's time.

Make sure you have a nice, long, and comforting bedtime routine. You can incorporate a wee bit of walking or rocking in it; just don't let it be the sleep crutch. A few minutes in the rocking chair while you read a book, or a brief stroll around the room saying good night to favorite toys is fine. Then put him down, drowsy but awake. If he wakes up, go to him quickly but don't walk or rock him. Sit by his bed and pat him, stroke him, whisper soothing words, but leave him in his cot. Whichever parent is least likely to cave in and rock him should be the one to do the cot-side duty the first few nights.

At fourteen months, Joshua was still getting up many times a night, and Carol was having a lot of internal conflict about the attachment-parenting model she had chosen for herself. Each time Joshua woke, it would take an hour or an hour and a half to get him back to sleep.

She and her husband, Daniel, tried everything – nursing, rocking, holding him. Nothing worked consistently. Making changes was difficult for Carol because she felt she had to hold and nurse Joshua all the time. She was at a total loss when it came to setting any boundaries or limits, and she felt very guilty if he cried. 'I was always putting that boob in his mouth. It soothed him, but it wasn't what he needed,' she said. 'I was a major rescuer.'

Carol knew she would have to make some difficult emotional adjustments if she was going to follow my advice, but she knew the time had come. She and Daniel were a wreck, and Joshua himself was a clingy, cranky, lethargic baby who got sick a lot. 'I just knew that wasn't his real personality,' Carol said. 'We wanted to get some sleep ourselves, and we wanted to get him functioning.'

Bedtime wasn't Joshua's biggest problem – middle-of-the-night awakenings were. When Joshua woke up, Daniel would go into Joshua's bedroom and sit next to him, pat the cot, and say over and over again in a calm, soothing voice, 'Night-night, time to go to sleep.' He stayed as long as it took for Joshua to get back to sleep. Joshua didn't improve the first few nights, but then his parents began noticing changes. He was still waking up, but the crying was tapering off, and he was going back to sleep faster. Within a few weeks, he was usually sleeping through the night.

Dummy (Pacifier) Withdrawal

Most doctors recommend weaning your child off the dummy by eighteen months to two years, but if your child is waking up a lot at night seeking his dummy, you might want to tackle it now. Be prepared for a few nights of unpleasantness. Comfort her and encourage the bond to a lovey. As you take the dummy away, say something like 'It's not dummy time, but Teddy Bear is here and wants to hug you.' That distracts her from the dummy and provides a security substitute.

If you don't want to take away the dummy yet, you should still be able to train your child to find it herself so you don't have to keep chasing it for her all night long. Leave a few dummies scattered around the cot so she can find at least one of them in the middle of the night while she's still half asleep. I do encourage restricting dummy use to sleeping, though, because research suggests 24/7 use can interfere with other aspects of development, including speech. Some families get rid of the dummy at night, but use it for naps.

At this age, however, a lot of babies go through the dummy-as-missile stage. They love to hurl it out of their cot and make you go after it. Ignore it. She may get very enraged if you don't go fetch, but if you pick it up, she'll just throw it again. (If you don't believe me, try it!) Wait until her complaints reach their crescendo, and when she seems like she's ready to lie down, tell her that if she lies down you will get her the dummy. You'll have to experiment a little to get the right rhythm for this little dance; the key is to discourage the throwing and to reward the calming down. (I worked with one family who no matter what we did their daughter continued to throw her dummy out and scream at the top of her lungs. The parents tried a cot tent. It worked − fast. It stopped her from throwing out the dummies immediately, and although she fussed about the tent for a few nights, she soon adapted and began sleeping through the night.)

Even low-tear-tolerance mums can often cope with this crying because they are tears of temper, not fear or despair. Even the calmest and happiest babies have occasional tantrums. Our task is to learn to distract and calm them instead of fueling their fires.

Early Birds

If your toddler is up at 6:00 a.m., cheerful and happy, it may be a strain on you, but it's not a crisis for her; 6:00 is a common wake-up time for young children. If she's up at 6:00 but cranky by 7:30, or if she wakes up consistently before 6:00, it may be a symptom of sleep deprivation. I know that sounds odd, but young children who go to bed too late wake up too early. Try getting her to sleep between 7:00 and 8:00 p.m., and ensure that she is getting enough naptime. You might move her morning nap later (in thirty-minute increments). This might help shift her whole body clock and help you conquer the early awakenings. Be careful and use your intuition. This is a dance between pushing her nap later but not postponing it so long that she is too wired to sleep.

But if she is waking up before 6:00 a.m., you are going to have to teach her to sleep later. After the first birthday, if early rising is an established habit that has gone on for a few months, it will probably take at least three to four weeks of parental consistency to change it. In some cases it takes longer, and it can be draining for you.

When she gets up, respond immediately. Your goal is to get her back to sleep quickly, not to let her scream herself into total awakeness. Give her the lovey and try to soothe her back to sleep without picking her up. No matter how much she protests, and she may protest a great deal, don't turn on the lights or let her out of the cot until 6:00 a.m. Be firm about it, or you'll find that if you get her up at 5:55 a.m., next it will be 5:45, then 5:30, and you'll be back to your undesirable starting point.

Sleep training at 5:00 a.m., when we are being pulled out of a dream sleep ourselves, is really hard. It's up to you whether you stay in the room or leave, and you may have to experiment to see what works best for you and your child. Some parents find that their presence stimulates the child into being more awake. In that case, soothe her a bit and then leave and see if she dozes off again on her own. You can come back in and make some checks if you want.

If you decide to stay in the room, keep the interaction minimal. Try sitting in a chair with your eyes closed or return to your Shuffle position. That helps you keep from engaging with her, and it conveys a message that it's still night-night time. Some parents who stay in the baby's room may even lie down on the floor or on a guest-bed mattress and be able to at least doze for a few minutes.

'The early rising is the area that took the longest to train, and it still fluctuates; he regresses,' Joshua's mum, Carol, said. 'If he woke up before six, we would go in and say, 'It's still night-night time.' Eventually we got to the point where we wouldn't go in, and he would go back to sleep or play quietly.'

If she's still awake when the clock finally strikes 6:00 – and it can seem like it takes forever – leave the room for a minute or two. She may cry, but try not to let it bother you; you will be right back in a minute. If you're already out of the room, now's your cue to come back. Put on a good-morning show when you reenter. Open the blinds, turn on the lights, sing a cheery morning song. You want to send a very clear message: 'I'm getting you out of the cot because it's wake-up time – not because you were carrying on.'

As I said, if it took your child months to get into this early-rising pattern, expect it to take at least a few weeks to get her out of it. You aren't going to feel very good at 5:00 a.m., dealing with a crying baby, so prepare yourself. Use cue cards, give yourself a pep talk, do whatever works. Having two parents take turns, so one isn't always exhausted and resentful, is also a good idea.

Early Risers

If your little one wakes up before 6:00 a.m., he's probably overtired. Overtired children don't sleep as well, or sleep as long, as well-rested ones. He may be:

- Going to bed too late
- Not napping enough
- Staying up too long between the end of his afternoon nap and going to bed (try not to let it exceed four hours)
- Going to bed when he's past that 'drowsy but awake' mark. If he's too drowsy, he won't know how to get himself back to sleep when he's more alert – including at 5:00 a.m.

Napping

When your child is taking two naps, the morning one should be about an hour (minimum forty-five minutes, maximum ninety minutes). The afternoon one should be about an hour and a half. A little variation is okay, but don't let her sleep so long in the morning that she can't go down in the afternoon. When she consolidates, the afternoon nap (which may be at midday for a while during the transition) is about two and a half hours up through eighteen months. Nap needs will slowly shrink to about ninety minutes by age three.

CREATE A GOOD NAP ENVIRONMENT. Keep in mind how hard it is for children to switch gears and get to sleep in daylight, particularly toddlers who are perpetual motion machines. In her dimly lit room, listen to some quiet music, read a book or two, or play some gentle games. Put her in her cot drowsy, even a little drowsier than she is at night, but awake.

FOLLOW THE SAME BASIC SHUFFLE RULES AS BEDTIME, and don't let her begin delaying games. If she stands up in the cot, put her down once; if she stands up again, ignore it. Don't feel obligated to feed her before every nap, particularly if you are working on breaking a food-sleep association. If you've been rocking or swinging her to bed, concentrate on phasing it out at naptime. Get her down drowsy but awake.

Sleep Lady Tip

To preserve that afternoon nap, which is the one she's going to keep through most or all of the preschool years (and occasionally longer), shorten the morning one. When she's ready to drop the morning nap, probably within a few months, you'll phase the morning one out and keep that afternoon snooze.

It's up to you whether you stay in the room doing the Sleep Lady Shuffle and soothe her or leave. If your presence calms her, stay. If your presence stimulates her, leave but don't go too far away and check on her every ten to fifteen minutes. Either way, don't converse; just say things like 'Sh-sh, naptime.' Resist picking her up unless she is about to reach that 'point of no return' hysteria, and then pick her up briefly and put her down as soon as she is calm.

GIVE HER AN ENTIRE HOUR TO FALL ASLEEP. She might cry the entire hour, and you'll hate it, but try to make yourself get through it. If you can't bear the full hour, you have plenty of company; don't push yourself beyond your limits. If she doesn't sleep in an hour (or even less if she's crying nonstop and you can't take it), leave the room and come back in and do your dramatic wake up, whether or not she's slept. Throw open the blinds and make a big deal about wake-up time.

If she did not sleep during the morning nap, try to get her down for her next nap earlier than usual, because she's going to be over-tired. Look for sleepy cues to know when to try again, maybe as soon as in about forty-five minutes.

TRY THE SAME APPROACH FOR THE NEXT NAP. If the afternoon nap doesn't go well either, trigger your *emergency backup plan*. You can break my no-motion sleep rule if you have to: Take her for a car ride, put her in the stroller, do whatever it takes but avoid returning to your original sleep crutch. She needs a nap one way or another; otherwise, she will be too overtired to go to bed at night and you'll be back to that downward spiral of sleep depri-vation generating more sleep deprivation. Go back to the nap training again the next day; eventually she'll get the message that when you put her in the cot, it's time to sleep.

CATNAPS. If she's a catnapper, sleeping less than forty-five minutes, attempt to prolong the naps. Also try to lengthen naps if she wakes up tired and cranky. If you hear her stir after twenty or thirty or forty minutes, she may be having a partial awakening, not a full awakening. You need to gently resettle her, and help her go back to sleep, which can be quite difficult for her. You want to respond quickly enough that she doesn't have time to awaken fully, but gently enough that you don't stimulate her into thinking naptime is over. It's a bit of a balancing act, but you'll get attuned to her cries and her rhythms.

Sleep Lady Tip

If your child is not yet sleeping through the night, work on that before you tackle the change from two naps to one. When she's slept through the night consistently for a few weeks, then you can begin altering the nap schedule if you see that she is ready.

When you respond, you can be in your Shuffle position in her room, or you can stay in the doorway. *Try to give her a full hour to fall asleep again, if you can.* Keep doing this every day, for both morning and afternoon naps if you have to. If she doesn't get more than a catnap, use your backup plan to make sure she gets at least one decent nap in the afternoon.

Adele had a good schedule for Alex, but it was a tough task getting him to follow it. It would take her at least thirty minutes to get him to sleep, and he had to fall asleep on her. Then she had to ease him into his cot so he wouldn't wake up. Nap training was really hard for her, 'grueling,' as she put it, but she knew that she couldn't put it off any longer. 'He'd cry for an hour in the morning, cry for an hour in the afternoon; we'd get in the car and drive him around.'

Adele chose not to stay in his room while he cried; he would try too hard to engage her in conversation or activity. She checked on him every fifteen minutes or so. Some mums find tears easier to deal with during daylight hours, but for Adele it was agonizing to be home alone with a crying child while her husband was at work. It took a month for Alex's naps to improve – but then they improved a lot, although they still ran on the short side. In retrospect, we learned that Alex was on the brink of consolidating his naps, and that probably made it even harder for him since Adele was trying to train him right as he entered that betwixt-and-between stage. Luckily, the transition itself went pretty smoothly.

Moving to One Nap a Day

The significant sleep event at this age is switching from two naps a day – morning and afternoon – to a single afternoon nap right after lunch. Consolidating naps is a definite physical and psychological transition, and almost all children undergo the 'one nap is too little, two naps are too many' phase. Many parents get very nervous about this transition, and even in the best-case scenario, you will probably have a little bit of crankiness and disruption for one, two, or sometimes even three weeks.

Your goal is to have your child's nap begin at around 12:30 or 1:00. It should last from two and a quarter to two and a half hours, although it will grow shorter during the next two or three years. As long as your childcare provider follows a basically sensible and healthy schedule, you should try to synchronize the home and childcare schedules. There's no sense in getting your child used to a schedule for weekends that will make her feel like she's jet-lagged the other five days a week.

Sleep Lady Tip

Your child is ready to consolidate to one nap when:
- she's about fifteen to eighteen months old (later is not uncommon, earlier very rare).
- she's sleeping through the night consistently – ten to eleven hours of uninterrupted sleep. If she's not, work on improving nighttime sleep before you tackle the nap change.
- she's taking longer and longer – and longer – to fall asleep for the morning nap, or falling asleep easily for her morning nap but then waking up from it quite early, or sleeping for such a long time in the morning that she won't take her afternoon nap (meaning you will have a very testy and overtired child by bedtime).

The trick is to know when your child is ready to shift to a single afternoon nap and to make sure that she doesn't get so overtired during the transition that she crosses the line between mildly cranky and totally sleep deprived. Be extra solicitous of her nighttime sleep while you are making this transition. If she's too overtired, her night-time sleep may get disrupted, or she may wake up earlier, which in turn will make her more tired and cranky in the daytime, which then will make it harder for her to nap. As you know, that's a recipe for sleep disaster. So as you adapt to new daytime patterns, *get her to bed earlier than usual, around 7 or 7:30.* Allow plenty of time to follow her familiar and soothing bedtime routine. Most children make the transition in about ten days, but it could take up to three weeks for her to fully adjust. Don't be alarmed if she has a bit of trouble napping or wakes up occasionally during the night during the transition. It's normal and temporary.

As you evaluate her daytime sleep schedule, remember that you are looking for a pattern, not just a one-day departure from the normal routine. Don't mistake one or two abbreviated morning naps or skipped afternoon naps for the sign that she's ready for the change; that might happen now and then as she gets older. But when her pattern becomes pretty consistent, the time is probably right to help her start the transition. If you aren't sure, keep a log of her napping and waking times for a week or two.

Once you've made sure that your child is ready for this change, make sure you are too!

CHOOSE A SENSIBLE TIME, just as you did when you started sleep coaching. Don't try to change her whole routine, for instance, the day before you leave for a vacation, or when you are under particularly intense deadline pressure at work.

PROCEED GRADUALLY, MAKING SMALL CHANGES EACH DAY FOR ABOUT SEVEN TO TEN DAYS. Don't go cold turkey and just scrap that morning nap. Instead, *push the morning nap a bit later.* Delay it until around 11:00 a.m. for two or three days, then 11:30 for a few days, then noon, and so on. Don't let it get stuck in late morning. *You want her on that early-afternoon schedule within seven to ten days*, although it may take another week or so for her body's wake and sleep rhythms to fully adjust. In other words, she'll have one nap starting at 11:00 and going until about 1:30. Then push it back some more, so she naps from about 11:30

to 2:00. Some kids can adapt quite quickly, adjusting to a noon start time. Others need to go a little slower. Just watch her; if by 11:30 she can't keep her eyes open, then she needs to nap. If she's perky and cheerful, try stretching the nap start time to noon.

IF SHE SLEEPS FOR ONLY ONE HOUR AND WAKES UP TIRED, WHICH IS COMMON DURING THE TRANSITION, try to soothe and resettle her back to sleep. (If you need more help, check out some of the napping tips in the chapters for younger babies and see if any will work for you.) If all else fails, use one of your emergency backup nap techniques, like putting her in the car or stroller, to get her some more sleep. Remember not to let her sleep past 4:00 or 4:30 p.m. Even if she naps later than usual, don't delay her bedtime. Keep it on the early side.

If you've been working on the one nap for a few days and you see that she is a bit 'off,' that she is too tired, *give her a 'two-nap day' to catch up*. I know I keep telling you to be consistent, but in this particular situation, your priority is to see that she's rested, to keep her from crossing into that exhausted but wired state. Keep the morning nap short, about forty-five minutes, so you can still put her down after lunch for the second nap. The next day, get back on the one-nap consolidation path.

Try to avoid consolidating naps when *you* think she's ready; wait for *her* to give you the signal. Doing this prematurely won't work. Remember, watch your child, not the calendar. *Also, avoid consolidating the naptimes in the wrong direction — getting rid of the afternoon one and keeping the morning one!* Parents may let a twelve month old take a two-or three-hour nap in the morning. The child will then refuse to sleep in the afternoon, but there's no way on earth she will make it from the end of that morning nap all the way until bedtime without melting down.

> *Despite Carol's valiant attempts to improve Joshua's napping at around fourteen to fifteen months, he remained a spotty daytime sleeper, particularly in the morning. She was relieved when the time came to drop that nap, at about sixteen months. 'We started skipping his 9:00 a.m. nap, which wasn't a good one anyway; it was so depressing. One nap worked so much better. We moved the 1:00 p.m. nap earlier (while he adjusted to one nap) and then pushed it back again,' she said. 'We try to keep 1:00 p.m. consistent, but you need to catch him at the moment he's tired, and if you miss it, it's gone. Sometimes he'll get tired at 10:30 and sometimes not until 2:00. I got better at picking up the signals – I can see it in his eyes. He blinks a lot; he just looks tired and lethargic.'*

Matthew

When Lizette and Carl watched newborn Matthew sleep peacefully in his cot, they didn't understand all the talk about sleep deprivation. Matthew slept through the night pretty often at three months, and just about every night by four months. But at five months, after a severe ten-day virus, his sleep deteriorated. 'During his illness, I got so used to running in there where I hadn't before; that was the beginning of the end,' Lizette said. 'Every time he made a peep, I'd run in.'

By nine months, they too were experts on parental sleep deprivation. They tried to Ferberize Matthew. But the baby just planted his sturdy little feet in his cot, pulled himself up, and gripped the top bar. He screamed bloody murder for ninety minutes the first night, even longer the next two nights. Lizette and Carl gave up. 'It tore my heart out, and I swore I would never do it again,' she said. Instead, they were in his room on and off all night, rocking him, giving him bottles, and replugging his dummy.

If he woke up three or four times before 11:00 p.m., they would bring him into their bed, where he would twist and thrash and keep them awake, until they tried to put him back into the cot, only to have him wake up and demand rocking, bottles, and a dummy all over again. 'You name it, we did it,' his mother said. Lizette and Carl convinced themselves that this was normal and adopted an attitude of acceptance.

At thirteen months and experiencing normal separation anxiety, Matthew felt his father's absence acutely when Carl's Coast Guard Reserve unit was called up and he could get home only once or twice a week. Lizette had trouble coping on her own, particularly with a child who didn't sleep well even when his dad was home. 'Carl's down in New York Harbor in some boat, patrolling, and I'm on the phone in tears. It got so bad.' She knew it was time to fix what was broken.

She consulted me and, after a few minor adjustments to Matthew's bedtime routine, began the Sleep Lady Shuffle. Carl helped on the nights he was home, and over time he took on many of the bedtime responsibilities. Matthew responded much more positively than Lizette had expected. The first two nights he fussed but did not cry as he had earlier when they left him alone. 'He kind of whimpered and wanted to know why I wasn't picking him up,' she recalled. 'He was complaining, but he never wailed; it wasn't like when we tried Ferber. I put my hands on the mattress and whispered, "Lie down, lie down."' Finally, he did.

Matthew rebelled on night 3. Kids often do that, once they figure out, 'This is for real!' 'He sort of said, "I'm not really digging this,"' his mum said, laughing. He threw everything out of his cot – the pillow, the five dummies Lizette was now putting in his cot, everything. Lizette put the essentials back in the cot, very discreetly because she didn't want him to think it was a game and do it all over again. He finally slept. The next three nights, as she moved the big rocking chair to the middle of the room, then toward the door, he protested, but it got milder each night. By night 12, she was sitting on the floor out in the hallway. 'I sat outside and verbally assured him. I said, "Sh-sh, night-night, Mummy loves you." Sometimes I would sing so he knew I was there. Having me there was the key.'

He continued to wake up at night, though less frequently, and she would return to her bedtime Shuffle position for that evening. He still needed his parents to touch base, but he no longer demanded that they come into his room or pick him up or rock him. As long as he heard one of them in the hallway, he was fine. Soon, he started sleeping all night, and even began looking forward to bedtime. 'He'd have both arms out, diving into his cot, wanting it, loving it, excited to go to sleep. I never thought that would happen.'

Simultaneously, Lizette worked on decreasing Matthew's use of the dummy, and switched him from a bottle to a cup. She started with a cup of water before naps, as she rocked him briefly. Then she switched to the cup for the rest of the day, and kept only one 120ml/4oz diluted bottle at bedtime, which he drank as they read books, before lights out.

Unfortunately, as nights improved, early mornings deteriorated, and Lizette found the process excruciatingly difficult. 'That was the hardest, having to get up and sit in the hallway at 5:00 a.m., but we had to do that,' she recalled. But that too improved over time.

Nap training was the low point of Lizette's day. 'I would get so exasperated; naps would take everything out of me.' Mornings weren't so bad; he took that nap pretty well. But afternoons were a misery. Lizette later realized that she had been reading Matthew's sleep windows wrong. 'He would go down in the morning fairly well. He'd wake up at 6:30 and nap at 9:00 or 9:30, but afternoon was a whole different story. I thought rubbing his eyes meant he was ready to go to sleep, when in fact rubbing his eyes meant it was too late! I had to look more at the clock and know that he needed to be asleep within three hours of waking up. I was underestimating how frequent and how early the naps had to be.'

Some days she couldn't get him to nap. He'd flail and resist and even strike her. Other days, he would sleep for just forty minutes, wake up, not know how to put himself back to sleep, and scream. Sometimes if she couldn't settle him back down she'd take him for a car ride, not a good long-term solution but an acceptable stopgap. The rides helped his body get into the rhythm of sleeping twice a day. Soon the afternoon nap became a habit, not a struggle.

No sooner did she get napping solved than she struck the dreaded 'one nap is too little, two naps are too many' phase. 'He was giving me a hassle about going down in the morning. He loved his morning nap. He was like Rip van Winkle, sleeping two hours in the morning, two hours in the afternoon, and going to bed at 7:00. Then all of a sudden, he didn't want to go to sleep in the morning. He'd play in his cot until 9:30 or 10:00, and not go to sleep until 10:30. That was late, so then he wouldn't go down for his afternoon nap.' Lizette recognized that this was his signal; he was ready to give up that morning nap. She began keeping him up in the morning, and putting him down at midday. Gradually, he made the adjustment.

Every once in a while, there is naturally still a bad nap or nighttime sleep, and some tears. But Lizette learned that it really helps to keep an eye on her watch. 'It may feel like he's crying a long time, but when I look at my watch, I realize it's only thirty seconds!'

10

One and a Half to Two and a Half Years Old

A *n eighteen month old on average sleeps eleven and a quarter hours at night and two and a quarter hours during one midday or afternoon nap. At age two, sleep requirements drop to eleven hours at night and two during the day. Over the next year that will drop to ten and a half hours at night and one and a half during the day. Remember these are averages but variations should not be huge. Watch your child's daytime behavior for clues to whether he or she needs more sleep.*

Toddlers and early preschoolers are a lot of fun, but bedtime can be a challenge. They are learning to follow simple directions, yet they also test our rules and their limits. Curious about their world, they are extremely eager to explore, leading to more limit testing and boundary breaking. They climb, crawl, crash, and clamber, standing on furniture, knocking down gates, trying to scramble out of the cot. Yet as they push their limits, they rely on their parents to keep setting boundaries, seeking safety, reassurance, and security.

Their language skills are blossoming, but they understand more than they can say, leading to frustration and tantrums. Their favorite words seem to be *no*, *I do*, and *mine*, and they are particularly possessive about their toys and their parents. As their language skills improve, they just love to stall, bargain, and negotiate, particularly around bedtime.

They may go through periods when they have the 'scaries' of the dark, thunder, monsters, and the like. Nightmares and night terrors may start, and be a recurring problem for the next several years. Potty training can complicate bedtime behavior, if you let it become a battle of wills rather than a cooperative venture. To prevent bedtime from becoming a war zone, make sure that you have a very consistent, predictable, and soothing routine. Clear rules and parental consistency are essential, along with plenty of love, cuddles, and kisses.

All too often, parents rush to get their child out of a cot and into a bed, as though it were a sign of achievement, maturity, or their guaranteed success as adults. One woman I worked with even reported an unspoken competition in her playgroup to see which baby could move first to a bed. Children who switch too young to a bed may experience sleep disruption and difficult bedtimes with tears and tantrums. Safety is also a factor. I worry a lot about a twenty month old roaming around in his room at night, pulling out drawers, unplugging lamps, exercising all that wonderful but potentially hazardous curiosity.

Even if the child is trying to climb out of the cot, I almost always advise parents to keep him in as long as possible, definitely until two and a half and preferably until three. By then, a child has the verbal skills to understand the 'big bed' rules and to communicate when he has got out of bed for the twentieth time that night.

This chapter is written with cot sleepers in mind, but I recognize that a few children do successfully transition to a bed at a young age, and some of you may have already made the switch before learning that it may not be ideal. So I include some advice here for children in beds, particularly on how to adapt the Sleep Lady Shuffle. You may also want to review the next chapter on older children for some additional insights.

One of the hardest aspects of sleep shaping for one and a half to two and a half year olds is that parents are a little skeptical that they can change deeply ingrained habits, and they are often so exhausted after two years of sleep deprivation that the required nighttime consistency is taxing. I've met parents who have literally fallen asleep on the floor in the middle of the night as they've tried to carry out these changes. But as you will see, children can and do learn to discard their sleep crutches; they give up their bottles, their midnight nursing, their need to be rocked, walked, or snuggled to sleep. They can become excellent sleepers, or at least reasonably good ones.

Developmental Changes

Separation Anxiety

Separation anxiety may have peaked at the first birthday, but prepare for another big wave at about eighteen months, and then spells of it throughout early childhood. A nice, long, gentle, predictable transition to bedtime, quality time with one or both parents who are really focused on bedtime rituals, and not on the telephone, washing dishes, or paying bills, helps soothe those worries.

At some point, your child may begin to articulate that he wants you to stay with him at bedtime. It can be heartbreaking to hear him plead 'Mummy, sit,' or 'Daddy, stay.' Be gentle but firm when the time does come to say good night. If your child isn't talking yet, she can probably still understand your verbal reassurances about how Mummy and Daddy love her and will be nearby. Many children find it easier to fall asleep if you stay in a nearby room, not on another floor of the house. They can't see you, but they know you are there.

Young enough to still experience some separation anxiety at

night, and old enough to suspect they may be missing excitement if they are asleep, children this age excel in stalling and delaying tactics at bedtime. I've heard some sleep doctors call these 'curtain calls' because they aim to get the parent to come back to the bedside over and over again .

When a child repeatedly seeks to be tucked in, kissed, given a blankie, and so on after normal, reasonable limits have been reached, the parent should respond once. Define what you consider reasonable limits for your child, balancing his separation fears with his gift for manipulation! Maybe you want to say good night once and that's it; maybe you don't mind going in three or four times. But once you set those limits, make them clear to your child and remind him, 'This is the last time.'

The next time, if there is a next time, your response should be neutral but firm. Say, 'Now it is time to go to sleep' or 'I love you, sweetheart, but you know it's time to go to sleep now.' A parent who says 'last time' better mean it's the last time, because children absolutely pounce on adult inconsistency.

Loveys

Loveys, usually a special stuffed animal or blanket, are very important for those children who are gaining independence but still need that extra helping of security. Loveys help with separation, with fighting the scaries, and with breaking lingering emotional attachments to bottles, cups, or dummies.

Even children who have spurned loveys in the past may embrace one now. They may want a lovey from a favorite book or video. With their blossoming imaginations, they also like including loveys in games, including bedtime and naptime rituals. For instance, if you look out the window and say good night to doggies or cars, have the lovey say good night to doggies and cars, too. Tuck the lovey in with her for bedtime and naps, and when she wakes up at night remind her that she has her lovey to snuggle.

However, if your child's lovey is a dummy, a bottle, a cup, or your breast, she may not accept a new lovey as easily. As you wean her from the bottle, or start to weaken the association between nursing and sleep, she will be more receptive to a new security object, but it takes time.

Parents may worry if their child wants to carry the lovey everywhere. If the lovey is a dummy, restrict it first to the house, then to sleep time. But if it's a toy or blanket, I don't regard carrying it as a problem before age two. At two you might want to restrict it to the house and car, or maybe a special occasion such as going to the doctor or an anxiety-provoking unfamiliar place or situation.

Barry at two and a half could not get to sleep or back to sleep without his bottle or twirling his mother's hair, a fixation he had formed when he was only six months old. Helene took Barry to one of those workshops where you can make your own teddy bear; they have them at malls and crafts shops. Helene made Barry a 'fireman bear' to match his fireman bed theme, while Barry made a pink 'wishes' bear for his mum. His excitement made it easy to weave the fireman bear into the bedtime routine, and ease out of the bottle drinking and hair twirling. 'Making it himself really got him invested in it,' Helene said.

Later Barry adopted a long-eared bunny as a lovey, and, yes, he twirled its ears to his heart's content. Barry, whose own hair was too short to twirl, still wanted Mum's hair when he was sick or particularly tired, even after she got a short, tousled cut. 'I don't know why he likes it so much; he is always telling me, "I love your hair." ' But while it still may be a habit, it is no longer a constant need that disrupts his sleep.

New Mobility: The Change from Cot to Bed

I like keeping toddlers in a cot as long as I can, but they sometimes have their own agenda. If your child starts climbing out, dissuade him by making the climb harder by lowering the mattress. Put pillows on the ground for safety in case he attempts Olympic-style hurdling. Remove large toys or stuffed animals from the cot that might serve as a launchpad.

If he does get out, put him right back in the cot with minimal interaction – except to say, 'No climbing.' Be firm, but don't yell at him. Try stationing yourself outside the bedroom door, out of his line of vision if possible, and peek in. When he starts to raise his leg again say, 'No climbing.' Sound like you mean it, and keep putting him back in the cot if you have to.

Sleep Lady Tip

If your child likes to climb out of his cot, put him to bed in a long T-shirt or nightshirt, which will make it harder for him to climb.

If your child still seems determined to get out, particularly if he's under the age of two, try a *cot tent*, a zipped mesh cover that lets him see out but not get out. That may buy you a few months before you switch to the bed.

Madison's parents noticed that she moved around a lot in her cot, and thought it might be too small for such an active sleeper, that she might sleep better if she had more space. They took her out of her cot at the unusually early age of fifteen months, and gave her a mattress on the floor. That gave her more room, but it didn't solve any of their problems, and it created a lot of new ones. She still tossed herself around, slept perpendicularly, and woke up a lot, but now she wanted her mum in her bed with her.

Children who move from the cot too early don't necessarily have the verbal skills to understand bedtime rules. Then they keep getting out of bed over and over again, and you may end up having to gate the doorway or even shut the door, which sometimes provokes the tears and tantrums that you were trying to avoid.

They may also miss that feeling of cozy containment in their cot. I know some families who regretted moving the child to the bed and managed to get him back to a cot, particularly if he was talking about his cot or trying to climb into a younger sibling's cot. That's not regression. It is listening to your child.

Some kids do hate cots and start talking about 'big boy' or 'big girl' beds. If they can articulate it, that's a reasonably good sign that they have the verbal ability to understand big bed rules. To make the transition easier, read the 'New Mobility: Switching to the Big Bed' section of the next chapter. Use a bed rail if he might fall out. Remind him that with the privilege comes rules – like staying in bed all night.

Sleep Lady Tip

Sticker charts can be wonderful behavior incentives for older children, and sometimes children this age respond as well. Children who don't yet understand a chart may like wearing a sticker in the morning.

Even as an infant, Ilan had never seemed to like his cot, perhaps because Zach, the much older brother he idolized, did not sleep in one. The summer before he turned two, and a few weeks before my first meeting with his parents, the family spent a week at the beach and instead of struggling with a portable cot that they knew he would never stay in, they threw a single mattress down on the floor. Elated, he slept better than he did at home – in other words, he slept poorly but not disastrously. He never tried to come into Joanne and Ken's bed at the beach, which is where he often ended up at home, although he did sometimes want Joanne to come into his bed.

The first few nights back home in a cot were miserable; he let them know loud and clear that he hated being back behind bars. That's when I met them. We talked about the pros and cons of cots and beds, but their instinct was to try a mattress on the floor like at the beach. He was only twenty-two months old, but had excellent verbal (and comedic) skills, as you'll see in a moment.

A few days earlier they had been in New York, where Ilan had been entranced by a huge line of fire trucks shrieking down Park Avenue, so when Joanne saw sheets decorated with bright-red fire trucks, she knew Ilan would be thrilled. They moved him out of the cot the same night they started sleep shaping with me. The timing was perfect. He embraced the bed, the fire-truck sheets, and the new sleep rules, figuring it was a package deal. Although it took a very long time to get Ilan sleeping consistently through the night, we solved several of his sleep problems in a matter of days, and he stayed in his new 'big boy' fire-truck bed all night long right from the start.

Eating and Sleeping

When our babies are little, we strive to get them to bed on a full tummy, hoping it will help them learn to sleep longer at night. That's no longer necessary. Those youngsters who are still breast-feeding may want to nurse briefly before sleep. That's fine, unless she must nurse in order to get herself to sleep at bedtime, naptime, or when she wakes up at night. (I'll talk more about how to gently modify night feeding when we address specific sleep solutions.)

In general, children this age should be able to go twelve, even fourteen, hours from dinner until breakfast, without a bedtime snack except perhaps a glass of water. Most pediatricians recommend limiting milk to 600ml/20oz a day maximum (a pint). Kids who drink milk (or juice) all day tend not to be hungry at mealtimes and don't get enough solid foods, or enough of a variety of solid foods, to meet their expanded nutritional needs.

Barring any unusual dietary or health concerns, children from eighteen to thirty months should have three recognizable meal-times, breakfast, lunch, and dinner, plus snacks in the midmorning and following the afternoon nap. Some will want a third nibble, but keep it very healthy if it's close to a meal. Remember that healthy childhood eating patterns help shape healthy eating patterns later in life. Toddlers and preschoolers begin to recognize and ask for sweets and junk food, but you should keep them as a special treat, not a staple.

If you haven't already introduced a cup, do so now even if you are still nursing. Offer the sippy cup, of water, milk, toddler formula, diluted juice, whatever your doctor recommends, at each meal. If he takes a bottle at night, switch to a cup, and if he takes milk at bedtime, switch to water. You don't want the milk bottle to become a sleep crutch, something he needs every time he tries to fall asleep. If you need more help with this, see Chapter 9, 'Thirteen to Eighteen Months.'

Joel was very small for his age and a poor eater. Dorothy worried about him a lot, and kept giving him bottles of milk when he got up at night long after she stopped nursing at nine months. 'My doctor said not to feed him all night, but I didn't believe him. I was just so happy to see Joel have the calories.' Dorothy also acknowledged to herself that as a working mother carrying more than her share of guilty feelings, she wasn't quite ready to give up that cuddly warmth of bottlefeeding her baby, even though she knew he was perfectly content to drink from a cup at child care.

Once I persuaded Dorothy that the bottle had to go as part of an overhaul of Joel's whole eating and sleeping routines, she found that he gave it up much more easily than she expected. The one odd side effect – and I've run into this with a few other children – was that he would no longer drink milk from a cup at home! He'd drink a cup of milk in daycare, he'd take it in his cereal, but he would not drink it from a cup offered by Mum, not even with chocolate! Dorothy took a very pragmatic approach to this, and instead of turning it into an issue, she made sure he got enough calcium from other foods.

The Scaries

Children at this age may get the *scaries*, conjuring up all sorts of gremlins and monsters at bedtime. Remember that the fear is real, even if the monsters aren't. Do what you need to console him, to convince him that there are no monsters. But don't let the monster business get so drawn out that it pushes bedtime back too long.

There are no hard-and-fast rules; trust your instincts and see what works. Try shining a flashlight into the closet, or under the bed. Enlist that lovey to help you look. 'See, your snuggly bear says there are no monsters under your bed, and now snuggly bear will get in bed with you and you'll both be safe and sound.' One of my clients found a 'boo-buster' ghost-fighting spray bottle on the Internet, and you could probably make your own with some pleasantly scented water. Maybe your child can help you decorate the spray bottle, making him feel a little more powerful against whatever is frightening him.

When Barry occasionally got scared and came looking for parental reassurance, Helene walked him back to bed and simply said, 'I'm right across the hall if you need me.'

Teddy, whom you met as a seven month old, slept well for many months but began experiencing some bedtime fears just shy of his second birthday. Although Teddy used to like to sleep in total darkness, Lisa now found that a small night light helped. 'He'll ask me, 'Mum, are monsters real?' and I'll say, 'Are there monsters? No, they are only in your imagination.' We have to go through this every single night.' He also clung to the book It's OK! Tom's Afraid of the Dark! *and she read it to him every night for many months.*

Potty Training

I don't see any problem doing sleep training and daytime potty training simultaneously, as long as the child is ready, able, and reasonably enthusiastic. Indeed, children often have a 'window' between eighteen and thirty months (later is not abnormal, so don't worry) when they are quite interested in at least starting toileting, and you should seize that moment or you might have to wait months for another chance.

I'm not going to get into all the different theories and techniques of potty training, except to recommend that you start with day training. At naptime give him a nappy or pull-up until he stays dry for at least a week. Leave nighttime for last. In fact, as far as I'm concerned, you can leave a nappy or pull-up on at night all the way up to age four or five. (I address bedwetting for older children in Chapter 15, 'Medical Problems.') Children often learn to stay dry at night on their own in time, and it makes no sense to expend all this energy teaching a child to sleep all night and then confuse him by waking him up to go to the bathroom! I do know one mum who put the little potty chair in the bedroom at night, so her son would have it nearby when he wanted it.

> ## Sleep Lady Tip
>
> Potty training is a major developmental milestone, so expect tempo-rary social, emotional, feeding, and sleep disturbances. You may occa-sionally hear about a child who trained in just a few days, but don't worry if your child takes months, which is perfectly normal. Be patient and celebrate achievements!

Ask your child to sit on the potty before naps and before bed (but don't insist). If your child starts using 'I need to go potty' as a stalling tactic at bedtime, bring him to the bathroom once, and only once. But keep it boring. No talking, no games, no show-and-tell. Don't let him do this over and over again or you will spend your whole night walking back and forth to the bathroom. Put him in a nappy or pull-up, reassure him it's fine to use the nappy at night, and get him to bed.

If he gets in the habit of having a dirty nappy at about 5:00 a.m., change him (change him in the cot if you are agile enough), but leave the lights as dim as possible and make it clear to him that it's not yet morning, that he gets up when it's morning time, not because he had a dirty nappy. Help him get back to sleep. (My section 'Early Birds' at the end of this chapter will help you.)

Creating a Schedule

Sample Schedule

(Shift earlier if your child wakes between 6:00 and 7:00 a.m.)

7:00–7:30 a.m.
    Wake-up and breakfast.

12:00–12:30 p.m.
    Lunch.

12:30 or 1:00 p.m.
 Start afternoon nap. Snack upon waking.

5:00–5:30 p.m.
 Dinner.

6:00–6:30 p.m.
 Start bath and bedtime routine.

7:00–8:00 p.m. (Sometimes 8:30, depending on age and nap schedule.)

Bedtime.

Children need regular naptimes and bedtimes, and reasonably regular mealtimes. Their bodies need the routine to regulate day and night hormone cycles, and their hearts and minds need the predictability to feel secure. But I believe in some flexibility. Sleep times are averages, but the variations are a lot less than many parents think, and your child may need a lot more sleep than he's getting.

Sleep Lady Tip

As toddlers turn into preschoolers, they may be able to skip an occasional nap without falling apart. Don't be fooled into thinking that she's outgrown naps completely. Most kids need about an hour or an hour and a half until age four.

Even when you do develop a workable schedule, you will experience some natural variations. Some days she will nap, or snack, a little more, and some days she will nap, or snack, a little less. As you learn to read her sleep cues and recognize her sleep windows, you'll be able to adjust the schedule more easily. Watch her daytime behavior. If she's easy and content, she's probably on a pretty good schedule. If she's fussy and demanding, she may need longer naps, an earlier bedtime, a later wake-up time, or all of the above.

Wake-up. Give her a *dramatic wake-up*. Throw open the blinds, switch on the lights, sing cheery good-morning songs, and start the day. Create morning rituals, just like you have evening ones, to reinforce her understanding of wake-up time versus sleep time. Any time between 6:00 and 7:30 is normal for this age group. If she sleeps much later than 7:30, start waking her up earlier to get her on a more age-appropriate schedule. Usually sleeping later just pushes the rest of her schedule out of whack, particularly if she attends preschool. With younger children I change wake-up time in ten-minute intervals over several days. At this age, do it faster because they adapt well. Either just wake her up at 7:30 and put up with a little crankiness for a day or two, or make the adjustment by about half an hour a day.

If your child is sleeping late because she is up several times a night and then has to fill up her sleep tank, shift her wake-up time earlier and follow my program for eliminating night wakenings. On the other hand, if your child goes to bed a little late, sleeps a little late, but still naps regularly and sleeps well at night, go ahead and leave it alone if it's working for your child, your family, and your preschool or child care.

Morning Nap. By eighteen months, most children have consolidated to one nap, usually afternoon or midday. If yours hasn't yet done so, don't worry; it's uncommon but not abnormal. Read the 'Moving to One Nap a Day' section in Chapter 9, 'Thirteen to Eighteen Months,' to make that rough spot a little less bumpy.

Lunch and the Afternoon Nap. Lunch is usually around noon, give or take a half hour. Afternoon naps for this age group usually start around 12:30 or 1:00, maybe 1:30. They'll cut back from two hours and fifteen minutes at eighteen months, to two hours at age two, and to about an hour and a half by age three.

A little variation is normal. Don't worry as long as the rest of his schedule is fine; tweak the napping schedule a bit if it's causing other sleep problems. For instance, if your eighteen month old naps for three hours but is cheerful and sleeping well, leave it alone. But if she's taking those long naps and then doesn't want to go to bed on time, gradually shorten the nap or move it a little earlier in the day (as long as it is after noon). Aim for about a four-hour gap between the end of the nap and bedtime for an eighteen month old; it will get closer to five hours as you near age three.

> *Barry, the hair twirler, took very long late naps, and then stayed awake until 10:00 p.m. After a lot of trial and error, Helene settled on a schedule that is later than most kids' but works for Barry's family, particularly since Larry gets home from his restaurant management job late. Barry goes down for a nap at about 2:30 p.m., and Helene wakes him up at around 5:00. Otherwise, he'd sleep another hour or so. Bedtime is 9:00 p.m., and he sleeps until 7:00 a.m.*

Dinner. Fight the temptation to keep young children up late so the whole family can eat together. Feed them around 5:00 or 6:00, even if that means eating without the rest of the family. The early schedule better matches their natural rhythm for eating and sleeping. If an early dinner means less family time, find other ways to compensate, such as building in a little more parental playtime in the morning. There's no reason you can't read good-morning books, as well as good-night books. And those stimulating games dads seem to favor, like space-rocket baby, are better suited for dawn than dusk anyway.

Bedtime. A soothing bedtime routine is a must, so allow plenty of time to prepare her for bed, physically and emotionally. By that

I mean leave time not just for bathing, toothbrushing, and pj's but also for calming down and getting ready to separate from you for the night. First, let's talk a bit about bedtime mechanics, the whens and wheres, including a few minor differences between being in a cot and a bed. Then we'll see how to create that calm, soothing transition to dreamland.

Bedtime, meaning asleep in bed, not thinking about going upstairs, should be between 7:00 and 8:00. Figuring out the exact time for your individual child is one part watching sleep cues and one part backward math. Start with her average wake-up time, and count back the hours she needs. For instance, if your eighteen month old wakes up at 7:00 a.m. and needs eleven and a quarter hours of sleep, she should be asleep by 7:45 p.m. Start putting her down at around 7:00 or 7:15, depending on how long her bath and bedtime routine take. If your two and a half year old wakes up at 7:00 a.m. and needs a tad less than eleven hours sleep, get her to sleep around 8:00 p.m., maybe a few minutes later, meaning you should probably be heading upstairs around 7:15 or 7:30. These are averages. Your child may need a half hour more or a half hour less. Watch her for signs that she is getting tired, and make sure she's in bed before she's overtired.

The bedtime routine should be in the bedroom, not all over the house, so she knows it's time to slow down and prepare for sleep. You still need to get her down drowsy but awake. As I mentioned, she no longer needs a feeding prior to bedtime, but some toddlers still like to nurse briefly or have a glass of water before bed. Just don't nurse her all the way to sleep or let her use her sippy cup as a sleep crutch. If you walk or rock your baby, keep it brief and keep it in her room. Keep any bedtime music very soft. Use it to cue her that it's time to sleep, but turn it off or let it run out before she gets into bed, or soon after. You don't want the lullaby to be a sleep crutch, so that she can't get to sleep or back to sleep without it. Ditto for toys with music and lights; phase them out before she falls asleep. At this age, toddlers often like a moment or two of deep-pressure hugging before you put them into bed.

Sleep Lady Tip

Either parent should be able to put the child to bed, and it's okay if two parents have slightly different styles. But both parents should put the child to bed at the same time, and should display a consistent response to such bedtime behavior as crying, throwing toys, and so forth. The united front sends a clearer, less confusing message that discourages such antics and lays the groundwork for all the coparenting to come.

The routine should be literally a routine. Young children are very ritual oriented. In fact, your child may well demand that you keep to the exact same routine each and every night. This may include singing the same song, playing the same game, or reading the same book over and over again. They get to the point where they notice if you try to skip a page or truncate a sentence!

Each of my kids had her own rituals at this age. Carleigh liked to kiss a flying cow she had hanging in her room. Later we made up a 'two things' game, where we talked about two things about her day. She liked to hear stories about my childhood, or about when she was a baby. Gretchen and I had our own silly little game. She liked me to kiss my pinkie and make it 'buzz' like a baby bee. The bee would then kiss her nose. I always told both girls that I would check on them again before I went to bed – a promise I made and carried out well into their school years.

Telling children what to expect, particularly as they get older and more verbal, helps fill their craving for predictability while underscoring the rules. 'Now I am going to tuck you in and give you a big hug, and then you are going to go to sleep and have wonderful dreams.' If they start stalling and negotiating, you might want to 'blame the clock' instead of getting into a power struggle. For instance, if they want to read three more books, point to the clock and say, 'It's ten minutes before eight, when we have to turn out the light. Let's see how many books we can read in ten minutes.'

Sleep Lady Tip

Starting at about age two, tell her how sweet and cozy she looks when she sleeps. Children love to hear that; it also reassures them that you are watching out for them while they sleep.

You may also try to make her feel invested in her bedtime, which becomes even more important in the next two or three years. For instance, Barry and his long-eared bunny like to watch the fish tank in his room, and Helene permitted Barry to decide whether the fish should have their little light on or not. Joanne always gave Ilan a two- or three-minute reminder before story time was over, and then she let him put out the bedside lamp by himself (at least, he thought his little hand was flicking that switch all by itself).

Talking about fun things that happened during the day, or about pleasant things to anticipate the next day allays bedtime anxieties. You can even make a list of sweet things to dream about.

Joanne made up two bedtime songs for Ilan. One, based on 'Skip to My Lou,' stayed the same every night, and included the names of his parents, brother, aunts, uncles, cousins, and grandparents. The other she adapted from a thank-you song he knew from a tot religious service. She kept some verses the same every night, for consistency and re-assurance, but the rest she improvised to suit his mood, the day's events, even whether he needed to eat more yummy vegetables.

If he was rubbing his eyes, she kept the song brief; if he was still pretty wide awake, she could throw in more verses and allow him more time to unwind. They did their snuggling at story time, but once the light was out, she gradually moved a little further from him as they sang their special songs together. That quiet time in the dark helped calm him down and get used to the darkened room while he still had his mother's company.

When Joanne had to work late, Ken would sing the same songs, and he would usually stay in a rocking chair in the room until Ilan fell asleep because the little boy got a little anxious when Mum wasn't home for bedtime. Ken could stay there because Ilan did not associate him as strongly with going to sleep or getting back to sleep in the middle of the night; his father was less of a sleep crutch.

Even if you do everything right at bedtime, your child may well go through phases where you put her down and she gets right back up again. If a toddler in a cot stands, put her down once. If she bounds up again like a jack-in-the-box, ignore it. She thinks it's hilarious, and if you keep responding, she'll keep doing it.

By eighteen months, most babies know how to get themselves back down from a standing position. If she doesn't, she will figure it out soon enough, even if her technique isn't particularly graceful. If she tries to climb out of the cot, lower the mattress and review the advice earlier in this chapter on keeping her in the cot.

If she's in a bed and gets out looking for you after good night, walk her back in a no-nonsense way. You don't need to scold, but don't play or interact or talk a lot, either. Tuck her in and do what you need to do to make her feel safe and comfortable, but do it quickly; don't linger. If she gets up repeatedly, put a gate on her door, or at least threaten to put up a gate if the threat alone suffices. This is common for children in beds at a young age. I'll talk about gates and the Sleep Lady Shuffle in a moment, and I go into more detail in the next chapter on older toddlers and preschoolers.

Ilan at twenty-two months had adapted beautifully to his new big boy bed and to an earlier and more structured bedtime routine. But soon after completing the Sleep Lady Shuffle, he went through a phase where he always had one pressing errand every night. Those same verbal skills that enabled him to stay in bed now became his vehicle for getting out of bed! He was always very matter-of-fact about his mission, and his parents and big brother, Zach, had a tough time reserving their laughter until Ilan was asleep.

'I go to McDonald's,' he said nonchalantly as he strolled to the bedroom door one night. This came as a particular surprise, as Joanne had never taken him to McDonald's. She put him back in bed and made a mental note to talk to Ilan's otherwise absolutely perfect babysitter about the fat content of french fries.

'I go to Max's,' he announced the second night, naming a kid-friendly restaurant he liked. Joanne briefly explained that you don't go to Max's in pajamas and put him back in bed.

The third night, he abandoned that restaurant strategy, and for the next few nights he tested a series of sporting events. 'I go play hockey' and 'I go fly kite, Mum' were particularly ingenious.

When the athletics didn't work, he got even more creative. He announced that he was doing whatever he thought his mum did in the evening, figuring that if it was a good-enough reason for a grown-up goose to be up and around, it should be an equally valid excuse for a toddler gander. 'I go check my e-mail, Mum' was one memorable example. 'I go spill water, make mess.' Next he aimed for tasks the family does in the morning, which must have made a lot of sense to him, because these were things you do when you get out of bed. 'I go get newspaper, Mum.' 'I go make coffee.'

When the coffee ploy failed, he knew he was defeated, and from then on he stayed in bed. Joanne put a gate up protectively, in case he had another spurt of imagination. He didn't mind the gate at that age, although at around age three, when Joanne used it only when he needed some reminders of 'big boy' stay-in-bed rules, the gate became an irritant. He would climb over it or body slam it out of the doorway until he finally learned to simply unlock it.

By the way, one other little stalling trick you see at this age: stripteases. If she pulls her nappy off, duct tape it! Or try a pull-up if it's harder for her to remove. I know some parents who have even taped zippers closed on pajamas, or put the pj's on backward to thwart attempts to take them off.

The Sleep Lady Shuffle

Many families use my Sleep Lady Shuffle, a gentle and gradual way of teaching children to fall asleep on their own. I explain my Sleep Lady Shuffle here for toddlers who are still in cots, but it's quite similar to the Shuffle for those in beds, and I outline the modifications below. As always, we try to minimize tears, but I can't promise to eliminate them completely. Don't rush to pick up a whimpering child during the Shuffle, but go ahead and pick him up briefly if he's really upset, especially the first night. Night wakenings taper off during the Shuffle, but they don't always disappear immediately, so *when your child calls for you in the middle of the night, resume the position you were in at bedtime that night as you calm him back to sleep.* It's okay if you briefly soothe him or pat him in his cot before you return to your bedtime position. We want a consistent response to all wakenings.

You should follow the Shuffle schedule, moving on to the next position even if your child has had a bad night or two, fussing or waking more frequently. Don't be surprised if there's a little regression or protest the first night of each new chair position. If your child gets sick during the Shuffle, you might want to pause and maintain your position until he feels a little better. You might even have to move a little closer during an illness to offer more comfort. But then resume the Shuffle when he recovers.

Nights 1–3. Once bath, stories, and songs are over, *sit in a chair next to your child's cot.* Stroke or pat him intermittently if he fusses or cries, but don't do it constantly or he will form a new sleep crutch or negative association and will need you to pat him constantly for him to sleep. (I'm a little more liberal about how much touching you do the first night, but by the second night make sure it's more sporadic.) Closing your own eyes conveys a sleepy-time message and makes it harder for him to talk to you or try to engage you, particularly at this age when he is probably going to try very hard to get you to interact. Stay there until he falls asleep. *Do this for each wakening.* If he stands up, pat the mattress and tell him to lie down. Once he does get down, stroke or pat him if he finds it comforting. This works better if you are sitting, not standing, by the cot.

Some children in this age group resist. That usually doesn't happen during the first few nights; it's more likely to occur a little way down the road when they realize this isn't a passing whim of yours, that it's their new reality. He might start throwing his toys out onto the floor. Then he'll want you to pick them all up and put them back for him. Then he'll throw them out again. It's both a way of expressing frustration at you for making new sleep demands and a way of engaging you. Don't fall for it. Let everything stay on the floor. If he throws out his lovey or dummy and then gets upset about it, tell him you will give it back as soon as he lies down. Make sure you read 'Some Extra Reminders for the First Three Shuffle Nights' in Chapter 7, 'Six to Eight Months.'

Be careful that you don't create new sleep crutches. One mother, using the Shuffle to teach her son to sleep without being rocked on and off all night, introduced a new song about the night sky, which immediately assumed the same psychological importance for him as the rocking had! Within a few nights, she found herself singing it three times, then four times and then five, because the instant she stopped, he roused himself from semislumber and demanded, 'Sky! Sky! Sky!' He also demanded the song each time he woke up at night.

Nights 4–6. Explain, particularly to an older child who can understand better, that because he has done such a wonderful job of learning to go to sleep you are now going to move your chair farther away but will still stay with him until he falls asleep. *Move the chair about halfway to the door.* (If the room is very small, or the cot happens to be very close to the door, you should instead move to the center of the room *or sit by the door in his room*.) Continue the soothing sounds, but stay in the chair as much as you can. Get up to pat or stroke him a little as needed, or make some of those same soothing sounds that you've been using. Try not to pick him up – but if he's really upset and you do need to pick him up, go ahead and do so, over the cot if possible. Hold him until he's calm, but keep it brief and don't let him fall asleep in your arms or on your lap. Sometimes a minute of deep-pressure holding will really help him calm down. Stay in the chair until he falls asleep.

Nights 7–9. Again, explain he is doing a great job and tell him that you are going to move the chair again. Sit close to him and hug him for a minute before you make that move, but don't get so entwined that you have to struggle to get loose. Then move the *chair to the doorway inside her room.* You should be dimly lit but still in his view. Continue the same soothing techniques, intervening as little as possible. He may cry a little bit but gently reassure him and he will fall asleep.

Time Checks

Sometimes we need to modify the Shuffle because a child is over-stimulated by the parent's presence by his cot or bed. He wants to engage and engage, and no matter how much you soothe and 'sh-sh,' he'll still keep trying to engage you. In this situation, you may want to try working with 'time checks,' a variant of what some call 'Ferberizing.' At bedtime, do your nighttime routine, getting your child calm and soothed before placing him down. Then kiss him and tell him you will check on him before leaving the room.

There is no magic rule about how often you should check on him, and you may have to experiment a bit. If you do it too quickly, he may treat it like a game and get even more stimulated. If you are away too long, he may get worked up and upset.

Start with every seven minutes, and gradually increase it, but trust your own instincts and make necessary adjustments. When you check on him, go directly to his cot and give him a quick reassuring pat. But don't linger: You will defeat the whole purpose if you stand there for a half hour patting him to sleep.

Nights 10–12. You are now going to move out into the *hallway with the door open enough so that he can still see you.* Explain this move carefully before you make it, and praise him again for what a good sleeping boy he is becoming. You can keep making 'sh-sh' sounds from the hallway – not constantly but enough to let him know that his parents are close by and responsive.

Night 13. Next you are going to stay in *the hallway or in a very nearby room, where the child cannot see you but can hear you.* You can make some reassuring 'sh-sh' sounds, not constantly but enough to let her know that Mum or Dad is close by and responsive. If she cries, try checking on her from her bedroom door – without going all the way into the room. Be calm and reassuring. Make some comforting sounds, conveying that you are not far away and that you know she can put herself to sleep.

A fair number of children start falling asleep and staying asleep by night 7 or 10 – occasionally even sooner – but most parents have to take one more step and leave the child alone for five-minute intervals. Tell him that you will keep checking on him until he is asleep. Leaving the child may seem like a radical change for you, but think about it: All that chair shuffling has given him nearly two weeks of preparation. He has given up some sleep crutches, and he has learned 'Mummy is right down the hall even though I can't see her.' Or 'Daddy is sitting on the floor right near my room, and he loves me.' Describe exactly where you will be sitting and explain that you will be close by even though he won't see you.

Don't go too far away. Stay on the same floor, maybe in a nearby room, maybe just read a magazine or a book for the first few nights. He may cry for a few minutes, but keep going back every five minutes to reassure him. You don't have to leave him more than five minutes, and, unlike the cry-it-out approaches, you don't keep making the intervals longer. In fact, I strongly encourage you to keep a close eye on the clock so you don't exceed five minutes and upset him more. They don't really understand what five minutes is, so for the older toddlers you can explain in terms of what I call 'job checks.' 'Mummy is going to change her clothes, and then I will be right back to check on you.' Or 'Daddy is going to brush his teeth, but I'll be right back.' (If your child gets stimulated and more awake each time you come to check, you may want to consider longer intervals, or you may want to start with five minutes and slowly lengthen it.)

He may cry a bit the first few nights, but very rarely do children cry for more than a few minutes after going through the chair routine. If he does cry, check on him from the doorway. Be reassuring but calm. Keep in mind, he has gained confidence that you are nearby and responsive. He's ready to learn this skill.

A few things to remember. Children get ritualized easily, like that boy with the 'Sky' song. Make the changes every three days – or less. Dragging it out makes it harder, not easier, for him. Give it more than three days, and he'll expect you to stay exactly where you are – and get mad or upset when you try to double that distance.

The Shuffle for Children in Bed

Children who move from the cot early don't necessarily have the verbal skills to understand 'big boy' or 'big girl' bedtime rules. That means the Shuffle may be a little challenging for children who are in a bed before the age of two and a half. Be patient and consistent. The basic Shuffle is the same, so read through the directions above for a cot sleeper. Sit by the child's bed, and keep moving the chair away every three days. If you've put his mattress on the floor, or if he's in a low toddler bed, sit nearby on the floor, not on a chair. Explain that you are going to move – that's even more important with toddlers in bed than in the cot, because you want them to understand that they must stay in the bed.

When the child gets upset, try to stay in your chair. Instead of reaching to touch him, try using soothing words and sounds. 'Night, night. Sh-sh. Mummy [or Daddy] loves you.' Don't talk too much; he'll suck you into a sleep-postponing conversation. Close your eyes if it helps. But if he gets really upset, get up and give him an occasional brief pat. If you absolutely have to pick him up, do it briefly, and do it close to the bed. When he calms down, put him back down and return to your chair (or floor). Don't let him fall asleep in your arms, and don't lie down in his bed, not even for a minute.

Like the cot sleeper, he may well throw toys and blankets at you. Ignore him; only return the lovey if he promises to stop. However, he may also get out of bed and come to you or try to crawl into your lap.

Give him a big hug and return him to bed. If he does it again, take him back to the bed. Don't talk, don't reason, don't explain, don't get exasperated. Just put him back, as many times as it takes. If he keeps climbing into your lap, you may have to move a little more quickly through the Shuffle – for instance, three days by the bed, three days by the door, and then the hallway.

When you get to the point where you are sitting in the hallway, where he can hear you but not see you, you might have to deviate from the basic plan a bit with a young child in a bed. Some kids will be fine with your position, but others will keep trying to come out and join you; they'll get really frustrated that you are close by but not with them.

Try putting up a gate and staying in the hall, and make sure he knows you are there even if he can't see you. If he sits or stands by the gate and cries, you may have to skip the step where you stay in the hallway and move to the next phase where you leave and do checks every five minutes. You have to find your own comfort level. If you don't want to skip ahead to the checks, explain that if he gets back into bed, you will tuck him in. Climb over the gate, give him a quick tuck-in, and then go back to the hallway. If he keeps demanding more tuck-ins until you reach the exasperation point, just stay in the hallway without any more tucking in. Stay there until he falls asleep, which may well be on the floor near the gate. You can move him to his bed once he is sleeping soundly; children usually give this up reasonably quickly. Use your intuition and your knowledge of your child's temperament to figure out which works best.

Some parents decide this is as far as they want to go for now, and they stay in the hallway a few feet away from the child's room. That's fine – as long as it's not taking an hour and the child doesn't need you in the doorway on and off all night long. Other parents gradually move away and phase out the checks. If you are using checks or job checks, always return as promised. Eventually, most families get to the point where they can say good night and the child won't call for them; they can dispense with those five-minute checks.

You might have to experiment a little until you find a 'job' that he doesn't find threatening.

Ilan did fine when Joanne reached the hallway stage in the Shuffle but resisted and cried when she tried to go to clean the kitchen or work at her computer. He would plead, 'No go computer, stay with Ilan.' One night she had a brainstorm. She said she had to go help Zach, Ilan's beloved big brother, with his homework. At twenty-three months, Ilan did not know what homework was but figured that if Zach did it, it had to be cool. He let her go without any tears or argument. That worked for about three months until he had a brainstorm of his own. 'No, Mummy stay with Ilan,' he said sweetly. 'Daddy go help Zachy homework.'

With the lovey and an earlier bedtime, Helene and Larry did a great job of laying the groundwork for Barry's Shuffle, but they had to do some improvising. They carefully explained to Barry that they had met the 'Sleep Lady' and she had helped them make new sleep rules. They made a sleep manners chart and told him they were going to do a better job now of helping him sleep. He was very forgiving. 'I am not mad at you for not teaching me how to put myself to sleep,' he said sympathetically.

Larry took on most of the sleep coaching because Barry associated his hair twirling and cosleeping with Helene. (If Helene tried to do the Shuffle, Barry would just get out of bed and giggle.) But Barry didn't like the Shuffle. If his dad wasn't going to engage him in his room, he didn't want him there. 'Go away,' he demanded, and he meant it. This is a great example of how a couple blended my framework with their instincts about their child. They skipped to the second part of the Shuffle, Larry sitting by the doorway in Barry's view for a few days, then out of sight in the hall, then 'job checks.' It went pretty well. Sometimes he would regress and get out of bed looking for one of them or asking for his bottle. But most of the time he fell asleep and stayed asleep.

Before working with me, it would take an hour and a half or two hours of all sorts of acrobatics to get Ilan to sleep, and then he would wake up repeatedly at night, often every hour or two. Through the Sleep Lady Shuffle and improvements to the household evening routine (difficult when both parents work irregular hours and there's a much older sibling who needs help with math homework while his baby brother needs a bath), Ilan's bedtime improved extremely quickly, and the night wakenings diminished. He also started napping well for his babysitter, and okay for his mum, despite having given up all but an occasional catnap when he was only ten months old.

But it took a very long time to get his night wakenings to go away completely. Joanne, who was always quite tears-averse in the middle of the night, partly because sustained crying just made it harder for both Ilan and her to get back to sleep, kept trying to shrink night-time intervention. She cut back and cut back until she was just sitting in the hallway and saying 'sh-sh.' Although Ilan was an extremely cheerful child without any unusual separation angst, it was very hard for him to give up that one middle-of-the-night Mum sighting. She just continued telling him he had to stay asleep in his own fire-truck bed, and devising new incentives as he got older and understood more.

She would finally get him sleeping all night, sometimes for several blissful weeks, but then each time he ran a fever, got an ear infection, or the family traveled for even a weekend, he'd get thrown off again. This continued to be a very stubborn pattern with Ilan. Sometimes retraining him would take just a day or two, but sometimes it took a few weeks.

Interestingly, when his much-loved babysitter moved on and he started preschool at two years and ten months, his sleep improved dramatically. A lot of kids regress when they start school or have a change in care. Ilan, in contrast, equated preschool with a new independence that carried into his sleep. This worked for two solid months – until the next break in his routine.

Problems and Solutions

Many experts who subscribe to the crying-it-out approach contend that once children learn how to fall asleep by themselves at bedtime, they somehow magically start sleeping all night. I have not found that to be the case. We have to address their night wakenings. If your child wakes up at night during the Sleep Lady Shuffle, it's important that you respond consistently from your bedtime Shuffle positions. Most toddlers will sleep through the night all or most of the time by the end of the Shuffle. However, these patterns may have been ingrained since birth, so I do see some toddlers and preschoolers like Ilan who acquired new bedtime sleep independence quite easily but still had a harder time applying it in the middle of the night. In this section, we'll concentrate on tools and techniques that help these children let go of their remaining sleep crutches.

Watch for negative associations – the bottle, the dummy, a music CD you had running at 7:00 p.m. but don't have on at 4:00 a.m. Rule out any medical factors, and make sure she is going to bed early enough, sleeping late enough, and napping enough. Overtired children wake up more at night.

Are you putting her to bed when she is a little too drowsy? If so, she is not getting the opportunity to learn how to put herself back to sleep at night. Put her to bed when she is a tad more alert (see 'Drowsy but Awake' in Chapter 2, 'Getting Started and Tips for Success') so she can become more adept at falling asleep on her own.

When a child does wake up and fuss at night, respond quickly. That helps reassure her, and makes her feel safe, secure, and listened to. It lets you serve as her 'secure base,' to use the vocabulary of attachment. It's also much easier on you. By going to her, you can reassure yourself that she hasn't got sick, her foot isn't stuck in a cot slat, the blanket isn't around her neck, the nappy isn't soaked, her socks haven't 'whoopsed,' as Ilan used to say when his slipped off. You can make sure her lovey is in reach. If she absolutely needs to be picked up, or hugged, then pick her up or hug her, but keep it brief and put her back down as soon as she is calm.

The goal is to get her back to sleep – not to have her scream herself wide awake. Hysterics makes everyone feel bad, and it's harder for both the child and the parent to get back to sleep. During the Shuffle, go to her quickly if you want and then return to your evening position. But if she's one of those children who is still waking up sometimes after the Shuffle, you have a few choices as to exactly how you respond. Strike a balance between what feels right to you as a parent and what helps your child learn to sleep:

- Sit by her side or in a chair in her room and comfort her. Don't lie down with her. Try to soothe her with loving sounds and phrases more than with patting and touching. However, if you sense that she is continuing to wake up one or more times every night in order to get you there, if just seeing you has become her sleep crutch, which is common, you'll have to back off a bit. Maybe sit in the hallway instead.

• Go to her room quickly to calm and reassure her, then sit in the doorway or hallway until she falls asleep again or gets drowsy enough for you to leave without setting off more tears.

• Go to quickly reassure her but then return to your own room.

• Let her cry if you think she'll get herself back to sleep quickly and you are comfortable with this approach. I've found that families usually know instinctively if and when they've reached that point where the child does a better job of getting herself back to sleep after a spurt of tears than they do when they rush in to rescue her. But in most cases, if the child could get herself back to sleep, you would know it by now!

Whichever method you choose, remember to interact as little as possible, and keep it soft and gentle. Don't scold. If your child is getting out of bed, walk her back to bed, tuck her in, and then choose one of the above strategies.

Sheila and Randy's daughter, Suzanna, was two years and four months old when they consulted me. She had been going to bed quite easily and independently since early infancy – but she was still waking up three times most nights. 'She just wanted to say, "Hi, Mum," ' Sheila said. Usually all Sheila had to do was go in and sit there for a moment or two and give her a pat, but it still disrupted everyone's sleep. Ignoring her to see if she could fall asleep again on her own made matters worse. 'She'd cry more and more. She was still in her cot then, and she'd be standing and would not sit down. Once it escalated, it would take much more time to get her back to sleep. She'd want to get out of her cot, we'd have to rock her, and then we'd put her down but she'd wake up again.'

Working with me, Sheila learned that Suzanna was too tired to sleep! We worked on her naps and her early-morning wakenings. Sheila also realized it was time to get her daughter off a nighttime milk bottle, and when she got a little older and moved to a bed, they made sure she knew how to reach the water cup, tissues, dummy, and teddy bear, right by her bed.

Suzanna was old enough to understand the new sleep rules that Randy and Sheila repeated to her over and over again, day and night, and she loved her sticker chart. When Suzanna woke up at night, one parent would go to her bedroom door and just say, 'You need to lie down.' They would reward her with a sticker in the morning when she put herself back to sleep. As she made up for her lost sleep, she became less dependent on seeing Mum at night. Her awakenings became less frequent, and then stopped. (See more about the sticker chart in Chapter 11, 'Two and a Half to Five Years Old.')

Eliminating Nighttime Feeding

A bedtime snack or milk will not prolong or improve children's sleep at this age. To the contrary, it may disrupt sleep by making them seek a cup, breast, or bottle every time they stir at night. That said, many kids do still have the nighttime milk habit, possibly because we as parents were so concerned about getting that last meal in them as infants that we haven't let go of it now that they are toddlers. In those cases, feeding and sleeping patterns may still be closely entwined. Let's talk first about nursing, and then about cups or bottles.

There's a subtle but important difference between nursing at bedtime and nursing to sleep. Some mums breastfeed until age two or older, and bedtime may be the nursing time they hold on to the longest. Avoid letting your child fall asleep at the breast. Either nurse until he's drowsy but still awake and then put him down or, better yet at this age, nurse him as part of the bedtime ritual but not as the last activity. In other words, nurse and then brush teeth, play a quiet game, read a book, or sing a song. Create a little space between nursing and sleep. Try keeping a light on while you nurse, so he is less likely to link breastfeeding with conking out.

With cups and bottles, you want to move from a bottle to a cup, from milk to water, from in bed to shortly before bed. How fast you make those changes depends on your temperament and your child's, but your end point is a cup of water before lights out. (Or no drink at all, eventually, but you don't have to push that.) Some kids switch in a day if you explain it to them, with no problem.

Others take it slower and may resist a little, but even a gradual transition should not take more than a week to ten days. The more they resist, the more emotionally attached they were to the cup or bottle.

If he now takes a bottle of milk at bedtime, switch to a cup, and when he adjusts to the cup, switch the milk to water. Alternatively, cut the amount of milk in the bottle in half before you switch to a cup, and then make the switch from milk to water. Give the cup at story time, not after the lights are out. Don't give him any milk during the night, either in a cup or in a bottle. He can have a cup of water if he's really fussy.

Once you weaken the food-sleep association at bedtime, night wakenings often – not always but often – stop by themselves. Once some toddlers realize they aren't going to get milk anymore, they don't bother waking up at night for water. However, if your child keeps waking up despite these bedtime beverage shifts, help him adjust his internal hunger clock. Encourage him to eat more at regular daytime meals. But you'll probably also have to tackle the nighttime wakenings more directly.

At this age, the best tactic is usually to stop the night feedings. Comfort the child when he wakes up wanting the breast, cup, or bottle. Explain at bedtime, or even during the day for a few days before you make the change, that he is a big boy now and no longer needs his milk at night, that he gets his milk during the day. Tell him he will sleep better and feel better if he doesn't wake up for milk anymore and that you will be very proud of him.

When he does wake up wanting that dairy fix, go to his room. 'Sh-sh' him, stroke him a bit, even pick him up for a moment for a big, deep, comforting hug. Keep encouraging that bond with the lovey, to replace the bottle. Then put him back down and stay quietly in his room until he falls asleep again. If you want to try more gradual approaches, try a set-time feed for three nights (outlined in Chapter 7, 'Six to Eight Months'). On the fourth night don't feed him at all and instead stay by his bedside an additional night and soothe him. It usually doesn't take more than a few days at this age to wean a child overnight, from either the breast or bottle.

The more gradual approach sometimes works at this age, or you may find that you'll need a more direct approach. But you'll be surprised at how fast they adapt.

Ilan had reflux as an infant and stayed on a newborn-style feeding schedule for months, since he could hold down only small amounts of food at a time and therefore continued to eat small, frequent meals pretty much around the clock. Even after the reflux diminished – his was pretty severe until ten months, and some problems lingered until he was almost three – milk at night had become a deeply ingrained pattern.

His parents switched him to water, but it didn't stop his night wakenings. And his bedtime water cups, much more than his stuffed bear, were his nighttime security objects. A stickler for symmetry, he clutched one cup in each fist to go to bed, and called them his 'one-two cups.' He needed water each time he woke up at night, often four or five times a night even as he approached age two. Joanne tried every gradual technique she and I could think of. Finally, she realized she had to just take away the water, not at bedtime, but in the middle of the night. He cried and protested and got mad at her but she sat with him and cuddled and soothed him, maybe a little more than she should. He gave up the night water in three nights.

Every few months, he would wake up demanding his water again. With a two year old it was hard to tell whether he was regressing and wanting the one-two cup security again, or whether he was genuinely thirsty after a little too much soy sauce in his broccoli that night. He also asked for water when he was sick. If he was quite insistent, and Joanne couldn't be 100 percent sure if she was dealing with a dry throat or a security pang, she'd usually give him the water. The next night, if he slept through, she knew she'd made the right call, that he really had been thirsty. But if he started the whole cycle all over again, getting up seeking his one-two cups, she knew she'd been outsmarted and she'd have to tackle it again.

Sometimes a little gentle coaxing would suffice or she could distract him with the lovey. But sometimes she would have to force the issue again. Each time she dreaded it, but it was always easier than she had anticipated, and it got easier each time they had to go through this drill. He would wake up and cry or yell at her once or twice, but that was it: no more plaintive cries at 3:00 a.m. for 'more water,

Mummy.' While she addressed the middle-of-the-night drinking, she never tried to flat-out break the bedtime water habit, because it never caused significant problems. At three, he learned to leave an ounce or two in his cup and entrust one of his stuffed animals to 'hold' it in case he wanted it later.

Phasing Out Walking and Rocking to Sleep

Many of us walk and rock our newborns to sleep, but after eighteen or twenty-four or thirty months, it gets a little old – and they get heavy. I often use the Sleep Lady Shuffle to break this association at bedtime. If you have been rocking him in the middle of the night, but not at bedtime, explain to your child that you will sit in his room and help him get himself back to sleep but you won't rock him anymore. Gradually phase yourself out of the room as in the Shuffle.

We aren't eliminating cuddles; we are eliminating cuddles as a sleep crutch. You can have your child nestle into your lap while you read stories or sing songs with the lights on. But don't let him fall asleep in your arms or your lap; he must fall asleep in his own bed.

> At twenty-one months, Madison, as her mother, Beth, put it, 'had every bad sleep habit in the book.' They had a nice, sensible 7:30 p.m. bedtime, but then it all fell apart. Beth and Vince would have to rock, walk, or 'bounce around' with her for about forty-five minutes every night to get her to sleep. She also demanded milk in bed, and insisted that her mum stay with her to get her to sleep. Like Barry, she had a thing about twirling her mum's hair, but rejected all the substitutes her mum offered, including dolls with yarn hair and blankets with fringe.
>
> She would wake up after three hours, and her parents would have to rock her for another forty-five minutes. Three hours later, when she woke up again, they were usually too tired to deal with another rocking marathon, so Beth usually ended up sleeping with Madison. But Beth did not get much sleep with a child who wriggled and moved all the time, and she missed sleeping with her husband.

A professional counselor who worked with teens, Beth knew a lot about what was wrong but didn't know how to make it right. She had tried Ferber when Madison was eight months old, with fairly good results. But when Madison got thrown off after being sick for a few days some months later, they were never able to get her back on track. A second attempt at Ferber failed dismally. Madison screamed for hours, and instead of crying herself to sleep, she would throw up.

Before we started the Shuffle, Beth switched Madison from milk to water at bedtime and stopped lying down with her to get her to sleep. She also made sure to keep her head out of hair-twirling reach. On the nights Vince put Madison to bed, long hair wasn't an issue.

They moved through the Shuffle quickly, changing every two days instead of three because Madison was easily ritualized. 'She's one of those kids that if she sits in a certain chair when she watches a certain TV show, she has to sit in that same chair every time she watches that show,' her mum explained. They didn't want her to get used to having a parent seated in a specific position and then get upset at the change on the fourth night. At first she still woke up once or twice at night, but all she needed now was for Vince to sit in her room for a few minutes. She didn't scream, she didn't request milk, and she didn't demand her rocking and snuggling. Her night wakenings did not go away 100 percent, but they became briefer and much less frequent.

Dummy (Pacifier) Withdrawal

If your child's dummy habit interferes with his sleep, particularly if he wakes up calling you to fetch it, the time may well have come to break the habit. Many pediatricians agree this is a good age to deal with it. Unfortunately, I haven't found any sweet and gentle ways to do this (although I do have a backup plan for the squeamish).

Tell him it's time to give up the binkie, dummy, or nuk, whatever he knows it as. Give him a little while to get used to the idea, and then pick a day to act. When he fusses or cries, calm him, soothe him, pat him, stroke him. Expect a few rough nights and naps. Make sure you work on strengthening his bond with his lovey. 'It's not dummy time, but Teddy Bear is here and wants to hug you.' That both distracts him from the dummy and provides a security substitute. Better yet, try getting him a brand-new lovey as you take away the dummy; the newness might further distract him. You could even try taking him shopping and letting him choose his own new bedtime pal.

If he's old enough, read some books about children who get rid of dummies, such as *Little Bunny's Dummy Plan* or *The Last Noo-Noo*. Some pediatricians have advised parents to keep cutting the tip of the dummy more and more until it's so mutilated the child no longer wants it. And I know one mom who had her son put it inside a Build-a-Bear and he slept with the bear! Whatever you do, once you send it away or give it away or throw it away, don't go out and buy another one after an hour of whining.

> *Sheila tried to get Suzanna to bond to a security blanket and encouraged the little girl to put all her dummies in a brightly colored envelope to send to a family friend's new baby. It worked brilliantly – for one whole day. Then Suzanna wanted her dummies back, and in an uncharacteristic moment of intermittent reinforcement, Sheila gave in and decided not to press the dummy issue at this time. Suzanna never did bond to that blanket, and Sheila may have made it harder to get rid of the dummy the next time she tries.*

Many parents do not feel comfortable taking away the dummy, preferring to wait and see if your child gives it up on his own. There's a good chance you will have to take it away eventually, but if you aren't ready now, I would restrict the dummy to bedtime and naptime. Don't let him keep carrying it around all day.

He's old enough to find it by himself by now if you put several dummies in his cot or bed with him, or in a little basket within reach. He should be able to grab one, and get back to sleep without calling for you. The first few nights, you might have to remind him from the doorway to reach for it himself. Don't get it for him – or if you do get it for him a few times, put it in his hand, and let him then put it in his mouth. Don't keep doing this; remind him at bedtime that he has to find it himself and if necessary show him again where it will be. You should still encourage the lovey; it is really more useful for him to hold on to at night than the dummy and will eventually help him give up the dummy.

Early Birds

Early rising, at 5:00 or 5:30 a.m., remains very common at this age, and children who get up very early are often exhausted and fussy by midmorning. It may sound counterintuitive, but early rising is often caused by a late bedtime. Rather than being up bright and early because they are so ready to start their day, they are actually sleep deprived!

Start by getting him to bed earlier. Shift bedtime a few minutes earlier each day, so that the child is going to bed between 7:00 and 8:00 p.m., which for most children remains a good target bedtime up until around age five. *Make sure he naps enough.* If early awakenings have been going on for months or even years, as is sometimes the case with children this age, it may take three to four weeks to change it.

Some families – not many, but some – have found that it has taken a few months until the child consistently sleeps in. *Parental consistency is hugely important. Consistency,* in this context, means utter consistency and a little more rigidity than other aspects of my program. Intermittent reinforcement at 5:00 a.m. is just not a good idea. Some parents give up trying to teach the child to sleep later, and instead are satisfied if they get him to stay in his room and play quietly until 6:00. That might work in some cases, but usually children do better and get less tired during the day if you can get them to sleep that extra half hour or hour.

Respond quickly when he wakes and calls for you. Letting him stew or scream will only make him more awake; you want to teach him to stay asleep. Go to him, saying, 'It is not time to wake up' or 'Mummy and Daddy are sleeping.' Don't turn on the light or raise the blinds. Give him his lovey and reassure him, including a hug if that's needed, but don't pick him up.

Have a response plan. With younger babies, I give the parents the option of staying in the room. At this age, I encourage you to leave the room (particularly if he's in a bed, not the cot), because your presence may stimulate him into trying to stay awake and engage you or to keep clambering onto your lap. Check on him every fifteen or twenty minutes, until he falls asleep again.

You may use a wake-up light, or with older toddlers music, to cue him to know when his day can begin. Either get an alarm clock with a CD player or iPod or attach an appliance timer (available at a hardware store) to a bedroom lamp. The wake-up light tells the child to try to go back to sleep, or at least stay in his bed, and when it's okay to get up and start his day. Set it for about 6:00 a.m., and once he sleeps pretty consistently until 6:00, you can gradually try setting it later. Keep anything electronic out of reach for safety, or to keep him from turning it on himself. Some families prefer the light because it's less likely to wake the child, on those days he does sleep, but it's your choice. With either the light or the music, be consistent. If you allow your child to get out of bed and start his day even fifteen or twenty minutes before the wake-up music or light comes on, he will not take the music or light seriously the next day.

If he gets out of bed and comes looking for you, take his hand and walk him back to bed. Remind him quietly but firmly that the 'wake-up light' (or music) is not on yet, that it's still 'night-night' time. You will probably go through this for several mornings. It's hard for them to learn this at this age. You might want to try a deep-pressure hug for a moment or two before putting him back in bed, but skip it if it makes him tug at and cling to you. If you are still doing the Shuffle, resume your chair position. If you've finished the Shuffle but still have early risings, leave the room.

If he gets out again and again, consider putting a gate on the door. You might want to sit or lie just on the other side of the gate, a compromise between leaving him alone and staying in the room. Children will sometimes end up falling asleep on the floor near the gate. Don't worry; he'll be fine. You are working on changing his internal wake-up clock, and when that occurs he'll naturally prefer his bed to the floor. I explore some of these issues for children in beds rather than cots in the next chapter.

If you really feel you need to stay in the room, go ahead and try it. If he calms down and goes back to sleep, great. But he may get more riled up if you keep putting him back in bed or ignore his determined attempts to engage you in conversation or activity. Whichever approach you try, and you may have to experiment a bit, don't lie down with him or touch, sing, or pat him completely to sleep.

Ideally, he will fall asleep again, and if you are lucky you can get some more sleep too. But often he will stay awake – and probably complain about it loudly. Keep him in bed, or at least in a dark room, until 6:00 a.m. When I say 6:00, I mean 6:00. I don't mean 5:50 or 5:40, or else you'll find that the wake-up time keeps getting earlier and earlier and you aren't making any progress.

At 6:00 a.m., if you are in his room, go out for a minute or two and then come back. If you are already out of the room, then 6:00 is the time to return. (If he's asleep, don't wake him, and if he's awake but quietly content you can wait until a little later than 6:00.) Go in and have a *dramatic wake-up* to start the day. Make a big deal about turning on the light and opening the shades. Or let your child turn on the lights with you. Sing a cheerful good-morning song like the one I have on my *The Sweetest Dream* CD.

Basically, you want to *have a good-morning ritual*, just like you have a bedtime ritual, although the morning one is more stimulating, of course. You want to convey the message that it's time for him to wake up because it's morning, not because he was crying or whining for you.

At some point in this age range, usually as they approach two and a half, try using the clock in one of several ways. Instead of having your child mad at you, blame the clock! 'The clock says it's not time to wake up yet, sweetie. You need to stay in bed until the clock says get up.' You might be able to teach him to recognize 6:00 on a digital clock, and not get out of bed or call for you until he sees that number. A variant is to set a musical alarm for 6:00, and tell the child that if he wakes up before the music starts, he has to stay in bed. A light on a timer can serve the same purpose, and it's quieter than music, so it won't wake other children or even wake him if he happens to still be asleep. These approaches are all a little hit or miss at this age; some kids get it, and others don't until they are three or so.

Once you get him sleeping until 6:00, you can try to push it back to 6:15 or 6:30 using the same techniques, but it may or may not work – 6:00 is a natural and common wake-up time for young children. Many early risers will begin to sleep later on their own in another year or two but there's no guarantee. Some tend to wake on the early side throughout childhood but will develop the ability to sleep in a little on occasions when they've gone to bed late.

Suzanna woke up much too early, sometimes at 4:30 a.m. Sheila and Randy tried several strategies and finally settled on the clock radio. When she awoke early, they gave her a very precise and consistent message. 'We'd go in briefly and say we aren't coming to get you until the music is on your radio. It's still dark out, and Mummy and Daddy are sleeping.' Over the next few months, as she became a better nighttime sleeper and napper, her mornings steadily improved. She stayed in bed until she heard her music, and later did not need the radio, sleeping until about 7:00 a.m. on her own. When she gets a little off track – for instance, after an illness or when the time changes in spring and autumn – her parents return to the clock radio for a few days. As she slept later in the morning, she awoke less frequently at night.

In many families, the toddler wakes up at 6:00 a.m. cheerful and happy – but the parent accustomed to sleeping until 7:00 or 8:00 is grumpy and not so happy. You can try training him to sleep later if you want, using the techniques I outline above for children who wake up too early. But you might have to accept it for a year or two more, and try to get to bed earlier yourself.

You can also try to teach him to stay in his room and play quietly or look at a book until you come to get him. Reward him if he does, but don't be mad or punitive if he doesn't. It's a hard skill to learn at this age. He wants to see Mum and Dad after being away from you all night, and he may also be hungry, wet, or in need of a little help reaching that bathroom light.

If he wakes up at 6:00 but is cranky and irritable by 6:30 or 7:00, then he is getting up too early. Consider it a sign of sleep deprivation, and use the advice above for early risers to train him to sleep for another half hour or hour. Make sure he gets to sleep between 7:00 and 8:00 at night, and that he naps enough during the day.

Early Risers

If your little one wakes up before 6:00 a.m., he's probably overtired. Overtired children don't sleep as well, or sleep as long, as well-rested ones. He may be:

- Going to bed too late
- Not napping enough
- Staying up too long between the end of his afternoon nap and going to bed (try not to let it exceed four hours)
- Going to bed when he's past that 'drowsy but awake' mark. If he's too drowsy, he won't know how to get himself back to sleep when he's more alert – including at 5:00 a.m.

Sometimes, your child is not an early riser until you embark on a sleep-coaching program. Before Joanne and Ken started working with me, Ilan woke up consistently between 5:00 and 5:30 a.m., demanding a bottle of milk or later a cup of water. Usually Ken, who had an easier time getting back to sleep at that hour than Joanne, would fetch him, Joanne would give him his cup, and they would all go back to sleep in the family bed. Ilan would then sleep until 7:00 or 7:30, sometimes later.

When we started sleep shaping, his bedtime got much easier, his napping improved, and his night sleep got significantly better, but the early risings got worse. That was very hard on Joanne. He would get up at 5:00, and she would sit in his bedroom instead of letting him come into her bed. She stayed in the room – he would work himself up into incredibly intense crying if she left – and sometimes she could get him back to sleep and sometimes she couldn't.

Joanne's own body clock never adjusted to a 5:00 a.m. wakening. She was one of those people who could function if she woke up at 6:00 but was a complete wreck if she was up at 5:00. Yet she had trouble getting back to sleep herself if she was up and around at 5:00; some switch in her brain was activated and wouldn't turn itself off. Sometimes Ilan fell asleep again; often he didn't, and he could make it a pretty unpleasant hour, demanding to get up as she tried to just gently get him back to sleep without responding to his determined provocation.

After three months, she tried letting him sleep with her after 5:00 in a guest bed in his room. That worked for both of them for a few days. Then he started waking up three, four, or five times a night again, demanding that they both get in the 'big bed,' a guest bed nearby. This is very common – and precisely why I warn you not to lie down with your child in the morning. Joanne gave up the morning snuggle and went back to sitting in the room and trying to calm him. Finally, he reset his body clock and began sleeping until 6:00 or 6:30 most of the time. And on those days he still woke at 5:00, he found it easier to get back to sleep.

About six months later, he began waking up at 5:00 again after the family's schedule had been disrupted by both travel and illness. Joanne tried sitting in his room with him but was so exhausted that she just fell asleep in the 'big bed' and he climbed in with her. He was older now, though, about two years and eight months. She very painstakingly explained that this was a special almost-morning big bed snuggle but that the rest of the time Ilan had to stay in his fire-truck bed. He had the language skills and the cognitive ability to get this abstract idea.

Once or twice when he woke up in the middle of the night and said, 'Big bed snuggle,' she said, 'No, Ilan, go back to your fire-truck bed. It's not time for our special almost-morning big bed snuggle yet.' It worked. He didn't wake up at night demanding her (at least not until the next time he got sick), and when he did wake up at 5:00 or 5:30, he'd call for her, and they'd both stumble into the big bed and get back to sleep quickly. This helped get him an extra hour or two of sleep a day, shielding him from that spiral of overtiredness that causes more early rising.

He began sleeping until 6:15 or 6:30 most of the time. On those days he still woke up earlier, they could both get back to sleep quickly. All of a sudden, in late summer, he began sleeping until 7:00 or even 7:30 and once even until 8:15. Naturally, that was exactly one week before big brother Zach started school, meaning the whole family had to be up at 6:00 or 6:30 and now had to tiptoe around and sacrifice using the coffee grinder to avoid waking up Ilan!

Napping

Most children this age have consolidated to one nap a day, or will do so shortly. (If your child hasn't, see 'Moving to One Nap a Day,' in Chapter 9, 'Thirteen to Eighteen Months'). Usually, they nap from roughly 1:00 to 3:00 in the afternoon. As you no doubt know, napping can be difficult for children, just as it is difficult for many adults to sleep during daylight. They need plenty of time to change gears. You should have a whole routine, shorter but similar to bedtime. Quiet stories or songs in his room are good prenap activities.

Sleep Lady Tip

If your toddler has already switched from cot to bed, you might have to gate the door. One mum who hated gates would read a book in the room across the hall from her son's room. If he came out, she'd meet him in the hallway and immediately walk him back to bed.

Children this age still need naps, even if they think they don't. You may have to train them – which as I've said before is my least-favorite aspect of sleep shaping. (See Chapter 7, 'Six to Eight Months,' for details of nap-training techniques.)

HAVE HIM STAY IN HIS COT OR BED FOR AN HOUR, whether he falls asleep or not. *Stay with him, sit right outside his door, or check on him every* ten or fifteen minutes or so, whichever feels right to you. Don't engage or converse, try not to pick him up, and do make him try to stay in bed, or at least in his room, for the full hour.

IF YOUR CHILD STILL HASN'T FALLEN ASLEEP AFTER AN HOUR, do a dramatic wake-up and get him out. But then use an *emergency backup* nap plan, such as a drive in the car, to get him to sleep. Motion sleep is not the most restful sleep, but it's better than no sleep while you are nap training. Try again to get him to nap the next day. Use nap stickers, logic, bribes, whatever it takes, but keep him in that room and coax him to sleep.

Sleep Lady Tip

Nap training is often very hard on a parent, who is home alone without support from another adult at that time of day. And even for those parents who cope with tears in daylight better than they do at night, nap training can seem incredibly time-consuming, and you'll have to stick around the house at naptime. If nap training is absolutely too much for you – or a child-care provider – then give yourself permission to give up for now. Keep using your backup temporary solutions so you don't have such an overtired child that bedtime falls apart again. Try nap training again in a few months.

Sometimes the child will learn to sleep for a parent but not a babysitter who may not be willing to do her share of the training. Sometimes the reverse is true, and the child naps angelically for the sitter, saving the napping power struggles for Mum.

CATNAPPING is less common at this age, but it still occurs.

Catnappers take several naps, each less than forty-five minutes. That's not a complete sleep cycle, and it's not refreshing. You want him to sleep about two hours (a little less by age two and a half). *If he wakes up after thirty or forty-five minutes, go to his cot or bed and re-assure him.* Tell him it's still naptime and he has to stay in his bed. Stroke him a little if that helps. Keep him in his cot or room for at least an hour, whether he falls asleep again or not.

If he sleeps longer than a thirty-minute catnap but his naps are still on the skimpy side, use these techniques to try to get him back to sleep. You want to stretch those naps out to ninety minutes or more, particularly if he still seems tired. On days when your child does not nap enough, try the backup nap plan and if he falls asleep late in the day, wake him after forty-five minutes or by 4:00 p.m. Get him to bed early, around 7:00.

Helene began a more disciplined approach to napping, including paying more attention to Barry's sleep window, catching him when he was tired but not too tired. Before, she had spent a good chunk of her day lying down with Barry, trying to get him to sleep. Sometimes she would put him in the car. Now, she would not lie down with him, and she made him stay in his room for an hour. Sometimes she would then have to take him for a drive, but he didn't wake up when she moved him into his bed.

Gradually, he adjusted to a better daytime sleep routine except when Larry, whose job running a restaurant meant erratic hours, was home. Barry would resist napping if it meant missing a minute of Daddy time. On those days, Helene and Larry tried to get him down but resorted to taking him for a drive if they saw he was determined to stay up. Getting him to sleep was more important than being a purist about how he slept. 'If he misses naps for two or three days he gets sick, and even he has begun to understand that,' Helene said.

Madison was another recalcitrant napper. She hated it if her mother left the room before she fell asleep and would cry hard enough to keep herself awake. So Beth stayed with her, and if Madison started to get out of bed, Beth would tell her to lie down again or else Mummy would leave. That usually worked, and she would fall asleep. Some disruptions in her schedule – a cross-country move, a stay at her grand-mother's house during renovations on her new home – disturbed her naps.

Later her preschool schedule also posed an obstacle. If she missed her 1:00 p.m. get-ready-for-nap window, she often failed to sleep. But on the days she attended preschool, she didn't get home until after 1:00. By the time she had a snack and settled down, it was 2:30. Either she couldn't fall asleep by then, or if she napped it was so late that it threw off the rest of her schedule and she was even worse the next day.

On those afternoons, Beth did enforce quiet rest time, which wasn't as good as a nap at that age but did help her keep it together. 'If she doesn't nap, she gets cranky at about 5:00, but it's a fifteen-minute meltdown and then she's okay until bedtime,' her mother said. Beth was also diligent about getting Madison to bed early on no-nap days.

Suzanna's nap was a challenge for Sheila, too, and it got even worse when she switched to a bed before turning three. This little girl had no intention of napping, and even less intention of staying in bed for a nap she wasn't going to take. Sheila tried gating the room but said, 'It made her more upset than it was worth.' Instead, Sheila allowed Suzanna to play in her room, while Sheila shut the door and read a magazine in the hallway. If Suzanna came out in pursuit, Sheila would calmly tell her to go back into her room or else Mummy wouldn't sit so close anymore. 'I couldn't force her to nap, so I let her play in her room. Sometimes she would just conk out on the floor,' her mom said. As Suzanna got accustomed to napping, maybe even understanding on some level that her body needed it, she gave up on the floor and went to bed. Again, the better rested she was by day, the better she slept by night.

Cosleeping

Many families who cosleep decide that they've had enough at this age, and the Shuffle can help end the practice. Similarly, some families who never planned on cosleeping find their toddler in their bed now that he's old enough to wander in on his own. Please refer to Chapter 12, 'Whose Bed Is It Anyway?' if you've been cosleeping since birth and want to stop, or if you've been taking your child into bed for all or part of the night because you think it's the only way you can get him to sleep. For those of you who choose to continue cosleeping, that chapter gives you some tips on how to improve the quality and quantity of sleep in a shared bed.

Joel

Remember Joel, the boy who wouldn't drink milk in a cup from Mum? I met Dorothy and Jack when Joel was nineteen months old. He was their first child, although he had a much older half-sister from Jack's first marriage who lived with them part-time.

Joel had never been a great sleeper, partly because he had frequent ear infections as an infant and Dorothy rocked and held him to sleep when he was sick. They had tried to let him cry it out, but he'd throw up if he cried too much, which was not exactly a soothing and sleep-promoting experience. Dorothy and Jack had agreed early not to cosleep, but at about sixteen months, an exhausted Dorothy, who was also dealing with guilt about being a working mum with a long commute to her engineering job, started bringing Joel into the family bed some of the time. Musical beds didn't solve the sleep problems, and it created marital friction. A move to a new house, job changes, and business travel for Jack added to the stress. 'We started a bad pattern. I felt guilty being back at work, and I compensated a lot. I'd come home, and I was tired and Jack was away, and Joel would get sick and I'd just take him into bed. I thought it would be just for a few days, but I couldn't reverse it; if I put him in his cot, he'd just cry and cry. And I tried letting him cry, but he'd throw up. And if he did fall asleep, he'd be up again in an hour and a half. Plus he needed a bottle all the time,' said Dorothy, who as you recall, was also very worried about his small size and nutrition.

Dorothy also disliked schedules. 'I'd come home late, I was tired, I wanted some wind-down time, I wanted to be with my baby. I didn't want to walk in and have it be bedtime.' She didn't like watching the clock or worrying about when to go upstairs. She often made an attempt to get him to sleep early with a bottle, but if that didn't work, she carried him around with her until trying another bottle around 10:00 p.m.

I helped Dorothy understand a little bit about sleep cycles and hormones, which made it easier for her to start keeping a closer eye on the clock and on Joel's sleep signs. She also realized it was finally time to give up the bottle, which was far easier than she imagined; Joel didn't need it as much as she thought he did, or maybe as much as she needed to give it to him. We began the Sleep Lady Shuffle, concentrating those first few nights on putting him into his cot while he was drowsy but still slightly awake.

The first two nights were difficult, and I'm not sure Dorothy would have stuck it out if she wasn't so afraid of admitting failure to Jack. Joel cried for more than an hour. But he didn't throw up; he never reached that point of complete hysteria. 'He was crying, but he wasn't completely inconsolable. It was different having me in there with him,' Dorothy said. 'He finally did fall asleep – people say babies can't fall asleep standing up, but he did.' Dorothy caressed him a little but was very mindful of my advice not to create any new sleep associations. 'He would reach out to me – he still does. That was hard. He was reaching out, and I wanted to hold and cuddle him, but I tried to comfort him with words.' She also kept some calm music running in the background, but that wasn't a problem because music is a mood setter, not a sleep crutch, for Joel. It helps him prepare for sleep, but he doesn't need it to stay asleep or get back to sleep at night.

The third night was much different, a good thing because the first two had been very hard on Dorothy. Joel cried briefly, but then fell asleep right away, this time lying down. I think part of the change was that Dorothy was getting much better at her new nighttime routine, at reading Joel's signals and getting him into the cot when he was 'really, really drowsy but still awake.' When she moved the chair farther away, he fussed a bit but not too much. He still woke up in the middle of the night, but as they went through the Shuffle they went in to quickly comfort him and then they could leave. 'It wasn't an ordeal; he went back to sleep in his cot, and we were able to go right back to sleep.' Gradually, he woke up less frequently. He still wakes up now and then, but not most of the time.

Even when Joel's schedule was disrupted – when Dorothy regressed (sleeping with him for a few days when he had a high fever), when a job crisis meant an eighty-hour workweek, when Jack was on the road again *and a frightening kook in the neighborhood was going around banging on everybody's doors at midnight – Dorothy managed to get Joel back into a good, sound sleep routine in less than two weeks. 'I learned that if I wanted to cuddle with him, I could still do that, but while we read books, not while I was getting him to sleep. I learned the difference between a tired child and an overtired child,' she said. 'I learned that even if I hate routine and consistency, even if I find them difficult, Joel needs them.'*

11

Two and a Half to Five Years Old

*B*etween the ages of two and three, average sleep needs drop to about *ten and a half hours a night, plus an hour and-a-half afternoon nap. Four year olds need eleven and a half hours at night, and most no longer nap daily, although they do need about forty-five minutes of quiet time each afternoon and possibly an occasional nap. Five year olds sleep about eleven hours a night, and afternoon quiet time is still beneficial.*

Preschoolers still need a lot of sleep, but they are immensely clever at devising reasons not to get it. They stall and evade with amazing ingenuity, which for parents can be frustrating, or comical, or both. They engage in philosophical discussions worthy of a junior Socrates, and they voice enough curiosity to rival a little Einstein. 'Why do bats fly at night?' 'Was the sky always blue?' 'What does God eat for breakfast?' Of course, none of these thoughts and questions hold any interest for them at 4:00 or 5:00 in the afternoon when they are busy playing, but become an all-consuming need to know as soon as they hear the word *pajamas*. I worked with one couple that dubbed their oldest daughter 'Captain Loophole' for her brilliance in delaying bedtime.

Sleep shaping for this age group requires a mix of the techniques you are already familiar with from earlier chapters and new ones designed for older and more verbal children. As parents, we need to inject some discipline into bedtime but still keep it warm and cozy. We need to help them with those bouts of the scaries that can make bedtime difficult even when they aren't turning stalling into a competitive sport. As they begin to cut back and eventually outgrow their naps, we have to keep tinkering with their sleep and wake schedules and introduce afternoon quiet time unless we enjoy meltdowns before dinner.

Solutions to ingrained problems that date back to infancy can take some time. You aren't going to undo four years of night wakening or dummy dependency in three days, so keep in mind my advice about patience and consistency. If some new problems emerge at this age, like a demand that you lie down with her at bedtime, address it quickly, before it becomes a long-term ingrained behavior. Luckily, from about age three on, sometimes even a few months earlier, children understand on some level that they need sleep, that sleeping poorly is a problem, that you are upset about it. They can then become an ally in your attempt to change things and begin to 'own' the solutions.

Developmental Changes

Separation Anxiety

Children this age often still experience lingering separation anxiety, which is why so many of them demand that you lie down with them at bedtime or they'll wander out of bed looking for you. If they have basically sound sleep habits, they can learn to settle down more easily with a lovey, a dim (four-watt) night light, and some reassurance. A good, comforting bedtime routine is essential. Don't rush through it, but don't let him keep stalling, negotiating, and bending the rules. A promise to check on him again before you go to bed is very reassuring. And if you say you are going to check on him, make sure you really do.

Sleep Lady Tip

Children love it if you tell them how snuggly and cozy and peaceful and beautiful they look when they sleep. I think they take it as a confirmation that you really are checking on them and watching over them while they are asleep, that you aren't that far away, that they are as safe and sound as you promised.

Loveys

Preschoolers and kindergartners shouldn't need to schlep around a security blanket, stuffed animal, or favorite toy wherever they go, barring perhaps exceptionally stressful or unfamiliar situations. But they are definitely not too old for a lovey at bedtime. I encourage it strongly. My own daughters had them for years. The lovey helps them cope with separation and nighttime fears. Some children are and always will be indifferent to loveys, but a lot of kids will get attached now, even if they spurned one toy after another when they were younger.

Include the lovey in your nighttime games, stories, and rituals. Be creative, and give your child a role in choosing her lovey. Go shopping together, or make a lovey together on your own or at a workshop at a local craft store. Some children switch alliances, first bonding to this bedtime toy, then latching on to that one. That's fine; it's their way of satisfying their own evolving tastes and needs. One little boy outgrew his baby lovey and started lining up all his macho action-hero toys around his bed to keep him safe at night. No monster would dare cross Spider-Man, Superman, and a big green Hulk!

If your child sleeps with the same lovey every night, make sure you tuck it in with her and say good night to them both. If she likes different loveys, let her make that night's selection pretty early in the routine or else it becomes another excuse for stalling at lights-out.

Each night Ariella would choose one of her baby dolls to sleep with. In a brilliant flash of intuition, Marcy used the doll to persuade Ariella to stay in bed. 'I would remind her to stay in bed, and tell her that baby doll Rachel needs her. 'If you get up, baby Rachel won't have anyone to be with her.' That made Ariella feel good and strong.'

Many kids this age have some kind of self-soothing ritual that involves the parent. They may want to twirl Mum's hair (surprisingly common!). They might do something a little more eccentric, like poking fingers in Dad's belly button. Try to transfer this habit to a lovey. One mother of a hair twirler went to a fabric store and made a lovey out of satin with a tassel. Others have found stuffed animals, blankets, and dolls with fringes or other twirlable features. She may not accept the substitute immediately, but ease her into it. Let her do her little ritual, like the hair twirling, for a few min utes while you are reading good-night stories, but then slowly start to move away, letting her gradually hold the lovey instead.

New Mobility: Switching to the Big Bed

Most children move out of the cot by the age of three, although I don't personally think there's anything wrong with keeping a child in a cot until the age of four. If you'd like to try to keep him in a cot a little longer, particularly if he does not yet have the verbal skills to understand big bed rules, review my tips on prolonging cot sleeping in the previous chapter. You might try a mesh cover called a *cot tent*. Some kids hate them, but others stay in the cot a few extra months with the tent. But if your child is climbing out of his cot frequently and is also talking about wanting a 'big boy' or 'big girl' bed, make the switch.

If you want to do it in several steps, start by leaving the cot railing down, with a stool at the side so he can get out by himself. You might want some extra pillows around on the floor for safety. You can either put a bed in his room with the cot or remove the cot and put the bed where the cot stood. You might want to put the bed in the corner of the room, so the child still has that sense of being safely contained. It's often a good idea to put up a bed rail so he doesn't fall out, and you might want to put some pillows or extra blankets on the floor to shield him if he does fall.

Putting a gate on the bedroom door, at least at the beginning, is usually a good idea both as a training device and as a safety measure. The gate delineates boundaries, helping a child understand that he has to stay in his bed. It also prevents him from wandering around and possibly getting hurt in a dark house in the middle of the night.

Let your child make a big deal about the transition to the big bed. Let him pick out some cool sheets. (No matter what design scheme you have in mind, there seems to be an inordinately high chance your little girl will want pink and purple and your little boy will want fire trucks. Just go with it.) Explain the privileges but also review the rules. Let him understand that you will still put him to bed, but then he's expected to stay there. Be consistent from the very start. If he gets out of bed, take him right back without any fuss. Reward him for staying in bed. Give him plenty of stickers and let him call his grandparents or aunts or cousins to brag about the new bed.

You met Suzanna, Sheila and Randy's daughter, in the previous chapter. Her sleep improved after I worked with them, but the little acrobat got very adept at scrambling out of her cot no matter what her parents tried. 'Every morning we'd wake up and she'd be standing at the edge of our bed,' her mum recalled. A few months before Suzanna turned three, she started showing a lot of interest in 'big girl' beds. She was sleeping well now, and had good language skills, so her parents decided she was ready for the switch.

'She knew a lot of her friends were in 'big girl' beds. When we went somewhere to play, she'd go to the 'big girl' bed to play, so I told her, 'You are getting your 'big girl' bed.' We put pillows next to the bed in case she fell out, and I got sheets with purple butterflies and flowers. She was very excited to have her 'big girl' bed,' said Sheila.

Sheila explained the 'big bed' rules very clearly and rewarded

*Suzanna with stickers for staying in her bed and not wandering out
to look for her parents. The transition went very smoothly.*

If you are about to embark on my Sleep Lady Shuffle or other
major nighttime changes, like taking away a bottle or dummy,
consider whether it would be easier if you kept him in the cot a
little longer. It keeps him in a safe and familiar environment while
you are changing other aspects of his sleep, and it may be simpler
if you don't have to worry about him getting up and out of bed
while you are trying to teach him how to sleep in it. Yet I have
also found that many of these older children do better if you change
everything at once. You give him the privilege of the new 'big boy'
bed, and incorporate the changed sleep expectations into the 'big
bed' rules. There's no right or wrong decision here. Trust your
instincts about which approach is a better match for your child's
temperament.

If your child, even up to age four, still likes the cot even with
the railing down, leave it alone. You can bring up the topic occasionally. You can look at beds and sheets, but there's no rush unless,
of course, your child's weight exceeds the cot's limit. He'll move
when he's ready, and he'll be ready soon enough. Some families
use toddler beds as an interim step, but I don't see a need for it. If
he really wants one, fine, but it's certainly not an essential invest-
ment. The one advantage is that they are usually too small for you
to fit into alongside him, which children often demand when they
move into a bed of their own.

Some preschoolers go through a phase when they don't want to
sleep in their bed; they want to sleep or nap on a little couch, or
a pad on the floor, or a beanbag chair, whatever. It may happen
right after the transition from the cot; it may happen later. You can
use some kind of system of rewards and incentives to lure him into
the bed, such as reading his favorite story together in the bed, or
giving him an extra back rub in bed, or something like that.

Probe whether something in the bed is frightening him. Maybe
he's afraid of falling off, in which case you can put extra pillows
on the floor or get bed rails for the side. But I would ask myself
if it's worth fussing over. If he's sleeping reasonably well in his room,

I wouldn't worry about it, and he'll probably move into the bed himself pretty quickly.

'I spent a fortune on custom-installed, room-darkening shades to get my son to nap,' one mother lamented. 'He did begin napping again – but only on the living room couch in the brightest room in the house!'

Eating and Sleeping

Children this age should have a regular meal routine: three meals a day plus healthy snacks in the midmorning and midafternoon – after their nap if they still take one. They just do not need a bottle anymore. Sucking on one at night is not good for their sleep, their teeth, or their overall nutrition. If your child is still using a bottle, go back and review my information in Chapter 8, 'Nine to Twelve Months,' and Chapter 9, 'Thirteen to Eighteen Months.'

At bedtime, she can have a cup of water, but no milk or juice in bed. I'd prefer you give her the water during story and song time, not after lights-out. If she makes you fill the water cup a zillion times at bedtime, set clear limits, explain them, and stick to them. You can leave a cup of water by her bedside overnight (I'd recommend a sippy cup or a sports bottle, not a baby bottle or an open cup, until she gets used to groping for it in the dark). But again, explain at bedtime that this has to last her all night; you aren't going to keep coming back to give her more. Remember how Joanne convinced her little boy to leave a few ounces in his nighttime water cup. Ilan gave it to a stuffed animal, his 'backup lovey' who slept near his bed but not in it, to hold for him in case he needed it.

Stalling and Curtain Calls

That father who called his eldest daughter 'Captain Loophole' pretty much summed it up. Children this age are brilliant procrastinators, and any separation anxiety or nighttime fears only hone their skills. The best defense is a sensible bedtime, a good routine, and the ability to gently disengage when they start to pepper you with all sorts of questions and requests.

Children this age are brilliant procrastinators, and any
separation anxiety or nighttime fears only hone their
skills.

If your child wants you to tuck him in three hundred times, try
to do it just once or twice. Tell him what you expect, when the
'last time' will be. Then stick to it. You can come back to his doorway
in a few minutes to quickly praise him for understanding and
following the bedtime directions. Once you've given him that dollop
of praise and reassurance, leave before he starts trying to engage
you all over again. Skip this step if it makes matters worse. Use
your judgment. Put up a gate if he insists on coming out of bed a
zillion times; he'll get the message.

Sometimes children know exactly which maternal anxiety button
to push. I know one little boy who got out of bed and told his
mother his tummy hurt. She was naturally solicitous and fussed over
him a bit as she got him back to bed. A half hour later he wandered
out again, this time declaring that his hair hurt!

> *'She stalls, stalls, stalls,' Marcy said of Ariella. 'She's so smart; she says
> she needs certain things, and she chooses things that push my buttons.
> It all seems so rational to me – she asks for such normal things. I'll
> ask her if she really needs a glass of water, and she'll tell me she didn't
> get that toothpaste taste out of her mouth. She'll tell me
> she needs a new nappy, she has pee-pee and can't sleep, so I go back
> in and change her. She'll say she needs that fuzzy blanket; it's a lot
> warmer. I try to plan ahead. I try to think of what she'll need at
> bedtime and set her up for total success. But she always manages to
> think of one last thing.'*

If a child says he is hungry, it's very hard for a parent to say
no and then guiltily wonder if he was truly hungry. If he's a picky
eater, or seems to have added epicurean demands to his stalling
repertoire at bedtime, just firmly say, 'No, you had dinner. We'll
have breakfast when you wake up tomorrow.' If it's a real aberra-

tion and you think he might genuinely be hungry, give him a quick, healthy snack but explain very carefully that you are doing this tonight but won't be doing it every night. The next night, consider a preemptive strike. Ask him if he needs a snack right before you start his bath and bedtime routine, and tell him he can have the snack now but not after bath and toothbrushing. Encourage enough eating during the day and have a sensible meal schedule.

The Scaries

Almost all children at some point in this age bracket experience vague fears in the evening: monsters, ghosts, shadows, or just things they can't quite put a name on. You need to acknowledge those fears, without allowing your child to turn them into an excuse to prolong bedtime, or to get out of bed repeatedly during the night.

Sleep Lady Tip

Make the lovey a part of the search team. The lovey can help you check the room and then snuggle into the child's arms and say, 'See, everything is safe and sound. There are no monsters, bears, ghosts,' whatever she fears.

Try not to ridicule the fears. They aren't ridiculous to the child. Tell her that there are no monsters, and then show her there are no monsters. Spend a minute looking under the bed or in the closet, if that's what she needs you to do. You might hold hands and check together, unless that seems to intensify her fear.

'Wes has never mentioned being scared of monsters or ghosts, but he's afraid of the dark. We use night lights in his room, the hallway, adjacent bedroom, and bathroom. He always takes a lovey and Blackie the bear to bed as security, which helps,' Amanda said.

At three and a half, Sam began saying he was afraid of voices outside. Nora thought he might be using it as a ploy to delay bedtime, but she gave him the benefit of the doubt. 'We reassure him that we've locked and double-checked all the doors, and that we are downstairs to keep anyone out. And when we're at my parents' house, we do the same thing and also tell him that their dogs won't let anyone in.'

Giving the child a physical prop to reassure himself can also help. Not a weapon, of course, but something he can see or hold or touch to know he will not be left at the mercy of the scaries. James, for instance, was a great sleeper but he started experiencing bedtime anxieties when he was three and a half. He was a small child with a very soft voice, so Ellen gave him a bedside bell. He could ring it, knowing that Mum or Dad would hear it right away. They even rehearsed during the day so he could see how quickly Mum and Dad would respond.

Other mums have found products like Monster Go Away! spray on the Internet, or you can make one out of a water spray bottle and some light, safe scent. Let your child help you decorate the bottle in a way that she feels confident will scare off those scaries. Spray the room together at bedtime and then leave the spray by her bed in case she needs it at night. You might also want to leave a flashlight in reach, unless you think she will stay up all night playing with it. Look through my list of recommended bedtime books to find stories that may help shake off her fears.

I gave my second daughter, Gretchen, a prop she could wear. She had used a blanket as her lovey since she was a baby, and even when she was very little she used to wrap it around her head. Naturally, this worried me and I would unravel her when I went in to check on her every night. Many children like some kind of pressure on them, because it is comforting, and when she got old enough to talk she would ask me to put the blanket on her head to make her feel protected and snuggled.

One December, when she was about three and a half, she saw a picture of a man with a sleeping cap in *The Night Before Christmas*. We decided I would design a cap for her, one that would give her that snuggly feeling but finally relieve me from all those suffocation nightmares. I took a rectangular piece of polar fleece, folded down the two top corners, and sewed it into an envelope shape. I would put it down on her pillow, and she would stick her head in the 'flap,' and snuggle with her blanket and stuffed animal. She still uses it now but not to ward off monsters. For a long time she would explain to me that it did a great job of keeping away monsters.

Sleep Lady Tip

If your child is one of those rare ones who can have you lie down with her once in a while without demanding that you do it all the time, go ahead and bend this rule, but be careful; try to get out of her bed before she's fully asleep because you are on a slippery sleep slope.

Obviously, if your child is truly terrified, give her the extra comfort she needs. It's usually better to sit by her and stroke her and hug her rather than lie down and go to sleep with her. If she really needs a lot of physical reassurance, hold her in your lap for a moment or two and then put her back down and continue patting her. You can also do a lot of snuggling and cuddling with the lights on, before the final stage of bedtime. You may have to spend a few nights sitting in the doorway while she falls asleep, rather than leaving her completely alone.

If your child has a nightmare, return her to bed and offer extra reassurance. Help her turn her thoughts away from the nightmare and to more pleasant images – 'rainbows and flowers,' as my older daughter used to say. Rita, whom you'll meet in a moment, used to circle four-year-old Isabel's bedroom saying, 'Bad dreams go away!' Occasional nightmares are normal; just about all kids have them. Read Chapter 14, 'Nightmares, Night Terrors, and Sleepwalking,' for more tips on coping.

Children's anxieties begin to expand as they become more aware of the larger world around them, especially in the early school years. They may begin to worry about personal harm, being hurt or robbed. They worry about one of their parents or grandparents getting sick. They start to worry about school, or their friends, or their pets. They can absorb far more than you may realize from even a brief glimpse of television news or a snippet of a radio report, and be quite worried about wars, earthquakes, hurricanes, and the like, however distant. In our post-9/11 world, many youngsters will also have explicit fears or perhaps a more vague unease about war or terrorism.

Assuaging anxieties can sometimes be as simple as talking to your child and getting the fears out in the open where they don't seem so terrifying. But the depth of childhood anxiety is often underestimated. Don't overreact – a little bit of fear and anxiety is normal at this age, and being afraid of a monster doesn't mean your child is going to grow up to be neurotic. But if your child seems excessively fearful, or phobic, talk to your doctor and her preschool or school teachers and consider if you need professional intervention.

Sleep Lady Tip

Sometimes a child who is not normally afraid will have a few days of palpable anxiety, and may have transferred that anxiety onto imaginary ghosts or monsters. Depending on her verbal skills, you may be able to tease out what's bothering her – a schedule change, a classmate being mean at preschool, an upcoming event that is worrying her.

Potty Training

I don't think there's any problem with working on changing sleep patterns at the same time you are potty training, as long as you don't turn potty training into a tug-of-war. Focus on daytime training, and leave a nappy or pull-up on at naptime until he stays dry for at least a week. At night, I think it's fine to keep a nappy or pull-up on until the age of four or five; they can develop overnight control on their own if you give them time. I just don't see any point in confusing your child – if you are trying to teach him to stay in bed, don't then tell him he's got to get up and out of bed in the middle of the night to pee! For more information on potty training, see Chapter 10, 'One and a Half to Two and a Half Years Old,' and for bedwetting in older children, see Chapter 15, 'Medical Problems.' Look at my resource list for book recommendations.

With a newly trained child, however, the potty itself can become yet another stalling tactic. When a child says he has to 'go potty,' you are of course going to let him get out of bed and go potty. But don't let him do this more than once a night, and do your best to make the trip to the potty brief and efficient. If he says he has to go potty again five minutes later, tell him that he's out of luck, it's too soon to go again, and he can wait until morning. Or you can direct him to go to the bathroom himself (or walk him there but don't interact, returning quickly and silently). If he's doing this constantly, you can tell him you'll put him back in nappies for bedtime. Remember to have him go potty before getting into bed in the first place – and remind him when he does that this is the bedtime potty call, and he can't make thirty more. If he's not stalling, if you think he's really not sure whether he has to go one more time before sleeping, let him know it's fine to use nappies or a pull-up overnight to be on the safe side for a bit longer.

Partnering with Your Child

Parents have an array of techniques available to them to help shape their toddler's sleep habits and routines. At this age, children can get vested in improving their own sleep and can feel pride and self-worth when they achieve it. Positive reinforcement goes a long way.

> At this age, children can get vested in improving their own sleep and can feel pride and self-worth when they achieve it. Positive reinforcement goes a long way for this age group.

The Family Meeting

Start with a family meeting where both parents sit down with the child and talk about sleep in an age-appropriate manner. Choose a time when your child is happy and receptive. Sunday morning after pancakes is a lot better than 5:00 p.m. on a weekday when she skipped her nap and is starving for dinner.

Tell her that you consulted (or read a book by) the Sleep Lady and learned about how children can sleep better. That way you can blame me for any changes or rules she doesn't like. For instance, if your child begs you to lie down with her, you can say the Sleep Lady said we can't do that but we can stay with you in your room.

Some children get furious with me. 'The Sleep Lady can't come over to play with me!' 'I don't like the Sleep Lady.' They may pick up this book and throw it! But when they succeed, when they start feeling good about their new sleep skills, they often want to call me on the phone and tell me how proud they are of themselves! They can even send me an e-mail at proudkids@sleeplady.com and I'll send them a certificate you can print out and decorate!

Keep the discussion upbeat and positive. You don't want your child to feel she has a problem, or that she's doing something wrong. To the contrary, you should portray it as your problem, your responsibility. 'Mummy and Daddy should have helped you learn to put yourself to sleep earlier, and we are sorry we didn't. But the Sleep Lady helped us understand that, and now we are going to help you learn.'

Sleep Lady Tip

You may be surprised at how sensitive children already are to sleep issues, and how quickly they pick up the lingo. Many children are relieved when parents bring this up. They know that something is wrong, that their parents are frustrated and want them to sleep differently. They are happy to know you are going to help them fix it.

Explain that children who go to bed without fussing and who sleep all night feel better in the morning and have more fun during the day. Encourage her to brainstorm about how she can participate, maybe by deciding what she can take into her bed to touch, hug, or twirl, or what extra game she will get to play in the morning if she uses her good sleep manners at night. You want her to have a stake in success.

If you think it will help, you can give your child examples, preferably of an older friend or cousin she looks up to. Say something like, 'We are going to teach you how to put yourself to sleep and sleep all night long in your own bed, just like cousin Johnny and cousin Jenny and Grandma and Aunt Rachel.' Be careful; you want to frame this in a positive way, not to make your child feel ashamed that she's not doing something you want or expect of her, or that other children are able to do.

At four, Isabel had trouble falling asleep, and seldom slept through the night. She usually ended up in a sleeping bag on the floor next to her parents. Her little sister Deirdre, in contrast, didn't mind just hanging out in her cot for a half hour or so until she fell asleep. Rita and Elliott put up with Isabel's problems until their third child, Rebecca, was born, and then it just got too hard to deal with three young children, two of whom were up half the time. Rita and Elliott convened a family meeting and learned that Isabel was already well aware of the problem. 'I told her that Daddy and I found out we were supposed to have taught her how to fall asleep by herself, like Deirdre. We said we talked to a lady who is an expert and she gave us some ideas. Isabel said she wanted to go to sleep like Deirdre. She was totally intrigued,' Rita remembered. Isabel was more aware of the problem, and more ready to make changes, than her parents had realized.

Explain clearly what changes your family will make so the child knows what to expect. Warn her about an earlier or more structured bedtime, or a new routine. 'Daddy is not going to lie down with you anymore, but Daddy will stay with you until you fall asleep.' Or 'If you come to our bed at night, we are going to tell you we love you and give you a big hug and take you back into your bed where you can snuggle with your teddy bear.' Adapt the script to the appropriate sleep challenge, but you don't have to give a lot more detail. Introduce a sticker chart to clearly define your expectations.

> Marcy said of her three-year-old daughter, 'Ariella is a real creature of habit, so I always prep her about change. If I do something one night, she'll expect it the next night. She'll say, 'Why don't you have your hand on my leg? You had it there yesterday.' I prep her all day long, letting her know about change in advance. I'll say, 'Tonight we're going to do this, but tomorrow it's going to be that.' If I don't tell her, she starts asking about tomorrow.'

Sticker Charts

Kids love stickers, stamps, and stars, and they work great for this age. As an extra incentive, you can let them choose their own stickers. Children can have toothbrushing sticker charts, potty sticker charts, eating-vegetables sticker charts, putting-away-toys sticker charts, not-screaming-for-a-cookie-during-communion sticker charts. And of course they have sleep sticker charts. But start with the sleep sticker chart. Later on you can introduce charts for other behaviors (or combine them – you can include toothbrushing as an item on the sleep sticker chart if you want). I don't want them to get a sticker for something relatively simple, or at least simple for adults to enforce, and then lack the motivation to earn another sticker by doing something much harder, like modifying years of sleep behavior. Nor do I want sleep modification to get tangled up with other power struggles – over cleanup, for example.

How elaborate your sticker scheme is depends on your child's age and temperament. Some kids, particularly younger ones, are perfectly happy to just get a star or a sticker stuck on a piece of paper or on their shirt so they can wear it and show it off all day. (Remember to remove them before you do the laundry!) Later you can create a more complex chart and your child can decorate it.

Sleep Lady Tip

I like to call it a *sleep manners* chart, instead of *sleep rules*. *Rules* implies judgment, or even potential punishment. *Manners* connotes expected daily behavior. It's a reminder that we want to incorporate manners in our life all the time, not just when we are getting stickers.

If you want, you can do a one-page chart for each week so he can see his track record and maybe get a little extra bonus at the end of each week. Ariella, for instance, got an assortment of stickers, but the special sparkly gold one was her reward at the end of a good week. To make a weekly chart, turn the paper horizontally, put the days of the week along the top, and the manners across the left, or short, side. You can even leave a little space to jot down a simple log: what time he went to bed, how long he slept, and so on.

Choose three to four manners that best apply to your child. You can change them over time if you need to, but not so often that you confuse your child about goals. Phrase the manners in positive terms – 'do's,' not 'don'ts.' Here are a few examples:

- 'Lie quietly in bed.' (This means no shouting or yelling; talking or humming quietly to themselves or their stuffed animal is okay.)
- 'Put yourself to sleep' or 'Put yourself to sleep without Mummy or Daddy lying down with you.'
- 'Put yourself quietly back to sleep during the night' or 'Put yourself back to sleep during the night without calling out.'
- 'Sleep or lie in bed quietly until 6:00 a.m.' (or whatever realistic time you choose) or 'Stays in bed quietly until the wake-up light (or music) comes on.'
- 'Go back to sleep without calling for Mummy or Daddy in the middle of the night.'
- 'Cooperate at nap or quiet time.'

In the beginning, include one relatively easy bedtime rule so they can always get some positive feedback. For instance, one category can be 'Cooperate at bedtime' a.k.a. 'Put on your pajamas without making Mummy have to chase you around the room!' This is a competence builder. It helps her feel she can live up to the new sleep expectations, that it's not too hard for her.

When your child becomes satisfied with that easy one, raise the bar. Tell her she is so very good at getting that sticker that she will now have to focus on a new manner. Get her invested in the new chart – give her a bunch of stickers as a 'graduation' present for that item, if it helps, or let her go to the store with you and select the stickers she will earn for the next task. (You can buy stickers online or from a catalog, or try your local pound shop.)

Hillary positively beamed with pride when she got her stickers, but after a good start in modifying her poor sleep habits, her progress stalled; she even regressed a bit. Her mum, Hope, changed the chart. She took off that easy 'Brush your teeth and put on your pajamas' and replaced it with 'No yelling out for Mummy and cooperate more with Daddy at bedtime.' Hillary was not pleased. She called out fifty-five times for Mum (Hope counted) that night. She finally asked for a book instead of Mum, and Hope gave it to her. She then fell asleep.

Give the chart some good, focused attention every night at bedtime, even if she appears to be ignoring you. You can talk about it during the day, too, emphasizing her successes, gently reminding her of expectations but not dwelling on failures. But the nighttime review is essential. In the morning, give out the rewards promptly, not just the stickers themselves but praise and hugs, which mean even more to her than those cherished stickers. Try not to make her feel that she is bad if she failed, just tell her that she can try again that night and that you know she can do it. Remind her of some other achievement that she is proud of, sleep related or not. If she's done a really good sleep job, you can give her an extra sticker for her jacket or her hand so she can show it to her grandmother, babysitter, preschool teacher, or the bank teller.

Give out the rewards promptly, not just the stickers themselves but praise and hugs, which mean even more to her than those cherished stickers.

Rewards

Some parents promise a reward, a gift, or trip, if the child earns a certain number of stickers. This isn't always necessary – the stickers, the praise, the hugs, the sense of accomplishment can be adequate rewards themselves. If you do want to give an extra reward, or if you've been using the sticker chart for some time and need a little extra pizzazz, go ahead and add a carrot, but start small and be realistic. If you promise a trip to Disney World, what are you going to do for a follow-up? With a small reward, you can withhold it if he regresses, but are you really going to cancel a trip to Disney World if he wakes up a few nights and climbs into your bed? You are probably better off just promising him a trip to the zoo!

Occasionally, children, particularly when they are a little older, need sticks in addition to carrots – although I'm not big on punishment, so maybe we should talk about 'twigs' instead of sticks. They may also need some privileges taken away to get them to change sleep behavior. It can be a little thing, like not letting her help you switch the kitchen light on in the morning if they woke you up before 6:00, or not so little, like taking away a favorite video, computer time, or morning TV if she still gets up in the middle of the night. I use this as a last resort, usually with older children, and I don't use it very often. And I never use the twig without the carrot. When I take away a privilege, I continue to offer a lot of praise and positive reinforcement for what the child is doing right.

Laurel ended cosleeping and improved Kerry's sleep when he was about two and a half, but a few months later he began getting out of bed repeatedly. She tried all sorts of solutions, but she wasn't a very good limit setter, and he knew it. We worked on giving Kerry many choices about things during the day – but making him under-

stand that he didn't get to make the rules at bedtime or naptime. Laurel eventually began taking a toy away from him when he wasn't cooperating. I suggested that instead of a toy, she take away an activity or privilege, like a favorite DVD or TV show. I also urged her to talk to Kerry about the consequences of breaking the rules shortly before lights-out – but not get into threats, recriminations, or even any discussion while he was misbehaving and getting out of bed.

Think of family outings and activities as rewards, instead of toys and games. Tell your child that if he earns his sleep chart, he can decide whether you are going out for pancakes Sunday morning or for pizza Saturday night. Treats can be free. Tell him Daddy will take him for an extra trip to the playground, or they can go sledging twice in one day. (Don't promise sledging in July; you want the reinforcement of a reward to come quickly after the behavior.) You can say Mummy will read three extra stories one afternoon or watch a special video with him twice. You have enough plastic junk in the house already, and time with you is more valuable to your child than anything you can get at the store.

Creating a Schedule

Scheduling isn't as elaborate or as difficult for these children as it is for younger ones, and the schedule may well be shaped largely by his preschool hours. Generally, you want your child to wake up between 6:00 and 7:30 a.m. Six is quite common and, unless they are tired by 7:00, perfectly acceptable. I'll address later how to help a child who persistently wakes up before 6:00.

Usually preschoolers need a midmorning snack, and then have lunch around noon or 12:30. If they are still napping, a common time is about 1:00 to 3:00 in the afternoon. When they stop napping, usually at around age four, they should still have some quiet time in the late afternoon.

As napping decreases, bedtime comes earlier. If your three year old has been going to bed at 8:30, when she eases out of the after-noon nap she'll probably need to go to bed at around 7:30. By age five, you probably want her to sleep from about 8:00 p.m. to 7:00

a.m. Adjust it, of course, depending on your family schedule and her school start time, but aim for at least eleven hours of unfragmented overnight sleep.

When you see her sleep window open, get her to bed. Common sleep cues at this age include yawning, rubbing their eyes, sucking a thumb or dummy, or just general fussiness. If she falls asleep on the floor, you probably missed the cue! Take note, however, that preschoolers are adept at hiding their sleep cues so you must also pay attention to the clock. If you miss the window and she gets that cortisol-fueled second wind, get her to bed a half hour or so earlier the next night. Avoid that vicious cycle where the less they sleep, the less they sleep. Similarly, if she dozes during her bedtime routine or falls asleep the very second you turn out the lights after story time, you are probably putting her to bed too late. Move bedtime earlier by fifteen to thirty minutes.

Kids themselves at this age learn to pick up on the sleep-window concept. Occasionally, they'll just say, 'Mummy, I'm ready for bed,' or 'Nye-nye,' or just crawl into bed by themselves. But that's not too common, even with much older children.

Perceptive children might pick up on the sleep-window concept and try to outsmart you. One night when he was about three, Ilan went to bed with unusual ease, and Joanne went to spend what she thought might be a few rare quiet moments with her husband before getting their older son, Zach, to bed. No sooner had she settled herself on the living room couch than a very small blond guy in blue baseball pajamas zoomed through the living room at about a hundred miles an hour shouting, 'I missed my sleep window, Mum!'

Bedtime Routine

For this age group, the bedtime routine is typically the most challenging part of the day. Now that your child is older, you may want to modify her routine a little but make sure it remains soothing and predictable. Bedtime preparations should be in her room (or perhaps the early stage can be in a younger sibling's room), not all over the house. Include stories, songs, or games that soothe, not stimulate. Make sure the rules for how many stories, or how long you will read, are completely clear and nonnegotiable. Avoid wild, fast-moving games and scary stories.

Leave plenty of time, at least a half hour, for her to unwind, and to get the attention from you she needs. If you rush it, she'll be more likely to run out of bed or stall or manipulate you into staying longer. If she starts bargaining for an even longer time with you, more stories or more songs, blame the clock. Tell her the clock says you have to stop reading at 8:00, so you have ten minutes. If two parents take turns at bedtime, you don't have to follow an identical script but you should have a similar routine, style, and response to bedtime power plays, fears, or manipulation.

'We used to have to go in his room for a half hour to play before we did our routine, but that's not necessary anymore,' said Amanda, who was able to reshape her son Wes's troublesome sleep after his apnea was corrected with adenoid surgery when he turned four, an experience you can read more about in Chapter 15, 'Medical Problems.' 'He goes into his room to play by himself and then we go in for ten or fifteen minutes. We read books, say a prayer, and have a quiet talk about our day. That's all he needs.'

Ariella is a champion negotiator who always tries to con Marcy into just one more story. It's a quandary for Marcy and Doyle because they know they need to be consistent, but sometimes if they don't succumb, Ariella gets so worked up and hysterical that it becomes that much harder to get her to sleep. 'It jacks her up; she gets more awake,' her mother said.

Recently Marcy has been using my advice to blame the clock. 'I started showing Ariella the time, and at first I thought it would be more stress and pressure, but I was wrong. It was a great idea. I can show her the time and tell her, 'You have to hurry or else you'll lose your book time.'' While most of Ariella's sleep issues are resolved and she generally sleeps through the night now, the stalling hasn't gone away completely, although it's not totally out of control, either. The clock promises to be another useful tool in containing it.

It's often a good idea to warn your children a minute or two before lights-out: 'We have a few more pages in this book, and then Mummy is going to turn out the light.' Sometimes they like to turn out the light themselves. It's another way they can 'own' bedtime. You might want to blame bedtime on the clock. 'Oh, look! The clock says 8:00. Lights-out time. We can't read any more books tonight. We'll have to get upstairs earlier tomorrow night so that we can read more books.'

If your child doesn't respond to the sight of numbers, you might try a clock radio or a timer. 'Oh, the music went on' or 'Oh, the bell rang, it's time for bed.' If the clock ploy doesn't work, feel free to blame me! 'It's 8:00. The Sleep Lady says we have to turn out the lights now.'

Some children will say, 'I can't do it; I can't put myself to sleep.' Explain that everyone has trouble going to sleep sometimes, even Mummy and Daddy, and then teach them some simple relaxation techniques and creative visualization. (See the 'Resource Directory' for some suggestions on age-appropriate guided visualizations and relaxation exercises.) Children have such wonderfully active imaginations, they are actually better at visualization than we are. They may not understand the word *visualization*, but they certainly get *pretend* and *imagine*. They can learn how to think relaxing thoughts at bedtime, how to close their eyes and imagine playing at the beach, building a snowman, taking a summer walk with their cousins in the woods.

Try to build on the images in their favorite illustrated book and

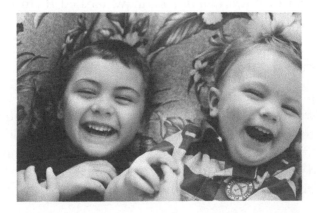

have them imagine entering the book to play with the characters (as long as there are no scary themes). My own girls loved playing 'in' *Angelina Ballerina*. The mouse house illustrations were so inviting and warm. Your children will come up with their own suggestions and will pleasantly surprise you with their creativity. I had one parent tell her daughter about my own girls' Angelina Ballerina game. They tried it, and then the little girl chose books of her own to 'go into.' She even had her mother call me on the phone so she could recommend it to my family.

You might also want to teach your child deep-relaxation techniques, the kind you do at the end of a good exercise class or before going into labor! Have her relax her toes, her feet, her ankles, shins, knees, and so forth, all the way up her body. If you don't want to do this yourself, you can play a relaxation CD (see my list of suggestions at the back of the book or try the Sleep Lady CD, *The Sweetest Dreams*, which has a relaxation exercise, available at www.sleeplady.com).

Children also like applying their imaginations to a dream agenda. 'Tonight I'll dream about playing basketball.' Or 'Tonight I will dream about building a sand castle.' Or 'Tonight I will dream about being a beautiful ballerina.' It helps them feel more in control of what happens to them after they fall asleep, particularly if they are worried about having nightmares. My 'Dream Cards' (also on my website) might help children feel in control of their dreams. The cards guide children through a progressive relaxation exercise and have several images for dream ideas such as a tree house, a beach scene, a field of flowers, and a rainbow. I based them on my experiences with creating dreams with my own daughters.

The Sleep Lady Shuffle

My Sleep Lady Shuffle is still a useful tool for this age group. But I'll warn you that it isn't as easy doing the Shuffle with a three or four year old in a bed as with a six month old in a cot. The Shuffle is gentle and gradual, but older children still get upset and fight the change. Don't get angry, but don't give up, either. Keep reminding him that he can learn to put himself to sleep in his wonderful 'big boy' bed without Mummy lying down with him.

Throughout the Shuffle we try to minimize tears, but I can't promise to eliminate them completely. Luckily, by the time our children are three or four most of us aren't as worried about tears damaging our children. We've inevitably had to listen to our share of tears by now, and we find it easier to cope with crying now that our children can also use words to communicate their wants and worries. To keep the tears in check, give plenty of reassurance, love, and praise. In addition to reviewing rules and expectations every night at bedtime, you should also pay your child some sleep compliments during the day. Don't dwell on his sleep failures, but keep praising his sleep achievements. (The directions here are for children in beds. If your child is still in a cot, follow the version of the Shuffle in the previous chapter, but do a little more explaining about each step, which helps an older child with better verbal skills buy into the Shuffle.)

If your child wakes up in the middle of the night, and he probably will at first, pat or soothe him briefly in bed and then return to where you were sitting at bedtime that night until he falls asleep again. We want to give a consistent response to every wakening. I give tips later in this chapter on ways of dealing with specific bedtime and middle-of-the-night sleep crutches.

Keep moving every three days, even if he had a bad night, woke up frequently, or protested a lot. Expect some regression or resistance each time you move a little further from his bed, but stick to it. Particularly with this age group, it's essential not to backtrack or give mixed signals. If he gets sick during the Shuffle, give him extra hugs and kisses and then maintain or 'freeze' your Shuffle position or sit closer if needed. When he starts to feel better, continue with the Shuffle. Try not to drag it out too long.

As you go through the Sleep Lady Shuffle with children this age, remember your biggest challenge will probably be that they will get out of bed and try to climb on your lap or hug or hold onto you. To make the Shuffle more successful and less stressful, remember:

- Children do better when they know what to expect, so explain things carefully.

- Review sleep manners and expectations every morning and repeat the explanations as you move through the Shuffle.
- Children respond well to positive reinforcement, so give them plenty of praise and encouragement.
- Allow plenty of time for bedtime routine; this isn't the time to rush.
- If your child wakes up in the middle of the night, go to him, calm him quickly, and then resume the Shuffle position you had at bedtime that night.
- They will test you – particularly if you haven't been consistent with them in the past.
- They may or may not still like sticker charts as a reward for good sleep behavior. Some kids outgrow them, while some will like increasingly elaborate sticker charts through the early school years. They may particularly dislike charts that encourage behavior – like sleeping on their own – that they don't want to do!

Nights 1–3. Once bath, stories, and songs are over, *sit in a chair or on the floor next to your child's bed*. Stroke or pat him intermittently if he fusses or cries, but don't do it constantly or he will form a new negative association and will need you to pat him constantly in order to fall asleep. You can be a little more generous with touch the first night, when the whole system is new to him, but be careful about creating difficult new patterns, starting on the second night. Children this age will almost certainly try to engage you. Try closing your eyes, which not only conveys an unambiguously sleepy message but also makes it easier for you to resist getting drawn into a conversation or philosophical seminar about the nature of the universe. Stay there until he falls asleep.

Some children get quite upset even on this first night if you won't lie down with them. In desperation some parents have put their head down on the pillow next to their child. Try not to do it, and if you do, please restrict it to the first night or you aren't going to make much progress. You will not be changing your child's ritual, or teaching him to learn new skills if you are sharing a pillow! Be careful to stroke, pat, sing, or hold hands intermittently, not constantly, at least after the first night. You will just be replacing one crutch with another. You, not the child, should be in charge of the touching. For instance, if he grabs your hand, gently remove it but then touch his hand sporadically. Close your eyes and 'sh-sh' him. Remember, in three more nights you won't be sitting next to him and won't be able to touch him constantly. You want to be able to fade out of his sleep picture, not add to his fury each time you make a change.

Nights 4–6. Tell him what a good job of sleeping, what a good night-night boy he's been, and how proud you are. Explain the next move. Tell him that you are going to give him a big wonderful hug, and then *move your chair to the door inside his room*. Reassure him that you will be able to see him and he will be able to see you. Promise him that you will still stay in the room until he falls asleep, but that once you turn out the lights, there's no more talking.

Once you are in the chair by the door, stay as quiet as possible, but an occasional soothing 'sh-sh' is okay. Stay in the chair, only getting up to pat or stroke him as little as needed. If he gets so upset that he needs some help calming down, go to his bedside, reassure him, and give him a deep-pressure hug. Remind him that you aren't going to leave him, that you'll stay until he falls asleep. Don't let him fall asleep in your arms or lap, and don't lie down with him in his bed. Keep telling him what a good job he's doing, and how proud you are of him. Return to your chair.

If he fights the Shuffle by getting out of bed and coming to you or trying to crawl into your lap, give him a big hug and return him to bed. If he does it again, take him back to the bed. Don't talk, don't reason, don't explain, don't get exasperated. Just put him back.

Usually they get tired and stay in bed, particularly if they become more confident that you are going to stay there until they fall asleep. But if he doesn't stop getting out of his bed, stand up and explain very clearly that if he keeps it up, you will have to leave. You can say something like, 'If you don't follow your sleep manners and lie quietly in your bed, then I am going to have to leave your room.' Remind him that if he does stay in bed and follows his sleep manners, you will stay there as long as he needs you to fall asleep, and that you will check on him before you go to bed.

Most children then stay in bed. If yours absolutely doesn't you have two choices:

- You can put a gate on the door and sit on the other side of the gate until he falls asleep. Tell him that if he gets in bed and stays in bed, you will come in and tuck him in. If he falls asleep on the floor near the gate, move him later when he's in a sound sleep.
- This is a little tougher, and it's an option for parents, not a requirement. If you choose, stand up (so he can't climb on you) and warn your child that if he doesn't get into bed and lie quietly that you will not sit in his room, you will leave and briefly close the door. Tell him he has one more chance to get in his bed and that if he is not in bed by the time you count to three you will leave the room and shut the door. Count to three. If he does not get back in to bed, you must follow through. Leave the room and close the door. Stand right outside the closed door and count to ten. Open the door and say calmly, 'Get back into your bed and I will come sit in your room.' Usually they make a mad dash into the bed; they want you sitting there.

Some preschoolers (especially if they are particularly alert or determined) will test you to see if you are going to follow through on your threat, particularly if you have not followed through on consequences in the past. If he does not get back in the bed, then repeat the counting to three and closing the door. Don't yell; be calm and firm but not exasperated or impatient. If closing the door gets your child overly upset and hysterical, stick with the gate.

Nights 7–9. Continue the praise, positive reinforcement, and clear explanation of what he can expect, and what you expect of him. Keep praising him on what a good sleeping boy he is becoming. *Sit in the hallway in view.* You can keep making those 'sh-sh' sounds from the hallway, not constantly, but with enough frequency to remind him you care. Some kids have trouble with this, and keep coming to you in the hallway and asking you to come back in the room. Tell him if he gets back into his bed *on his own* you will come in and tuck him in. If this happens repeatedly, you will have to put a limit on the number of tuck-ins. If it gets excessive, consider the options above, either putting up a gate in the door or trying the count-to-ten door-closing exercise.

Nights 10–12. Go through the same routine – praise and positive reinforcement, and an explanation of the next step. Now you will be *sitting in the hallway, but out of his view*. Leave his door open a crack or a few inches. Tell him you will be nearby, and use your voice intermittently to reassure him of your presence. If he comes out of bed, go through the same recommended options that you've used the last few nights.

Night 13. A fair number of children start falling asleep and staying asleep by the end of two weeks (it takes longer with older kids) – occasionally even sooner. But most parents have to take one more step and leave the child alone for five-minute intervals. Tell him that you will keep checking on him until he is asleep. When you check on him, just go as far as the doorway; don't go into the room where it will be easier for him to reengage you or tug at you all over again.

Children don't really understand what 'five minutes' means, and it may seem like a very long time to them lying in bed. It helps if you explain exactly where you will be and describe what you will be doing. Some parents sit down the hall out of sight for a few nights. Others do what I call *job checks*. Tell him that you will check on him in a few minutes after you've brushed your teeth, or changed your clothes, or some other brief but comprehensible task that helps him understand that you will be back quite soon. They sometimes like it if your 'jobs' have to do with getting yourself ready for bed, too. *Always return as promised.*

Leaving the child may seem like a radical change for you, but please remember that he's had nearly two weeks of preparation. He has given up some of his negative associations and gained quite a bit of sleep independence. He is old enough to understand that you are close by even if you are out of sight. Don't go too far away – stay on the same floor, in a nearby room, and just read a magazine or a book for the first few nights. Gradually, you can move a little further away. If he cries, you'll be back every five minutes to reassure him. Try not to go in more than that; he'll just get more stimulated and more upset if he has to say good-bye to you every two minutes.

Unlike the crying-it-out approaches, you don't keep stretching out the intervals for longer than five minutes. The only exception is if you sense that five minutes is too brief for your individual child, that having to see you but separate again every five minutes is making him more agitated. Then experiment and see if he finds it less disturbing if you check on him every ten or fifteen minutes. Parents often resist this idea; they are so worried about harming their children by being away from them, they have trouble adjusting to the idea that certain children actually need a little more distance to calm themselves down and fall asleep.

He may well cry a bit the first few nights – he may even cry a fair amount for one or two nights. But very rarely do children cry persistently during the full Shuffle. If he does cry, check on him from the doorway. Remind him to hug his lovey. Be reassuring but calm. Keep in mind, he has gained confidence that you are nearby and responsive. He's ready to learn this.

By the way, if you do use the gate, or close the door briefly, and it's hard for you, feel free to blame it on me! 'The Sleep Lady told us you are so used to waking up during the night and getting out of your bed that you are forgetting your sleep manners. She told us to put up the gate so that if you wake up tonight and get to the door, it will help you remember your sleep manners and stay in your bed.' A preschooler may not get this right off the bat, but repetition is key at this age. Stick with it (and keep blaming me!). You may also consider some kind of incentive – either taking a privilege briefly away from your child (if that's your parenting style) and then restoring it as soon as he follows his sleep manners. Or once he's been making progress for a week or so, consider giving him some kind of reward, either extra stickers or a special activity or time with you. (I'd rather you give of yourself, not buy him a material reward or junk food.)

You could also try to portray the gate as a treat, not a threat. It doesn't have to be horrible. A mum I know decorated the gate with colorful ribbons so her little girl loved having it up at bedtime. I worked with one little boy who just loved his gate. He decided it was like an entrance to his own apartment, just like *The Wiggles* had on television.

Cliff slept reasonably well until he was about two, when a series of changes, including a new baby sister and the start of child care, threw him off. Dislocation because of home remodeling was the last straw. The family stayed at Cliff's grandmother's house, with mum, Hailey, sleeping upstairs with the baby, Janice, while Cliff and his dad, Harry, camped out in the living room, one on a cot, one on the couch.

When they went back to their own home, Cliff was much clingier. He also experienced night terrors sometimes. His parents let him stay up until 9:30, by which time he was overtired but wired. It took forever to get him to sleep, and Harry often fell asleep in Cliff's bed before Cliff did. 'Hailey would come in at 11:30 or midnight and tap me on the shoulder and say, 'Come to bed — he's asleep now!'' Harry recalled.

About two months before his third birthday, Hailey and Harry told Cliff that the 'Sleep Lady' had given them new bedtime rules. 'I don't like the Sleep Lady,' he declared. They began taking him upstairs between 7:30 and 8:00 p.m., for a shorter and more structured bedtime routine. They still snuggled, but now they snuggled during the lights-on stage of the bedtime routine.

When they started the Shuffle, Cliff, whom Harry described as a 'very spirited child,' was not at all pleased. Cliff did okay the first few nights, when Harry was beside his bed. He tried to coax his dad into his bed, but he acquiesced when Harry declined. But the further Harry moved away, the unhappier Cliff got. 'When I moved the chair, he would plead; he would look sad and cry quietly. That was worse for me than having him screaming mad at me.' But because they had shifted his bedtime and improved their routine, Cliff still fell asleep an hour earlier than usual.

When Harry neared the end of the Shuffle, standing by the door and then leaving to make checks, Cliff screamed and ran out of the room. Harry said it felt like he ran out a million times, but in fact it was only about three. Then he'd go to bed. Within a few weeks, he stopped protesting at bedtime. His father made checks every five minutes for a while, and after about two weeks, noticing that the checks sometimes caused Cliff to stir when he was almost asleep, Harry switched to one check after five minutes, which Cliff liked, and then he wouldn't come back for another twenty minutes, by which time Cliff was almost always asleep.

'Big Kid' Bed Tips for the Sleep Lady Shuffle

1. *Don't get into a power struggle. Doing the Shuffle with a child who is in a bed, not a cot, can be a challenge.* If she sits up in bed, ignore it; if she gets out, pat the mattress and encourage her to get back in. Do not chase her around and put her in bed.
2. *You can reach over and stroke, pat, rub your child intermittently in her bed.* But don't caress her constantly until she falls asleep or it will become her new sleep crutch. Stop the stroking when she is starting to fall asleep. (Some children don't like to be touched as they fall asleep; follow their cues.)
3. *The parent controls the touch.* Don't let your child fall asleep grasping your finger or hand, for example, because she will wake up when you move and it will all start all over again. Pat or stroke a different part of her body or the top of her hand. If she keeps putting her legs on yours, or persists in trying to touch you, scoot your chair away. You can still lean in to touch or reassure her.
4. *If she becomes hysterical, hug her in her bed to calm her, but don't lie down in her bed.* Don't let her fall asleep in your arms. Hysteria is not common at this age, although the toughest nights are probably later in the Shuffle when you are sitting in the hallway but still in her view.
5. *Return to your Shuffle position and follow these rules each time she awakes at night.* Go to her bed, give her a kiss, encourage her to lie down if necessary, and sit in the chair. Do this at each awakening until 6:00 a.m. Remind her of her wake-up light or music.

Cliff's night wakenings also decreased during the Shuffle. When he did wake, Harry checked on him quickly to make sure he was okay, and then reminded him to snuggle with his special blanket and stuffed animals. He'd tell him, 'The Sleep Lady says you have to sleep all night.' It didn't make Cliff a fan of mine, but he listened! Soon, all that Cliff would need when he woke up was a quick reassuring look at his father, then he'd roll over and go back to sleep.

The first week of the Shuffle, Cliff woke up two or three times each night. The second week, he woke up only two times during the whole week. The third week saw a little regression; he slept through three nights and woke up once or twice the other nights. That was it; he began sleeping through pretty consistently, except of course if he was sick. Some mornings he did talk about having been up briefly but was very proud that he could get himself back to sleep. He'd say, 'I didn't cry out for you, Daddy,' so Harry knew that Cliff had woken up, taken his blanket, and gone back to sleep. 'I gave him lots of praise for that,' his father said.

Children get ritualized easily. Make the changes every three days – or less. Dragging it out makes it harder, not easier, for him. Give it more than three days, and he'll expect you to stay exactly where you are and get even more frustrated and angry when you try to double that distance.

Some parents decide to stop the Shuffle at the point when they are sitting in the hallway a few feet from the child's room. If that feels right to you, go ahead and try it, as long as it's not taking an hour and the child doesn't need you to come back to the doorway on and off all night long. Other families continue to make the five-minute checks for weeks or months, if that's what makes everyone comfortable. That's okay as long as he's sleeping through the night and falling asleep reasonably quickly, that he's not using those checks as an excuse to keep himself awake so he can keep seeing you. But most families do get to the point where they can do their bedtime routine, say good night, and leave.

'Even now I can't go downstairs until Wes falls asleep,' Amanda said, months after Wes sailed through the Shuffle and began sleeping beautifully. 'I can be somewhere else on the same floor, but I can't go down and do the dishes. Luckily, there's always enough for me to do upstairs, believe me. But he likes me to go in and check on him from the doorway; it's very reassuring to him.'

Sometimes even children who have 'graduated' from the Shuffle and sleep well regress a little. Routines get disrupted, illnesses occur, or they experience normal waves of fear or insecurity. Don't return to whatever prolonged and convoluted bedtime techniques you used before the Shuffle. Be particularly wary of relapsing into cosleeping. Instead, sit quietly in the doorway for two or three nights, where he can see you. That allows you to be present and comforting, without abandoning all your progress. Then move on to the final steps of the Shuffle. It should go pretty smoothly.

Problems and Solutions

Many sleep experts maintain that once children learn to fall asleep by themselves at bedtime, they will sleep all night. In my experience, that is often but by no means always the case. I have found that night awakenings become much briefer and less frequent in one to three weeks after starting the Shuffle, and that the children go back to sleep much more quickly with less help from us. But the awakenings don't necessarily totally evaporate, particularly with older children whose sleep problems may date back a few years. In this section, I will help you address specific middle-of-the-night sleep crutches that may linger after bedtime problems dissipate (or that you may want to understand better as you go through the Shuffle).

Your child may still want you to lie down with her at 3:00 a.m., even if she no longer needs that at 8:00 p.m. She may want to be snuggled or given yet another cup or bottle when she wakes up at night. She may still be sending you scurrying to find that dummy under the bed. Dealing with the normal nighttime fears and worries of the preschool years, a child may just wake up to say, 'Hi, Mum, just testing! Just checking to make sure you're where you're supposed to be!'

We want to give our children enough comfort so
that they feel safe and can go back to sleep, but not
so much reinforcement that they have no incentive
to give up these awakenings.

I believe in responding when our children need us. Leaving them to scream in the dark does not promote good sleep for them or for us. Checking on them makes them feel better, and it makes us feel better. (You do need to make sure she's truly awake before you rush in to 'rescue' her. If she's whimpering or crying out briefly during a partial awakening, don't charge in with parental sirens blaring when she's about to drift back into a deeper sleep on her own.) But we don't want to overdo it. We want to give our children enough comfort so that they feel safe and can go back to sleep, but not so much reinforcement that they have no incentive to give up these awakenings. Make sure she's going to bed early enough, and getting the naps she needs at her age. Overtired children are more likely to wake up at night.

When your child wakes up at night during the Shuffle, give her a brief reassuring pat and return to the position you were in that night at bedtime. Sometimes after children have finished the Shuffle and are sleeping well, something may throw them off and you may have a few night awakenings. If she gets up, quietly return her to her bed, and sit in a chair or stand in the doorway. You might want to start in the chair, and then after a night or two move to the door, similar to what you did during the Shuffle to fade yourself out of her middle-of-the-night picture.

Remember – do not engage her. Bore her. Do not take her into your bed. Do not get into her bed. Do not pick her up and walk around the house. Do not criticize or scold or talk about consequences or punishments or disappointments at this particular time. In fact, do not talk at all except for a few soft phrases like 'Night-night' or 'I love you. Go to sleep.' Hand her the lovey and give her a quick hug and a kiss, but don't do too much hugging, patting, and cuddling or she'll keep waking up every night wanting her fix of snuggles. Leave as soon as you can without engendering hysterics.

The exception to the rule: Some children do better if we don't respond, if we do let them cry – not for hours but for a few minutes. These are kids who get more awake, more stimulated, when you come in at night. Occasionally, I've come across couples so utterly convinced that their child can't get back to sleep without them that they have trouble recognizing when the opposite is true, when the child actually goes to sleep better without them in the room. But most parents know instinctively when they should leave their child alone and when they do belong at her side, or at least in her doorway.

Bells and Whistles

Occasionally, children sneak into your bed during the night but you don't even notice until much later. Hang a plastic kitchen utensil or a bell from your bedroom door and close the door enough so the child has to push it to enter. The bell or spoon will probably make enough noise to wake you up. Warn her that you are going to do this, and let her hear what it sounds like, so it doesn't terrify her in the middle of the night.

One mum said it didn't really bother her if her two and a half year old sneaked into her bed – she didn't even notice, and everybody slept. She had second thoughts after the night her daughter crawled into bed with some unsuspecting houseguests.

Gates and Doors

Some parents use gates on the bedroom door, either to keep children from popping out of bed repeatedly at bedtime or as a safety measure to prevent nocturnal wandering. Some kids respect the gate as a boundary; they like the visible limit. Others climb over it, knock it down, or figure out how to unlock it. A few families I've worked with have even put up two gates, if they are dealing with particularly agile climbers or future safecrackers.

Some kids detest the gate so much that their parents don't even have to use it; they just say, 'If you get out of bed again, I'll put up the gate,' and that does the trick. Or instead of threatening, they entice. They put up the gate but say, 'As soon as you lie down quietly in your bed and stay there, I'll take down the gate.' Or 'If you follow all your sleep manners tonight, we can take the gate down tomorrow night.'

Parents may choose to sit or lie down on the other side of the gate as a transitional step once they have reached the hallway stage of the Shuffle. That enables you to reassure your child that Mum or Dad is there, while reinforcing the message that she has to stay in her room after lights-out.

Sam had been a pretty good sleeper for more than two years. His mum, Nora, a labor and delivery nurse, found Dr Marc Weissbluth's explanations of infant sleep cycles helpful, and she successfully followed his crying-it-out technique with Sam at four months. But in his second year, Sam had all sorts of changes: a lot of travel, some separation from his father due to a job change, then a move from Washington to California, and yet more travel. His mum also discovered she was pregnant during all this transition, so Sam had both a new home, a new routine, and a little sister on the way. His sleep deteriorated, and even though Nora as a nurse knew a whole lot about newborns, Sam's nighttime problems stumped her and she didn't think leaving him alone to scream was going to help.

He was just about three when we did the Shuffle. It was successful up to the point where they left him alone in his room. Two seconds later, he would appear. They tried to reason with him but – guess what? – reason didn't get them very far. So they made up the 'two-strikes' method. The first time Sam came out of the room, they told him, 'Strike one,' and returned him to his room. When he marched out the second time, they'd say, 'Strike two,' and put up two gates, one on top of the other because he was an incredible climber. But he wasn't able to get around the double barrier. 'He could climb over one, but he was a little gun-shy about climbing over two,' Nora said. He sometimes would fall asleep on the floor with his pillow by the door, and they would put him in bed later.

His sleep improved, but another round of holiday travel to relatives and the birth of his sister threw him off. By now, he literally had worn out the gates. Nora shut the door. 'I held it shut, and he wigged out. My husband was freaked out that my son was freaked out. I held it for about thirty seconds, and you could tell I made my point.' All she had to do after that was threaten to shut the door, and he'd hop back into bed.

But in the next few weeks after Lizzie's birth, Nora's instincts told her to compromise – but to have a definite plan for ending the compromise. Lizzie is cosleeping with her parents, so Sam gets to come into Mum and Dad's room, too. He isn't allowed in their bed; he has a special little sleeping place on the floor, and he brings his special fleece, his stuffed pig, and some water to drink.

As soon as Lizzie gets to the point where she's only nursing once a night, she'll be out of their bed, and Nora will put both kids in Sam's room. She knows that Sam might then require a little refresher course in sleeping, but thinks this arrangement is best for him right now, and doesn't anticipate that retraining him will be all that hard, especially with his little sister in his room. 'I'm letting him sleep near us because it's finite. Then there will be no kids in our bedroom until morning. That's easier than having different rules for different kids,' Nora said, adding, 'I think he'll like being in the room with her. He loves her, loves her, loves her; once she's in there, things might take care of themselves.'

Eliminating Nighttime Feeding

If your child still takes a bottle, it's definitely time to get rid of it. Explain that she is a big girl now and doesn't need a bottle. She may well realize this herself by now. Offer her a cup of water during story time, and if she cries for her bottle, soothe, comfort, and distract her but don't give her the bottle. In fact, you should get the bottles out of the house or at least out of sight (or adapt some of the strategies overleaf for getting rid of the dummy). Focus on strengthening her attachment to a lovey as you remove the bottle, or let her choose a new lovey as an incentive. Alternatively, you could try the bottle-to-cup advice I give for younger babies in Chapter 9, 'Thirteen to Eighteen Months.' If you plan to continue nursing, try to separate it from sleep. Nurse with a light on to weaken that sleep association.

If she is emotionally attached to the water cup and it has become a sleep crutch, help her learn to go back to sleep without it. Go to her when she calls for it in the middle of the night, but either just quietly point to the cup you left by her bed and encourage her to take a sip or two and go back to sleep or try to soothe her into going back to sleep without it. Don't refill the cup. It will probably take a few nights, and you'll probably have some tears, but you can sit with her, stroke her intermittently, 'sh-sh' her, and comfort her like you would a younger child. As a reward, offer her an extra sticker instead of her cup!

Phasing Out Walking and Rocking to Sleep

By this age, children aren't usually rocked like they were as infants, but some still like to be lulled to sleep on their parents' laps during or after story time. Use the Shuffle to try to break that habit, just as you would for a child who wants you to lie down with him. Rock or hold him during the bedtime routine, while you read books and sing your songs, but don't rock him to sleep after lights-out. If he tries to climb out of bed and get in your lap, just put him back to bed and soothe him. If he wakes up at night wanting to be rocked or held, return to your Shuffle position.

Sleep Lady Tip

I have very rarely encountered a child who still wanted the rocking in the middle of the night after learning to do without it at bedtime. If yours still wakes up, soothe him but don't let him get onto your lap again. (And try not to fall asleep in his bed either at story time, or he'll expect you to be there all night.)

Dummy (Pacifier) Withdrawal

If you still aren't ready to get rid of the dummy, at this age definitely restrict it to sleep. Hide it or at least keep it by the bed but out of reach during the day, except at naptime and bedtime. If your toddler wakes up one or more times during the night summoning you to help her find her dummy, put several in and around her bed, or leave a spare in a little basket or bowl where she can find it herself. If she demands that you get it for her, go to her and gently remind her where they are and reward her for learning to do it by herself. If she absolutely cannot find it herself, then as an interim step you should retrieve it but hand it to her and make her put it into her mouth by herself. Try again to teach her to retrieve it herself when she's a few months older. Most kids over age three can manage this. Add this to her sticker chart.

Now that your child has pretty good verbal skills, consider eliminating the dummy completely. Talk to her about the decision; she's old enough to be part of it. Choose a time when she's relatively rested and relaxed – not right after she's been sick, when you've been traveling, or she's in her first week at preschool. Work on transferring some of her attachment to a lovey, and expand the lovey's role in bedtime rituals.

If you haven't already restricted the dummy to bedtime and naps, do that first before you get rid of it completely. You'll get a little resistance, but distract her and praise her for not using it. When she adapts to not having it during the day, take it away at bedtime, but let her keep it for a while longer at naps. Pick a 'big day' when she will no longer have the dummy. Give her a few days to get used to the idea. She may agree to it – but then get very upset when the big day arrives. Get the dummy out of the house; she can't demand them quite as much and you can't give in if they just aren't there anymore. If you yield when she cries, she will learn that you don't really mean it, and the next time you try to wean her from the dummy she will cry and fuss even more.

Sleep Lady Tip

I've heard lots of creative ways to get the child to invest in getting rid of the dummy, like mailing it to a new baby, or leaving it by the chimney so Santa can take it for the reindeer. Some kids wrap it up in a box and save it for their own children, although that can be a little abstract for most preschoolers. I even heard of one child who gave hers to the goat at a petting zoo, although I'm sure that could not have made the zookeeper very happy.

Once you have disposed of the dummy, brace yourself for a few rough naps and bedtimes. She will probably cry. Give her that lovey and offer extra reassurance. Cuddle a little longer before the lights go out, or sit by her bed until she falls asleep. Don't do this for more than a week, or you will be stuck by her bedside indefinitely. If you've been sitting by her bed for several days, you might want to do a truncated version of the Sleep Lady Shuffle again to get out of her room. If it's the second (or third!) time you've done it, move through it quickly: just one or two nights in each position or go straight from her bed to the doorway. Use your instincts and your judgment, but try to do it on the speedy side. Offer plenty of praise and keep encouraging attachment to a lovey.

I worked with Charlotte's twins, Ethan and Nathaniel, when they were just a few months old, and you can read about their experiences in Chapter 13, 'Helping Twins and Siblings Sleep.' But Charlotte and Ed decided at the time that they didn't want to get rid of the dummies – a decision that they later regretted! After spending three years chasing two sets of dummies, Charlotte finally got rid of them around the boys' third birthday. 'They didn't have pillows yet, but they saw a friend who had a toy under his pillow and they wanted one. I said sure, you can have a pillow and put a toy under it, but you have to get rid of the dummies first. They were fine with that – for about ten minutes and then they wanted the dummies back. I said, 'I'm sorry, it's too late.' That was it. They weren't pleased. There were rough nights, and rough naps, but I stuck with it. One of them screamed really hysterically for two weeks straight, and then he sort of said, 'Okay, never mind, I'm going to sleep.' The other was really sad and hung on and almost stopped napping, but eventually he got used to it.'

Thumb Sucking

If your child is still sucking his thumb, I don't think he'll outgrow the habit on his own. I've even met a few teenagers who still suck their thumbs, braces and all. Age four or five is a good time to address it because your child now has the language skills to communicate with you about what can be a several-month process. He also may be getting a little self-conscious about his habit.

My daughter Carleigh was a determined thumb sucker, and I decided to address the habit when she was five, already in kindergarten. She had sucked her thumb since she was six months old, and had the callus to prove it! She had a lovey, a small pillow she'd used since she was a baby, but instead of being a substitute for the thumb, it was a companion. When she snuggled against that pillow, the thumb went right into the mouth.

I enlisted her dentist's support in encouraging her to stop sucking her thumb because she was going to get 'big girl' teeth soon and we wanted them to grow in straight and strong and beautiful. Use whatever words and images will reach your child and get her invested. Her father and I empathized a lot and told her we knew it was very hard and were very proud that she was going to try. We also enlisted other people, including her grandmother, to share their memories of how they stopped sucking their thumbs as children, and how proud they felt.

Praise and encouragement will, however, get you only so far. Bribery will get you the rest of the way. We asked Carleigh what she wanted as a prize or reward. Her first choice was pierced ears, but I managed to dodge that bullet for a few more years. I let her talk me into her second choice: adopting the class hamster at the end of kindergarten. I wasn't thrilled, but at least it wasn't a class snake. We found a picture of a hamster that we pinned on her bulletin board so she could see it from her bed. I also talked to her about the hamster a lot, and of course she had the hamster in class as an additional reminder all day. We found an unexpectedly large selection of hamster books at our local library, and I think we read them all.

We started by giving up daytime thumb sucking. Children are often not even aware that they are sucking, so she agreed to let me point it out to her by gently removing her hand. I noticed patterns: Carleigh was much more likely to rely on her thumb when she was frustrated, upset, overstimulated, or overtired. Once we had cut down on daytime sucking, we got rid of the thumb sucking at naptime – she still needed an occasional nap at five and a half. (I usually recommend getting rid of thumb sucking at bedtime before napping, but I reversed that with Carleigh because at that age her naps were sporadic, while bedtime was daily.) When she napped, and later when she slept, we put bandage tape not just on her thumb but on all of her fingertips. Carleigh, a partner in this process, suggested that herself because she thought she would suck other fingers if we taped just the thumb.

As I expected, the first night in the thumb-free zone was the hardest. Carleigh was generally an excellent sleeper, but I recognized that falling asleep without the familiar association of thumb and lovey pillow was a struggle that night. She snuggled with her special pillow, looked at books, and talked to me about what she wanted to dream about. I told her I would check on her a lot that night, which I did. I reassured her that she could do this, that she would love having a hamster. It was hard for me as her mother to watch her that night, but she eventually did fall asleep.

We kept the tape for several weeks and slowly reduced the number of fingers being taped. Carleigh told me which fingers she would be most likely to suck at night. We then went tapeless but still didn't bring the hamster home until she was no longer sucking any fingers when we checked on her at night. Her callus disappeared, the nail changed shape, and she even said her thumb no longer tasted as good! (Someone once told me a sucked thumb does taste different from an unsucked thumb; it has something to do with the oils in the skin. But I confess I don't recall seeing any scientific confirmation of this phenomenon.) We finally celebrated Carleigh's accomplishments and brought home the hamster. (That hamster, alas, died, as did two of his successors.)

Although this plan worked for Carleigh, it took several months. We might have been able to do it faster, but I think it would have meant more tears, more trauma, and probably a higher risk of failure. Be patient and be creative. Involve your child, and respect her insights; she may know well what will help. I can't imagine doing this with a younger child, or one who lacks good language skills.

Early Birds

Early rising is a little more complicated once children switch from cot to bed because they can get up and try to begin their day whether you like it or not. It is a hard pattern to change, and it usually takes three or four weeks of very consistent coaching, longer if she's had early wake ups for more than six months. Children sometimes wake up too early because they are actually overtired. Remember that sleep-begets-sleep idea we talked about in Chapter 2, 'Getting Started and Tips for Success'? She may find it easier to sleep later if you make bedtime earlier by a half hour or so.

Sleep Lady Tip

If a child wakes up early but acts fine all day and doesn't doze off in late afternoon or in the car, she may need less sleep than average. Slowly move bedtime later and see if she sleeps later in the morning. But this is rare, so don't rush to try it unless you are quite certain that your child has below-average sleep needs.

Remind her at bedtime every night that she has to sleep until at least 6:00 a.m. You may use a wake-up light or music to cue her to know when her day can begin. Either get an inexpensive alarm clock that plays CDs or an iPod or attach an appliance timer (available at a hardware store) to a bedroom lamp. That tells the child to try to go back to sleep, or at least stay in his bed, and when it's okay to get up and start his day. Set it for about 6:00 a.m., and once he sleeps pretty consistently until 6:00, you can gradually try setting it later. Keep anything electronic out of reach for safety or to keep him from turning it on himself. Some families prefer the light because it's less likely to wake the child, on those days he does sleep, but it's your choice. With either the light or the music, be consistent. If you allow your child to get out of bed and start his day even fifteen or twenty minutes before the wake-up music or light comes on, he will not take the music or light seriously the next day.

You can blame the wake-up rules on the clock: 'The clock says it's still night-night time,' or simply remind her that the music or light is not on, or you can blame it on me: 'The Sleep Lady says you will feel better if you sleep until 6:00.' Sticker charts help a lot with early awakenings. Keep reminding her that she can't get up because Mummy and Daddy (and brothers and sisters) are still sleeping. She'll feel better if she knows she isn't missing a party!

If she gets up at, say, 5:00 or 5:15 and comes looking for you or calling you, get her back to bed with minimal conversation. Remind her that it isn't morning time yet, that her wake-up music or wake-up light hasn't gone on yet. Decide whether you will stay in her room until 6:00, or whether you will leave and check on her every ten or fifteen minutes. Base your decision partly on which approach is more likely to get her back to sleep – or even get her to stay in her bed. You don't want her chasing you every thirty seconds if you leave, and you may need to gate her door. Nor do you want her to keep talking and chatting and trying to engage you if you stay in her room.

You can try both approaches for a day or two to get an idea of which will work, but don't keep switching back and forth. Choose a system and stick to it for a while. You may find a two-stage approach works best. Stay in her room in the morning for a while, maybe a week or so to communicate that she has to stay in bed. Then leave the room to give her more space to fall asleep again on her own.

Ideally, she should get back to sleep until 6:00 or later, and you can snooze in a chair, lie on her floor, or get back to your own bed. If she does go back to sleep, wake her up at 7:30 a.m. If she doesn't get back to sleep, wait until 6:00. Then come back into her room (if you are already in the room, leave for a minute or two but explain you'll be right back) with your dramatic wake-up and morning routine. Convey the message that she is starting her day because it's 6:00 a.m. and her wake-up music or light has come on – not because she cried, fussed, and screamed.

Early Risers

If your little one wakes up before 6:00 a.m., he's probably overtired. Overtired children don't sleep as well, or sleep as long, as well-rested ones. He may be:

- Going to bed too late
- Not napping enough
- Staying up too long between the end of his afternoon nap and going to bed (try not to let it exceed four hours)
- Going to bed when he's past that 'drowsy but awake' mark. If he's too drowsy, he won't know how to get himself back to sleep when he's more alert – including at 5:00 a.m.

For children who wake up at 6:00 and are perfectly content, you'll probably have to live with it. It's a common and appropriate wake-up time for young children, even if you'd rather have them sleep later. You can try to teach her to stay in her room and maybe put out some special toys that she gets to play with only in the morning if she stays in her room and is quiet. However, if she wakes up at 6:00 but is cranky and miserable by 7:00, then she needs to sleep later. Try putting her to bed earlier in the evening or use the early-bird techniques described above to teach her to sleep later.

Some children naturally start sleeping later as they get a little older and outgrow napping. If that happens, it will happen on its own; you can't force it. You should not take away or shorten naps in the hopes of persuading her to sleep later (unless her naps are much longer than typical for her age). That usually backfires, and you just end up with an even more overtired child, who will still wake up early and be even grouchier.

> Even when they stop napping, quiet time in the late afternoon or before dinner is a must for four year olds, and a wise idea for five year olds, unless you actually like watching your child melt down.

Napping and Quiet Time

Sleep needs shift year to year for this age group. As their naps shrink and disappear, they need to sleep a little longer at night. You'll have to adjust bedtime, unless they naturally begin to sleep in a little later in the morning. Even when they stop napping, quiet time in the late afternoon or before dinner is a must for four year olds, and a wise idea for five year olds, unless you actually like watching your child melt down.

With the two and a half or three year old, you still need to be vigilant about daily naps. He can skip an occasional one, but put him to bed earlier that night. Naps also remain essential for older children who aren't sleeping through the night or who are obviously tired during the day. You may have to nap coach.

You can do a Shuffle for naps in this age group, or you can just put him in his room and check on him every ten to fifteen minutes. Every day, promise that you will come get him as soon as his nap is over. Make him stay in his room for an hour, every day. He may protest, and you may have to put a gate on his door. Some parents sit outside the gate at naptime with a book; it helps the child stay calm and get to sleep. Don't let him nap too late. Leave at least four hours between the end of the nap and bedtime or he'll have trouble falling asleep. (Nap training is hard. If you need more encouragement and advice about backup plans, read about napping for younger age groups.)

You may find that your child no longer needs a daily nap but still needs a 'nap day' every three or four days. Carleigh napped daily until age five, and slept every other day after school for the first few months of kindergarten. That's longer than most children, but I could tell by her behavior that she still needed that extra sleep in the afternoon. My second daughter, Gretchen, in what was probably a more typical pattern, stopped napping at home when she was about three and a half but still napped at preschool.

Sleep Lady Tip

The simplest way to tell whether a preschooler or kindergartner needs a nap is to watch him. If he gets a lot of nighttime sleep and is cheerful and easygoing during the day, he probably doesn't need to nap. If he is cranky or teary or frequently melting down, he probably needs at least a few naps a week. Car behavior is also a good clue. If he conks out every time you start your engine, he probably still needs that afternoon snooze.

After they moved, napping was a struggle for Sam, and Nora never found a wholly satisfactory solution. His bedroom overlooked a school with indecently loud and frequent bells, so she let him nap in her room, which she knew was not ideal. 'Once I got him to sleep, he'd often sleep for three hours,' she said, which is really too much for a three year old. But she had a hard time getting him to sleep. 'It was a fight at naptime. He'd tantrum and wear himself out. Even when I gave him time, he still needed some tantruming to get out that last bit of energy and fall asleep.'

If your child is getting about eleven hours of unfragmented sleep at night and seems well rested during the day, it may be time to go from naps to quiet time. You might want to cut out naps every other day, rather than eliminate them completely, or you may find that he naps great on the days he's with his sitter or at preschool but won't nap on days he's with you (or vice versa). Children who were good nappers but who now take a very long time to fall asleep in the afternoon may also be ready to phase out the nap and start quiet time.

When Kerry was two years and nine months, Laurel abandoned her struggle to make him nap on the days he was home with her, but he still napped beautifully on the days he had a sitter. A few months later, Laurel noticed that he was much more difficult at bedtime on nap days. 'I'd put him to bed, and he'd be up and out of bed six times. It more than made up for the nap,' she said. 'Everybody would be angry – I felt so bad for him.' Although I usually urge families to continue the nap until around three and a half or four, in this case Mum's instincts were right. When they cut out the nap, bedtime became simple and pleasant. 'We can shut the light and say good night, and he goes to sleep,' Laurel said.

Quiet time is exactly what it sounds like, about forty-five minutes of structured, solitary play, preferably at about the same time every afternoon. It's a time for children to rest their bodies and, to a lesser extent, their minds. It helps pave the way for a peaceful dinner hour and easy bedtime. Good activities include looking at books, watching an age-appropriate, calm children's video (leave fast-paced, action-packed cartoons for another time), coloring, or playing in their room with dolls, trains, trucks, or the like. The activity should not need a lot of adult interaction or supervision, so make sure the child is in a safe place.

Cosleeping

Some of the families in this chapter coslept with their children for at least part of the night, and, as you've seen, the Shuffle can help end that practice. But cosleeping is a complicated subject, so I've devoted a separate chapter to it. Please refer to Chapter 12, 'Whose Bed Is It Anyway?' if you've been cosleeping since birth and want to stop, or if you've been taking your child into bed for all or part of the night because you think it's the only way you can get him to sleep. If you want to continue cosleeping, I can help you teach your child some sleep independence at naptime that will help him when he does eventually move into his own bed.

Isabel

When Rita and Elliott had that family meeting with Isabel, they faced a daunting agenda. Isabel was four and had been a poor sleeper since birth, waking up every night and resisting napping anywhere but in a stroller. For the past year, her parents had had to sing and dance her to sleep, making up all sorts of silly Isabel songs and doing their own customized adaptation of 'Kumbaya.' Even with all that, she still ended up sleeping on the floor of their bedroom or sometimes crawling into bed with them, even though little sister Deirdre slept peacefully in her cot.

Rita had tolerated this until her third daughter, Rebecca, was born. 'We had learned to live with it; if she wants to live in a sleeping bag on the floor, fine. But now with one child on the floor and a newborn screaming in our bedroom, it was too much.'

They held their meeting, made their chart, decorated it with little illustrations of her goals, and began the Shuffle. 'Instead of singing I told her I'd keep her company until she was having a good dream. We talked about things that were nice to dream about,' Rita said. Isabel resisted the Shuffle only two or three nights. Mostly she was 'really excited and pleased in the morning' when she put her stickers on her chart.

At first she still woke up some nights and came to them. 'We'd walk her back to bed. We'd sit there if she needed us to. She was just so tired, all she would do was crawl back to bed and fall asleep. If she was really awake and distraught about something, I would end up staying with her.' But within a few weeks, she stopped waking up.

Juggling three little girls in four years, Rita is ecstatic to have a 'blessedly simple and short' bedtime. She gives Isabel and Deirdre their dinner and bath, then reads them books, with baby Rebecca on her arm. She puts Deirdre, the easier sleeper, in her cot first and says good night. Then they go to Isabel's room, and she gets to pick out a few books of her own for Mum to read. 'She gets into bed, gets a big hug and kiss, and I say good night. She likes me to leave the door open, but she doesn't need me in the room anymore.' No more singing and dancing.

Mary Catherine

Mary Catherine did the Shuffle in stereo – two daughters at once. Ashley, like her much older brother, had been 'Ferberized' as a baby, and slept reasonably well until she moved into a bed too early and her sleep fell apart. Then her baby sister, Mimi, was born. Mary Catherine had not coslept with her first two children, but her whole life was different now; she was a stay-at-home mum and wanted to have her kids around her all the time. She coslept and nursed the baby, but Ashley figured out that little sister was upstairs in bed with Mum and Dad, while she was stuck by herself downstairs. Eventually, she joined the gang in the family bed. They all went to bed at around 9:00 p.m., Mum in the middle, one girl on each side, both girls twirling Mum's hair. Dad usually ended up in the guest room. Mimi also had a dummy. A poor sleeper who seldom napped after the first year, Mimi was often overtired.

After about a year, Mary Catherine realized this was not a truly restful experience. 'The girls were getting bigger and kicking and thrashing around. They were both very light sleepers. When I would get up to go to the bathroom, they would follow. If the TV was on, they were watching. If I was reading in bed, they were awake. I was suffocating and getting very frustrated.'

Their pediatrician recommended that she separate the girls, 'put locks on the doors on the outside, and let them cry.' That was way too much for Mary Catherine and Keith, so they tried all sorts of bribes – even a brand-new bunk bed for the girls. When Mary Catherine found Keith in the bottom bunk and the girls still in her bed, she knew they had hit rock bottom. She called me and took charge.

They had a family meeting with the girls, now three and five, and explained the new sleep scenarios. Mary Catherine introduced the new tasseled satin pillows she had made for them to use as loveys they could twirl instead of her hair and explained that they would have each other for company in their shared room. She also bought some material like curly sheep fur (her own hair was very curly) as a backup. Brand-new Barbie sheets were an extra incentive, along with sticker charts and a system of rewards. Ashley understood the sticker chart; Mimi didn't quite get it, at least not enough to make it work for her at first.

Mary Catherine began the Shuffle sitting between the girls, first comforting one child and then the other. She also rolled up some blankets and put them on the sides of the bed to make the girls feel more snuggly and nest-like as they got used to sleeping without two or three other bodies in bed. The first five nights were hard, particularly on Mimi, and Mary Catherine felt sad about her daughters' obvious distress. In a stroke of unfortunate timing, Ashley had just started asthma medication that made her heart race and inhibited sleep. But Mary Catherine stuck it out, knowing that she needed to make this change, and knowing that the girls were getting a lot of comfort from each other. 'Ashley became a little mum and would reassure Mimi,' she said.

The Shuffle went reasonably well, although she had some problems when she reached the hallway. One or both girls would want to come out after her, and Ashley fell asleep in the hallway a few times. If they got out of bed later or tried to make their way into their parents' bed, Mary Catherine would silently return them to their room. On a few very rough nights Mary Catherine threatened to close the door, and that definitely motivated them to stay in their room.

It took three weeks before both girls slept through the night – Ashley, who started to twirl her own hair, would have done it earlier, but Mimi would wake her up, sometimes crawling into her big sister's bed.

It's now been three years, and the girls sleep well, but Mary Catherine is still careful to enforce clear rules, including no sweets after 6:00 p.m. 'Bedtime routine is not as strict as it was when we were laying down the law, but we're still consistent.'

Part Three

Part Three

12

Whose Bed Is It Anyway?
Making Choices About
Bedsharing and Roomsharing

When I work with expectant parents, the subject of cosleeping, or the family bed, inevitably arises. Cosleeping or bedsharing has been a hotly debated child-rearing topic in recent years, one that can push intense emotional buttons. Some people argue that sharing a bed is the right and natural way to raise a child, that they have stronger bonds and a more secure attachment. Others will tell you just as forcefully that it's risky, ridiculous, or simply not what they want for their family.

My task isn't to make that decision for you, but to help you figure out the right and comfortable sleep-enhancing decision for both you and your child. I also want to suggest an alternative, a middle ground that's become known as 'roomsharing.' That's when the parents keep a new baby in their room, but not in their bed, for a few months or even a year. I mentioned this option in earlier chapters of this book, and I am giving it more emphasis here because I have found it really is a good solution for many families. Having the baby in a cot right next to you, in a Moses basket that you can reach over and touch, or a cosleeper sidecar cot that can actually attach to your bed (www.armsreach.com is one brand) may well be the best of both worlds. It's easy to feed the baby at night, you have the peace of mind of having her literally at your fingertips, but you don't have to worry about the safety challenges of bedsharing, or get yourself committed to a shared-bed arrangement that you may have trouble changing a year or two from now. It may also be a very helpful solution to women who have had C-sections and will have difficulty getting up and moving around a lot at night for the first few weeks. When you decide you want to move the baby out of your room, you can follow the advice I give later in this chapter for families who wish to stop cosleeping. (If she will be sharing a room with a brother or sister, you might want to check out my advice in Chapter 13, 'Helping Twins and Siblings Sleep.')

I'm going to spend a lot of time in this chapter on bedsharing, not because I think it's bad but because so many of the parents I work with have had difficulties stopping it when they want to. I want to be very clear that I'm not predicting that you will have problems too; countless families cosleep for at least some portion of time safely and happily. I think it's important for those babies to learn how to put themselves to sleep, too, and I'll offer some suggestions about how to help them even in a family bed environment. But my task in this chapter is also to offer help for those of you who want to make a change, who ended up bedsharing without intending to, or who have found that, as I said earlier, it's all 'co-' and no 'sleep,' and everybody is an exhausted wreck.

I encourage you as parents to make a decision about the shared bed before the baby is born, reserving the option to change your minds without any guilt if your decision turns out not to be the best one for *you*. It's important to understand that cosleeping is not magic. Although some proponents of the family bed would disagree, I have worked with numerous couples whose babies did not necessarily sleep deeper or longer because they were in bed with their parents. In fact, some parents found that their child slept longer and woke less frequently when they stopped cosleeping and moved her into her own cot.

I can't tell you how strongly I feel about finding a solution that feels right for you, even if it wasn't what you planned, hoped, or expected. If you are constantly exhausted, you can't be the mother or father you want to be, and you aren't going to be as adept at reading your baby's cues and responding to her needs. And you have a higher risk of ending up depressed, which isn't good for you or your child.

Cosleeping Categories

I divide cosleeping into three categories: the committed cosleepers, the short-term cosleepers, and the 'we didn't plan it this way' cosleepers.

The committed cosleepers are couples (also a lot of single mums) who choose the family bed as a philosophy and lifestyle. Many are influenced by the *attachment parenting* philosophy popularized by William Sears and Martha Sears. These parents consciously decide to have the baby (or, later, all the children) sleep with them until he expresses a desire for his own bed, even if that takes several years.

The short-term cosleepers want the baby with them the first few months, although the first three months are the riskiest time to bedshare (see the Appendix, 'Safe Sleeping Recommendations for Babies'). They like the bonding, and they like the convenience of having the newborn right there when they are nursing frequently. As new parents are often anxious parents, they may also feel less worried if the baby is by their side. These parents may do well by choosing roomsharing as an alternative because it satisfies the need for closeness and minimizes the safety risks. (In the interest of full disclosure, I initially planned on cosleeping with Carleigh for the first few months, but I was so terrified that I'd roll over on top of her that I didn't sleep a wink. She also made a lot of noise, even as a tiny baby. We put her, and later her sister, in her own room early on.) I recommend that if you choose to cosleep short-term with your newborn, plan to transition to the cot at about three months. (You may choose to keep the cot in your room for another few months, i.e., switch from bedsharing to roomsharing.)

During the three months in which you are cosleeping, you should have the baby nap in his cot, cosleeper, or Moses basket consistently. Having him sleep on his own at naptime will make the eventual switch to nighttime sleep in the cot much smoother. It also makes it much easier for him (and you) to master the self-soothing skills for newborns I discuss in Chapter 5, 'The Right Start for Newborns and Infants.'

The 'we didn't plan it this way' cosleepers are also called *reactive cosleepers.* These parents end up with the baby in the bed part or all of the night, not by choice or philosophical commitment but because it's the only way they can get their baby to sleep at bedtime, or back to sleep in the middle of the night. Some started out as short-term cosleepers but never figured out how to stop it. Others put the baby in the cot at bedtime but take her into their bed when she wakes up at night. And there are those who are ambivalent and either can't decide where they want the baby to sleep or are conflicted, with one parent advocating the family bed and the other wanting to put the baby in the cot. Disagreement usually results in a mishmash of cot sleeping and cosleeping, which can make even a very young baby confused about where and how she is supposed to fall asleep. Even the most enthusiastic proponents of bedsharing don't promote reactive cosleeping.

What's Right for You

When you are deciding whether long-term cosleeping is right for you, an array of practical and emotional issues bear consideration. Think about your own childhood, your nighttime fears, your feelings of closeness to or isolation from your parents. Mothers working outside the home need to consider whether they want the extra closeness at night because they feel guilty or are afraid they are hurting the baby by being away during the day. I don't mean to imply that all parents who cosleep do so out of guilt. But understanding your motives can often clarify your decision. Ask yourself too whether nighttime physical proximity is really the key to a secure bond or attachment with your child. As a mother and as a family therapist, I am not convinced that it's a requirement; most of our bonding, our attachment, and our interaction take place during the day. How we touch our children, care for our children, play with our children, listen to our children, respond to our children, and laugh with our children when we are awake seem more essential to the formation of our relationships than where and how we choose to sleep.

You also need to think carefully about how having a child in bed with you all the time will affect your marriage. Think too about how you will deal with a growing family. Will you have two or three children are in bed with you? If you are a single parent, consider the implications of integrating a new partner into your life when your child is sharing your pillow.

Keep in mind that cosleeping is a long-term commitment, a practice that you will need to continue until the child *chooses* to transition to her own bed. Sometimes that takes a year or two, sometimes seven or eight. Reid and Julia, for instance, coslept with their first two children, and it was easy, pleasant, and emotionally gratifying. Both children quickly transitioned to their own beds. Then along came Todd, their third child, who was a very disruptive cosleeper and didn't want to move until I helped them ease him into his own room at fourteen months.

Also take more mundane matters into account. How light a sleeper are you? Will a wriggling baby keep you up at night? Will you worry more if he's with you or if he's away from you? Will you miss being able to read in bed with the light on, or watch television late at night?

If you change your mind during the first three or four months, the transition isn't much of a problem. After that it gets harder, but it's not impossible. I've worked with many families who have practiced cosleeping for two years and then decided that they needed to change their sleeping arrangements. I will give you advice on how to transition a two year old into her own bed as smoothly and gently as possible, but I must emphasize that I don't recommend letting a child sleep in your bed for two years and then abruptly sending her down the hall to her 'own' bed. After all, she thinks your bed *is* her bed. And I definitely don't encourage abruptly ending cosleeping with one child to make room for a new baby in your bed. (I'll have some suggestions later in this chapter for coping with that situation.)

Safety Concerns and Precautions

As you consider the pros and cons of the family bed, you should be aware of some safety issues. Some studies have found a higher risk of sudden infant death syndrome in babies that bedshare. The American Academy of Pediatrics and the U.S. Consumer Product Safety Commission (CPSC) have formally recommended against cosleeping with a child under the age of two because of the possible risk of death or injury. In the U.K., to reduce the risk of cot death, the Department of Health recommends you should not share a bed with your baby if you or your partner have been drinking alcohol, taking drugs or medication, or if either of you smokes. You should also refrain from cosleeping if you feel very tired or if your baby was premature.

In a January 2003 bulletin, the CPSC cited concerns associated with the cosleeping of adult and baby that include suffocation of an infant who becomes entrapped or wedged between the mattress and another object, suffocation due to airway obstruction when the baby is face-down on a waterbed mattress, and strangulation in rails or openings on beds that allow a baby's body to pass through while entrapping the head. First Candle (www.FirstCandle.org), an organization devoted to reducing sudden infant deaths, cites published research that suggests the toll is higher, that up to 80 percent of sudden infant deaths occur when the baby is sleeping with a parent or other adult. Similarly, some research shows that SIDS rates are lower when parent and infant sleep in the same room, but not in the same bed.

Quality Sleep in the Family Bed

Those of you who are cosleeping happily and healthily may still benefit from steps I outline here that can improve the quality of everyone's sleep. You can help your baby develop good sleep patterns and at least a degree of sleep independence even in a family-bed setting.

If you decide to cosleep, talk to your doctor about the most recent safety recommendations and do everything you can to reduce the hazards. Some experts recommend placing a firm, smooth mattress or futon on the floor away from all walls. Use well-fitted sheets that can't be easily pulled off. Don't use any pillows or blankets in the early months, and make sure the baby can't get stuck in a mattress pad. Never use waterbeds or any other soft and flexible surfaces. Make sure there are no crevices or soft spots where the baby can get caught or smothered.

If your mattress is not on the floor, use well-designed guardrails that cannot entrap a baby. If your bed is next to the wall or other furniture, make sure there is no place the baby can get stuck or smothered. Or move your bed away from the walls.

Some experts, including Elizabeth Pantley, author of *The No-Cry Sleep Solution*, recommend placing the baby between the mother and the wall or rail, not between the two parents. She believes that fathers, grandparents, older siblings, and babysitters don't have the same 'instinctual awareness of a baby's location' and won't respond as well to the baby's needs and positioning. Pantley also says that mothers who are very deep sleepers, who won't wake up at the baby's subtle cues, might want to refrain from cosleeping.

Do not sleep with your baby if you are very overweight, or if you have been drinking alcohol or using drugs or medications. I've included a full list of child safety rules – for *all* babies, not just cosleeping ones – at the back of the book. Please read it.

As I mentioned, I very strongly recommend having the baby nap in his Moses basket or cot and restricting the cosleeping to nighttime. (An occasional exception of a parent-child nap will not create a problem.) Not only does this promote better sleep habits for the child, but it also gives the parent a lot more freedom. If your child knows how to fall asleep on his own, you won't have to lie down with him for every nap, or go to bed at 7:00 every night.

Some couples who cosleep but also want to foster a degree of sleep independence in their baby and a little early-evening freedom for themselves put the baby down in her cot at bedtime. Then they move her into the family bed when they get ready for sleep themselves, or the first time she wakes up at night.

Sleep Lady Tip

Napping with your baby is a great idea sometimes, particularly during those tiring newborn months, but you won't want to be locked into napping with him all the time for several years. It can also create a big child-care napping problem if you go back to work or want to get out of the house now and then. It gets really complicated if you have two children napping at different times, or one who needs you to lie down with her and a slightly older one who isn't napping at all anymore and needs your supervision and attention. If she's in a cot, you also have a little more freedom to move around your home. You don't have to stay in the room every minute to make sure she doesn't get smothered by your bedclothes or, when she gets a little older, roll out of bed.

Remember that sleep is a learned skill, regardless of whether your child is in your bed or her cot. Helping her develop the ability to fall asleep without being nursed, held, or rocked each and every time is an important foundation. Try to put her down drowsy but awake at least once a day. Review some of my sections for newborns and infants, especially Chapter 5, 'The Right Start for Newborns and Infants,' and Chapter 6, 'Newborn to Five Months.' The morning nap is usually the easiest time. This prevents reactive cosleeping and reduces a baby's need to be nursed back to sleep at each partial arousal.

Try not to sleep with your baby latched onto your breast all night. Even if you are feeding on demand, realize that your baby might not always be demanding to eat. She might be perfectly content with other ways of being soothed and comforted if you give her a chance. If it's too hard for you to break that pattern, sleep in a T-shirt or try letting Dad do more of the snuggling and comforting. Remember that your breast is not the only tool in your soothing repertoire and review the suggestions on soothing in Chapter 5, 'The Right Start for Newborns and Infants.'

If your baby is eating much more at night than during the day, keep track of her nursing patterns and then try to shift them. Consult the appropriate age chapter in this book for techniques on cutting back on nighttime nursing, even if you don't want to eliminate it completely, and adapt those strategies to the family bed. For instance, if your child were not cosleeping, you would nurse her before putting her to bed and keep some separation between the two activities.

If you are nursing in bed, you have to find subtler ways of creating that separation. Feed her, unlatch her while she's still awake, and pull your shirt down. Then place her facing away from you, and put a lovey in her arms. You might also want to create a little space between you and the baby as she falls asleep after nursing. Comfort her to sleep but don't let her have your breast again until a predetermined interval has passed – two hours perhaps until a very young baby needs to be nursed again, four hours for a slightly older one. If she wakes up wanting the breast again sooner than that, use one of your other comforting techniques to help her get back to sleep. If that proves too hard, Mum might sleep in another room between nursings for a few nights, letting Dad comfort and share the bed with the baby.

Moving Out of the Family Bed

Many of the couples who consult me started out committed to cosleeping and later found it didn't quite work out for them. I also encounter a lot of 'we didn't plan it this way' couples seeking help in finally breaking the pattern. These families end up missing their privacy, or they are just not getting very much sleep. Babies can be very noisy, squiggly sleepers, thrashing around or burrowing down to the foot of the bed, where you then worry about them being smothered in bedding. Some babies may not learn to sleep very well in bed with their parents, nursing frequently because the opportunity is always present, or because they are too stimulated to sleep much of the night simply by being so close to their parents. It can be a bit of a jolt for a couple who opted to cosleep because they believed their baby truly needed their constant presence, only to find that this particular child sleeps better without them.

Although I told you my preference is that you make an informed decision about cosleeping early on and stick to it, if you find it isn't working, do not hesitate to make a change. Don't feel guilty, and don't let anyone else make you feel guilty – or incompetent. You can and will have a strong and healthy attachment with your child even if you don't cosleep. I'm going to share several families' stories to demonstrate how some couples have dealt with what can be a difficult transition. The switch goes pretty quickly for babies who are less than three or four months old, and I'll guide you through that. For older children, expect the adjustment to take at least three weeks, and then give it another two or three months until you can be confident the change has really taken root.

The one time I do not recommend ending cosleeping with your child is with the birth of a new baby. It's not ideal to move one child out of your bed to make room for the next, particularly since fears, rivalries, and feelings of displacement are so common even without making dramatic changes. I know a few kids aged three and older who have graciously got up and out of Mum and Dad's bed to accommodate the new baby, but that is really asking an awful lot of them. Either complete the transition a good three to six months before the new baby comes, or keep the older child in your bed for a few more months. You can put the newborn in a Moses basket or cosleeper sidecar nearby. Then simultaneously transition both children to their own room or rooms. Some couples divvy up the cosleeping tasks, with the mum in one room with the newborn and the dad in another room with the older child. They usually do that for a few months, until the newborn is sleeping through the night, and then end cosleeping with both kids.

When you do move a child out of your bed, you must be completely consistent. You mustn't cave in and take her into your bed sometimes, not even when it's almost morning, or you are going to confuse her. This can be emotionally difficult for a parent who still enjoys aspects of sleeping with her child. If you miss that little baby head curled against your neck, find another way to satisfy that yearning with some extra cuddling throughout the day.

After a baby has been in your bed for months or years I suggest making changes in several stages over several weeks (though not every family goes through every step): daytime acclimation to her room, daytime napping, sleeping with the child in her room, and the Sleep Lady Shuffle, my multistep program for teaching sleep independence. I'll explain each stage in more detail below.

If your child is old enough, try to prepare her by talking through the imminent change. Even a one year old may comprehend more than you realize, and certainly from eighteen months or so they can understand a good deal. Letting them know what is coming – and making it sound enticing and exciting – often helps the transition. For an older child, sticker charts and rewards are great incentives.

Stage 1: Daytime and Playtime

Start by getting your baby used to his room awake and in daylight. In fact, he shouldn't just be used to it, he should like it. Play with him there, change him there, hug him, and kiss him there. If he needs some incentives to venture into the unfamiliar room, buy him some fun new toys or take some books and tapes out of the library. (You can skip this stage if your child is already playing in his room or napping there.)

Stage 2: Napping

If she's not already napping in her bedroom, start now. Spend a week or two getting her accustomed to napping in her own cot or bed during the day, before you make the nighttime transition. Go ahead and nap in her room with her for two or three days if your intuition tells you she needs that extra assistance. Then if she has trouble falling asleep in her room, sit with her for the next few days but try to be a fairly neutral presence. Calm and soothe her a bit, but don't let her constantly engage you, or all the interaction will be an excuse for her not to sleep. After a few days, you can try the Sleep Lady Shuffle to help her learn to nap on her own.

It is up to you whether you want to address the napping first or napping and nighttime sleep simultaneously – it doesn't matter if you are sitting in exactly the same position day and night at this point. Instead of the Shuffle, you have the option of trying to settle her in for a nap with her lovey and then leaving the room, checking on her every four or five minutes if she's crying. If that feels too abrupt to you, remember that either approach is fine and that you should choose the one that feels best for you and suits your child. Read the chapter for your child's age for details on the Shuffle and nap training.

Stage 3: The Sleep Lady Shuffle

When he's ready for night training (and it will be clear – we're talking days or weeks, not months), you should start the Sleep Lady Shuffle, my method of gradually teaching the baby or child to put himself to sleep without you.

With most babies, you start the Shuffle by sitting right next to the cot or bed. With cosleeping, I add one more preliminary phase. You can spend a few nights cosleeping in his room with him, to create a bridge between the family bed and independent sleep. Throw a mattress on the floor, drag in the guest bed, whatever is safe and comfortable for both of you.

Now you are ready for the heart of the Shuffle. Begin by sitting next to your child's cot or bed for three nights to soothe him. If the thought of leaving your child once he is asleep feels too abrupt, you can sleep in the room in a makeshift bed for two to three nights so you can attend to him quickly when he wakes. *But stay only two or three nights.* Any longer and he will become accustomed to having you there, and it will be harder for him when you try to leave. If he is in a bed and not a cot and he gets out and tries to join you during the night, simply put him back immediately, without a word. If he does this repeatedly or if you wake up at night and find he has joined you in your bed, remove the makeshift bed the next morning and stop sleeping in his room. Continue with the Shuffle from a chair.

Every three nights move your Shuffle position a little further away so that he can gradually fall asleep more independently. Move across the room, then to the doorway, then out the door into the hall. Within about two weeks, you will be able to leave him alone while still checking on him and reassuring him frequently. The fine points of the system vary a little bit by age, so please review my directions in the relevant age chapter.

Cynthia (Four Months)

Jayne and Paul were understandably nervous new parents. Cynthia was six weeks premature and spent some time in the newborn intensive care unit and on a home monitor. She was a colicky, fussy baby, requiring her parents to pace with her for three or four hours every night to calm her down. She fussed when they put her in a Moses basket, and she balked when they tried to get her into the cot, so mostly she slept with Jayne – or, more accurately, she slept on top of Jayne. 'I was a nervous new parent, and I couldn't sleep. I had to lie on my back with this baby on top of me,' Jayne recalled. 'I was exhausted and grumpy. It was taking up half my day to walk her to sleep and hold her when she was napping.'

When they consulted me, Cynthia was four months old. Our first task was to get her into the cot. To prepare, Jayne revised what had been a far too late nap schedule. Cynthia had been napping from around 4:00 to 7:00 p.m., meaning she was overstimulated, tired, and fussy earlier in the afternoon when she should have been napping, and then up way too late at night. Jayne started having Cynthia nap much earlier in the afternoon. She'd nurse her, and put her in the cot drowsy but awake. To make the cot feel more cozy and less vast to a little baby used to being snugly held, Jayne rolled up two receiving blankets, fastened them with ponytail holders, and placed them at the top and bottom of the cot, under the bottom sheet of the cot where they couldn't pose a smothering threat. (If you do this, review the exact position with your doctor or healthvisitor.)

As Jayne expected, Cynthia cried at first when her mum put her down for her nap. Earlier Jayne hadn't been able to cope with any tears, but now she was more comfortable with letting her cry a little bit. In fact, once Jayne decided tears weren't lethal, she ended up having a higher tear tolerance than many mums I work with (and you don't have to tolerate as many tears as she did if it's outside your comfort zone). Jayne found that if she stayed in the room with Cynthia but did not pick her up and nurse her, Cynthia threw the newborn equivalent of a hissy fit. She screamed, and none of Jayne's assiduous attempts to comfort her did any good. But Jayne found that if she worked on soothing and calming and preparing Cynthia for her nap, and timed the nap right, she could put the baby down in her cot and leave the room. Cynthia would cry for a few minutes and then fall asleep.

Having a schedule was a godsend for Jayne. The structure suited her, and she had intuited early on that it would suit Cynthia's temperament. But until we sat down and talked about feeding and sleeping needs and patterns for newborns, she hadn't really known how to establish a suitable schedule. 'Cynthia wasn't a 'go with the flow' kind of baby. She couldn't cope when she was tired; she'd just be fussy. I desperately wanted a schedule. I wanted to know: This is when she's going to nap, this is when she'll eat, this is when I can make plans,' said her mum.

Jayne and Paul also revised the evening routine. They fed her at about 6:00 p.m. – when a few weeks earlier she had still been napping. They'd give her a bath, change her, and read her a little book. (Some newborns like books; some don't.) Then they put her down in her cot, sat by her side, patted and comforted her – and she did cry. 'I thought this was horrible, it was going to scar her for life, but my husband reminded me that no, it wouldn't, that she needed to sleep, this is something she needed to learn how to do.' They ended up leaving her alone but checking on her about every fifteen to twenty minutes. It's not an approach that all families I work with like – it's not all that different from Ferber – but it felt right for them because Cynthia actually did better left on her own than with a parent in the room.

Jayne and Paul's goal at this point wasn't to get Cynthia sleeping through the night. It was just to get her sleeping in the cot. So when she woke at night, Jayne nursed her right back to sleep but then put her in her cot, not in her parents' bed. By the end of the week, she was going into her cot *without screaming, and was sleeping up to five hours at a stretch. Jayne was ready for stage 2, cutting back on the nighttime nursing and encouraging Cynthia to sleep all night. They went from three to two nighttime feedings, and then at six months eliminated the feedings completely. 'I thought she couldn't go that long without food, but once we took the feedings away, we realized she could,' Jayne said. If she woke up early, before 5:00 a.m., they would go in and pat and soothe her but not feed her or take her out of her cot until 6:00. They still go through stages when she wakes up on the early side, but in general she's a 'supersleeper,' going to bed at 7:00 p.m. and staying asleep for twelve solid hours.*

Cosleeping Transition for Babies Under Six Months

For babies under six months, you don't need the Shuffle or many preliminaries. You can put her down 'drowsy but awake' in her cosleeper and soothe her from your bed. When she learns to fall asleep there with little help from you, you can move her into her cot and sit by her bedside and soothe her to sleep. Don't pat or stroke her constantly. Give her enough contact to feel loved and secure, but not so much contact that it becomes a sleep crutch – that she needs you to be there stroking her all the time at bedtime and during the night. You can then gradually move further away, in a modified version of the Shuffle, or you can try just putting her down in her cot, offering some love and assurance, leaving, and coming back to check on her every few minutes.

After she gets accustomed to sleeping in her cot, keep your bed strictly off limits for three months or else you'll start the whole cycle all over again, which is not fair to her. Snuggle – but not in your bed. Find a comfy chair or couch somewhere, and don't let her fall asleep in your arms. After three months, it's okay to let her snuggle in your bed sometimes, but don't let her fall asleep there.

If your child has been going to bed in her cot but ending up with you in the middle of the night, you can't ease out of this habit gradually. You have to stop it, and stop it consistently. You can stroke, soothe, whisper, murmur, and pat your baby when she gets up and expects to come to you, but don't give in, not if you really want to end the cosleeping. That means you have to keep her in her cot every time – at 2:00, 3:00, 4:00, and 5:00 a.m. If you reassure her but make her stay in her cot at 2:00, 3:00, and 4:00, but take her into your bed at 5:00, you have confused her and possibly trained her to cry longer and harder next time. Babies can't tell time. She can't understand why you take her into your bed sometimes and not others. It's a classic example of intermittent reinforcement, and it's only going to make life harder for both of you.

Kevin (Eight Months)

Heidi and Steve were 'we didn't plan it this way' cosleepers. Although Kevin was born a big, hearty nine pounds and certainly didn't need to eat all night long, at eight months he was still getting up almost every hour wanting to nurse. His parents ended up keeping him in their bed because it was so much less disruptive to their sleep than having to go to him and nurse every hour. Kevin did nap in his cot, which helped the eventual transition. But once Heidi decided to stop nursing him at night and keep him in his cot, it was easier than they expected, using the Shuffle.

The first night didn't go too well. Kevin cried and Heidi, sitting by his cot, interacted a lot, which is fine the first night, but you have to be careful about not letting him make a habit of it. She rubbed his back, talked to him, and slipped her arm through the cot bars so he could fall asleep hugging it. The next night she patted him and whispered more sporadically, and gave him more space to fall asleep on his own. By the fifth night, he went to bed much more easily, with Heidi sitting in a chair halfway to the door. He woke up only once that night. When he did wake up, she would soothe him but make him stay in his cot. She would not nurse him. They let him keep his dummy, but when he demanded it at night, they would try to remember to put it in his hand without saying a word and leave.

Over the next two weeks, the nighttime awakenings steadily tapered off, until they were the exception, not the rule. When Kevin did wake up, Heidi or Steve would still go in to comfort him, but as he got older, they found that if they went in, he would only wake up more, interact, and stay up longer. If they let him work it out himself, he would cry for one or two minutes and then go back to sleep. 'I can tolerate the tears now – I know it's not going to damage him forever,' said Heidi. 'It's two minutes – and then he's asleep.' If he cries much longer or more sharply than that, which is highly unusual, they assume he needs them and they respond.

Candice (Eleven Months)

At eleven months, Candice had a severe aversion to her room. She had been cosleeping with her mum, Patty, while her dad, Don, afraid of squishing her, had been sleeping in another room. When Candice was six months old, her parents had made an attempt at reclaiming their bed and tried to 'Ferberize' her. It was a disaster. Candice cried and cried, and the more she cried, the more awake she became. The experience traumatized her so badly she would not even go into her room anymore, not even to play, not even accompanied by parents. She went back into their bed – and Don went back into the guest room. Five more months passed, and her parents finally decided something had to give.

The first step was to reacquaint Candice with her room. Patty put a lot of enticing new toys there, and the two of them played there together each day. This went on for two weeks. We actually altered the usual order. Instead of working on naps, which were difficult for Candice, we addressed bedtime. Patty put Candice in her cot, while she slept on an air mattress on the floor. When Candice protested or awoke in the middle of the night wanting Mum, Patty was near her, but would not pick her up. Patty would reach through the cot slats to pat and reassure her daughter.

Then Patty and Don did the Sleep Lady Shuffle. Patty noticed that Candice was beginning to develop her own techniques for soothing herself to sleep, twirling her hair, playing with her cot, and using her dummies not only to suck on but to play with.

Finally, it was time for the big move – leaving Candice's room so she could fall asleep on her own. When Patty was ready to leave, she told Candice where Mummy would be, and what she would be doing. There were some tears for four or five nights, but she never got so hysterical that she couldn't calm herself down, nor did the tears ever get so intense that Patty and Don couldn't tolerate them. During those nights, they would check on her from the doorway every five minutes, and if they sensed Candice needed a little more reassurance, Patty would give her a quick hug. That was the last hurdle.

Then just when Patty and Don thought they were done, Candice got sick. They handled it well. Instead of taking her back into their bed and ending up at square one, Patty would sit in a chair in Candice's room until the baby was very calm and drowsy, but not completely asleep. When she recovered, they checked on her from the doorway for a few nights. Candice quickly became an excellent sleeper. Soon Patty and Don could even leave her with a sitter and go out for dinner. 'It's a totally different world for us,' her mother said. 'Now she loves to sleep in her cot.'

Todd (Fourteen Months)

Julia and Reid were committed to attachment parenting, and had enjoyed cosleeping with their first two children, now both in school. In addition to believing in the family bed as part of a child-rearing approach that fosters bonding and security, Julia also felt she slept better just having to stir briefly to nurse without having to get out of bed and go into another room.

With their first two children, both girls, they coslept from birth, but as the girls began settling into more regular sleep and feeding patterns – without much of a nudge from their admittedly schedule-averse mother – Julia and Reid began putting them in their own cots, with age-appropriate bedtime rituals and routines. If they woke up needing a feeding while Julia was still awake, she'd nurse them in a rocking chair and return them to their cots. But when the girls would wake up at about 2:00 a.m. for a feeding, Reid would quickly fetch them and bring them back to the family bed. Julia could nurse without having to wake up completely, and everybody then slept contentedly together until morning. As that middle-of-the-night feeding time got later and later, the cosleeping window shrank. Eventually, the girls just slept all night in their cots, by nine months with one daughter, twelve months with the other. The shift was gradual and easy. Then came Todd. He was fourteen months old when his family consulted me. All was not well.

Todd had a number of health problems, including allergies and one prolonged and severe ear infection that led to surgery to insert tubes. Although those conditions aggravated Todd's disjointed sleep, they didn't fully explain it. And once his ears were better and his allergies addressed, he still didn't sleep any longer or better. He nursed much more frequently than his sisters had, slept more poorly, and had a less malleable temperament. 'Todd wasn't an easily detached baby. We even had to leave a preschool because he didn't separate well,' his mum said.

Getting so little sleep with him in their bed, they first tried to move him to a cot at eight months. It didn't work. Instead of Todd napping in the cot, Julia ended up taking thirty-minute walks around the house with the stroller. 'It gets pretty boring making endless loops on those hardwood floors,' Julia said.

Bedtime was a struggle. They had to rock and nurse him to sleep, and he didn't stay asleep unless he was in their bed, nursing and snuggling. 'We had to add all these layers of shenanigans on top of all the rituals,' Reid recalled. At the same time, they were dealing with two other young children with their own bedtime needs and demands. So they put Todd back in their bed and tried to make the best of it.

Julia and Reid knew that Todd was capable of sleeping all night and in a cot if he wanted to. He had proven that when Julia had surgery for kidney stones and pumped so Todd could have breast milk in a bottle. Todd didn't like bottles, so he just slept all night, albeit not very happily. 'That worked until those breasts were back in his world, and that's what he wanted,' she ruefully recalled.

When I saw them, we talked a lot about their parenting styles, what changes they would be able to make, what changes just weren't realistic given their personalities, values, and lifestyles. 'I am not a schedule person – you give me hours to follow, and I come unhinged,' Julia said. She identified which tasks she could accomplish and which she had to turn over to Reid. She agreed to work on limiting feedings to six times a day and to try comforting techniques other than nursing, not an easy task with an agile and determined fourteen month old who, whenever he got distressed, would try to climb up his mum, lift up her shirt, and wriggle himself underneath. They also switched the dinner hour from 6:00 to 5:00, so they'd have plenty of time to eat as a family and to start Todd's bedtime routine at 7:00 and have him asleep by 8:00. Before, he had gone to bed at 9:00 or 9:30, too late for a one year old.

At night, as we began the Sleep Lady Shuffle, we wanted to create a distinct separation between nursing and sleep. Julia nursed downstairs in the sunroom at about 6:30. (Most families I work with nurse in the child's bedroom, being careful not to nurse the child into a deep sleep. In Todd's case, we thought additional separation was warranted.)

Julia knew that she wouldn't be able to cope with the initial phase of sleep training, so Reid took charge. Todd went down more easily than they *expected the first night, with his dad sitting by his side. But he woke up at 11:00 p.m. and again at midnight. The second time was the worst. He screamed furiously for an hour and twenty minutes. Reid sat next to him, calm and consistent. 'I knew it was okay to touch him but not to hold his hand. I knew to pat him on the back and then stop, or to pat the mattress gently. It was almost more difficult for me than for him, because you want to reach out – you want to take care of your kid. But I knew I couldn't start out holding his hand because I would be moving further away in a few nights, and I wasn't going to be able to hold his hand when I was five feet away,' Reid said.*

Julia sat outside the bedroom and tried to empathize through the door until she finally realized that she needed to stop listening, ignore the baby monitor, and try to get some sleep for herself.

The second night, Todd got mad. Reid, who is pretty laid back, remembered thinking, 'Oh, my God, I've got a demon child in the cot!' Todd threw things out of the cot and tried to crawl out. They put a really big nightshirt on him so he couldn't get a leghold.

'I just kept repeating the same reassuring words. I just kept repeating them like I was teaching a dog a trick. 'Todd, you can do this, go night-night. You can do this, go night-night.' By three days, I just shortened it to, 'Night-night, night-night,'" Reid remembered.

The third day Reid saw an improvement. It still wasn't easy, but looking at his log, Reid could see that Todd had cried for twenty-two minutes. 'That felt like a lot – until I looked back and saw he had cried one hour and twenty minutes the first night. It was bumpy and not a lot of fun, but it was getting better.' Reid and Julia were still having doubts and second-guessing themselves at this point, but decided to stick with it and gave each other moral support.

By the time Reid reached the point where he had to leave the room, he was feeling much more optimistic. 'I realized the next step didn't have to be a big step. I was confident he could do it.' Reid came back and checked on Todd every five minutes or so. The nights Julia took bedtime duty, she made less frequent checks because Todd would get furious if he saw her but didn't get to nurse himself to sleep. 'It was tough for a few nights,' she recalled. 'But we knew he was pulling it together.'

Julia says she still believes in attachment parenting, and turns to Sears and Sears for child-rearing advice. But she is a little more open to modi-

fications and alternatives based on her children's temperaments, less afraid that she will hurt her children or weaken her bond with them, if she doesn't do everything by the attachment-theory book. 'I was a Sears devotee, and I still tend to be,' she said. 'But what I found is that before we started sleep training, I had a sweet, wonderful, tired little boy. When we finished, I had a sweet, wonderful little boy who wasn't tired.' He wasn't less secure, less attached, less loving, or less happy. He was only less exhausted.

Partly because they were still a little ambivalent about the cosleeping and partly because the family experienced a lot of changes and adjust-ments in the next few months – Reid lost his job when the high-tech bubble burst, and the family spent several months traveling around trying to decide where to relocate – they were not always completely consistent. Sometimes Todd didn't cry at all at bedtime, and sometimes he'd cry for four or five minutes, but never longer than that and never as ferociously as he had those first two nights. Among Todd's first full phrases was, 'Mummy, lie down, bed.' And sometimes one parent did give in and lie down with him, particularly while they were traveling or going through one transition or another. 'We've had some recidivism,' said Reid. 'And then it takes a few days to get back. The lesson to be learned is the more you get into a routine and stick to a routine, the easier it is for the kids to know what to expect.'

Months later, Todd was generally restricting his bedtime screaming to hotel stays with his sisters. And, his father confided, 'He only does that because he thinks it's a riot.'

Sleep Lady Tip

Children often sleep in positions that look uncomfortable to us – but feel fine to them. Unless there's a hazard, you are better off not trying to resettle them. If they're really uncomfortable, they'll let you know it! (Do run an unconventional sleep position by your doctor, though, just in case it's linked to apnea and he's adopted that posture to keep his airways open. Read Chapter 15, 'Medical Problems,' for more information.)

Alex (Fifteen Months)

Adele and Geoff read every book and tried every technique with Alex before they came to me. By then, he was fifteen months and very confused about what he was supposed to do to get to sleep. 'Everything worked a little bit, but nothing worked completely,' Adele said. They had 'Ferberized' him earlier, and while it helped him fall asleep, it didn't keep him asleep. Eventually, they tried letting him cry it out for those middle-of-the-night awakenings too, but it was intolerable; he cried and cried, three or four hours at a stretch. 'I couldn't take it. It was 2:00 a.m., he was in there crying, showing no sign of stopping, and just crying himself more awake. That panicked me. So I went back to nursing him to sleep. That would work; it would only take five minutes. But I'd have to do it three or four times a night.'

Later she weaned him at night, but it was a slow process, taking about six weeks, partly because he got sick several times around then and Adele would nurse him again while he wasn't feeling well. By age one, the night-time weaning was over, but he was still waking up all night and she wasn't about to put up with all those tears anymore. Desperate, she started taking him into her bed. 'He'd go back and forth, shuttling between the cot, and the bed. It was horrible and I felt like a complete failure because I had been so anti–baby in bed.' Adele and Geoff realized that they couldn't confuse Alex with any more partial solutions. They decided to do the Sleep Lady Shuffle and stick with it. It didn't take long.

Before we started, we made sure he got good daytime sleep so he wouldn't be overtired at bedtime. He napped in his room, and we limited the naps to an hour in the morning and ninety minutes in the afternoon. We wanted to time naps to maximize his readiness to sleep at bedtime. We wanted him tired but not overtired, rested but not so rested that he would fight sleep. We also cut the holding and rocking at naptime in half, right from the start, particularly for the morning nap.

To prepare for the Shuffle, Geoff slept on the floor in Alex's room with Alex in the cot. There, he could comfort Alex when he woke up at night, without bringing him into the family bed. Geoff also took bedtime duty the first few nights of the Shuffle because Alex, like many toddlers, tended to cry less at night with his dad than his mum. But after that, because of work and wake schedules, Adele took weeknights and Geoff took week-

*ends. 'We moved every three nights. It was three nights sleeping on the floor,
three sitting by the bed, three in a chair near the door, three in the doorway,
three just outside the door. By the time we got to just outside the door, he
really didn't wake up for very long and he didn't really cry. He'd fuss and
I'd go in and say 'night-night,' and he would lie down. His head would
pop up like a turtle to see if someone was still there, but it was very sporadic.
Some nights I'd hear him fuss briefly, but he'd go right back to sleep,' his
mother remembered.*

*When Alex woke up at night, Adele and Geoff didn't take him out of
bed, and they were very consistent about not taking him back into their
bed. 'I would go in and say 'Night-night' or 'Night-night, go to sleep' and
pat him on the back. I'd hand him his animal, and, during the first week,
I'd sit in his room or lie on the floor,' his mother said. Although he did
cry during the night, it wasn't the three- and four-hour jags they'd experienced earlier. The absolute longest he ever cried was thirty minutes, and
he always had a parent in the room with him comforting him. 'He's a crier;
he's a screamer. But he quickly learned that crying wasn't going to cut it
anymore. He wasn't coming into our bed. He had to sleep.'*

*When Alex woke up at night, he'd often do his screaming standing up.
Adele would pat the mattress and encourage him to lie down, but she didn't
keep intervening and putting him down. 'He was standing, then he'd be
sitting, and he'd fall asleep sitting up and fall over like a tree.' That didn't
wake him, and Adele and Geoff quickly learned to leave it alone. At some
point in his sleep cycle, he would wiggle himself into a more conventional
sleeping position. But if they tried to lay him down and straighten him
out, it would backfire. He'd be wide awake again.*

Kerry (Two and a Half Years Old)

*Laurel and Richard were classic 'we didn't plan it this way' cosleepers.
Kerry slept in a cot − except when he didn't. When he fussed and wanted
his mum, Laurel slept with him in the family room or guest room. He was
quite young when he moved into a toddler bed where she couldn't fit alongside him, but when he got out of bed, as toddlers often do, they often ended
up asleep together on the floor.*

*Philosophically, she didn't object to sleeping with him, only neither of
them slept very much. 'If I had to sleep with him − well, okay. But sleeping*

with him wasn't even resolving the issue. He was extremely restless. He would be perpendicular in the bed, kicking me in the head, rolling around a lot. I was so worried about him rolling off, he was moving so much, I couldn't sleep,' said Laurel, a therapist who knew about behavioral modification with older children but found it was 'a lot different when you are dealing with your own emotional stuff and your own child.'

Shortly before he turned two and a half, I urged them to dismantle the toddler bed and leave the mattress on the floor because that's where he was accustomed to sleeping. Before starting the Sleep Lady Shuffle, we tweaked his bedtime routine to change, but not shorten, his snuggle time. They did the bath, toothbrushing, and so forth, and then Laurel and Kerry snuggled up to read books on a little couch in his room. To earn his last story, his special reading of Toy Story, he had to get into bed. 'That was the incentive; we could entice him into bed,' Laurel said. They also used a star chart for good bedtime behavior.

After reading to Kerry, Laurel turned off the light and began the Shuffle, sitting by his side on the floor. The first night, she kept her hand on him because she knew he was going to need that contact. By the second night she was careful to make the hand touching more sporadic lest it become another sleep crutch. She returned to his side and patted his hand, without lying down with him, each time he woke those first nights.

Since Kerry was on the floor and was used to having Laurel there as well, she never used a chair. She sat on the floor, but she moved through the Shuffle, to the end of the bed, the doorway, then out in the hall. But since he was used to having the door closed, she sat in the hall on the far side of a closed door. 'He knew I was right on the other side of it. He didn't really care one way or another; he was already drifting off to sleep on his own.'

Kerry had progressed nicely, in less than two weeks. But he was still getting up at night to look for Mum. She would take him back to his room silently. Resisting the impulse to lie down and sleep with him — and it can be a strong impulse when you are tired and want to get both you and your baby back to sleep quickly — she would assume whatever position she had been in at bedtime that night and sit there until he drifted back to sleep. The night wakenings tapered off. There were some bumps, because he'd regress each time he got sick or traveled, but the overall progress was good.

I stayed in touch with the family for several months, and as Kerry got closer to the age of three, I suggested that Laurel, who sometimes had trouble setting limits, be a little stricter. I advised her to give him plenty of choices during the day but to enforce extremely well-defined limits around bedtime behavior. That meant an occasional bedtime tantrum, but Laurel learned to set rules and age-appropriate consequences without ever slipping back into cosleeping.

Two Children (Dylan, Five Years; Leila, Fifteen Months)

While earning her master's degree in education and working with at-risk preschoolers, Shauna had studied cross-cultural child rearing and become convinced that cosleeping was the right and natural path. When she and Nick had children, they were drawn to attachment parenting. Shauna nursed Dylan on demand, breastfeeding until he was almost two and a half. She carried him in a sling and coslept, including lying down with him at naptime. Although they had been trying to transition him to a bed, it was not very successful, and he usually stayed with them. That's where he was at four, when Shauna went into labor with his little sister, Leila.

Shauna didn't initially bring Leila full-time into an already crowded bed. Instead, she placed her in an adjacent cosleeper for six months, and then brought her into the family bed. In the meantime, they worked on shifting Dylan into his own bed. They managed to get him out of their bed, but one of the parents often ended up sleeping in his bed! Or they'd get him to sleep, and he'd crawl back in their bed, or someone, somewhere, would end up sleeping on the floor to be near someone else.

Exhausted by this routine, Shauna set goals. She wanted Dylan sleeping all night in his own bed. She wanted Leila to stop nighttime nursing and be in her cot at fifteen months. With my help, she and Nick tackled both children's sleep issues simultaneously, with Nick concentrating on Dylan and Shauna on Leila, who was still being breastfed at bedtime and during the day.

They called a family meeting for Dylan, who was now five, and explained their expectations. They made him a star sticker chart with five sleep manners. If he earned all five stars for a whole week, he would get a treat. He also had both moral support and a little peer pressure in his preschool where another little girl had worked with me. She became his sleep buddy as they compared their star tallies.

They began the Sleep Lady Shuffle. 'He cried at the beginning. He'd say, 'I want Mummy.' Then he would be really proud of himself for quieting down and falling asleep,' Shauna said. If he came to them at night, one of them would quietly walk him back to his own room. 'We'd sit in a chair outside the door of his room where he could see us, but there was no talking. If he was having a bad dream or he was scared, we would help him think of happy things,' she said.

After five years of cosleeping and emotional ambivalence about ending it, they were not always consistent. They knew it was unwise to lie down with Dylan, but they relapsed, sometimes because their hearts tugged their heads toward their little boy's pillow, sometimes because they were just too tired to do anything else. They had become a sort of hybrid of backsliding 'committed cosleepers' and 'we didn't plan it this way' cosleepers.

When Nick traveled overseas, Shauna, by then pregnant with a third child, allowed Dylan to have a 'sleepover' in Mum's bed. 'He was getting up and walking in, and I just let him — I couldn't deal with both his and Leila's sleep issues while I was pregnant and Nick was away. It was just too much for me to handle.' She knew there would be sleep consequences but decided to face them, believing she would be able to cope better when Nick was back home and she could get more rest.

Meanwhile, Leila was making progress, partly because Shauna was determined to improve Leila's sleep before the next baby came. Nighttime weaning took only two nights. Shauna still nursed her before bed, but during the night she would offer her a cup of water; Leila wasn't all that interested in it, so Shauna stopped. Then she would pat Leila and hold her until she fell asleep without anything in her mouth. At the same time, she introduced a lovey to distract Leila from touching Shauna's hair as she fell asleep.

Leila had sometimes spent at least part of the night in a cot, but it was in her parents' room. Now they moved the cot to her own room. Shauna and Leila slept on the floor together for one night, but Leila kept trying to sleep on top of Shauna's chest. Although Shauna's own style and preference were to be very slow and gradual, something told her not to sleep on the floor too long, that Leila would start expecting to sleep this way. The next night she nursed Leila until she was drowsy but still awake and then put her into her cot and began the Shuffle.

Leila accepted the changes reasonably well during the first few nights when Shauna was sitting by her side, but once Mum moved that chair away, Leila stood up in her cot and let everyone know she was mad. Shauna at first tried to be a calming, soothing presence, but by the end of a week realized that Leila did better if her mum just left the room. She cried for three minutes – tear-sensitive Shauna clocked it – and then put herself to sleep and pretty much stayed asleep. She woke up too early, 5:00 a.m., so for the first few mornings Shauna lay on a mattress on the floor, and her presence helped Leila get back to sleep. Later Shauna would go in and pat and reassure Leila if she woke up too early and then leave the room as Leila drifted back to sleep.

Leila's sleep for the next six months or so was good but not perfect, partly because the family went away for a month that summer shortly after the Shuffle. Leila potty trained early, which has its advantages, but she would yell, 'Potty, potty, potty!' wanting to get out of the cot at night. She slept through the night for a while, but then began waking up again in the early morning, between 4:00 and 6:00. She also tried to climb out of her cot before age two, but Shauna stopped it. 'I wasn't ready for her to get out of the cot. I had just got her in it!' Like many toddlers, she also went through those spells of separation trouble at bedtime, and Shauna experimented with how to ease those fears. She found that at times Leila sought her presence but not her touch. She sat in a chair in Leila's room at night, and knew that soon she would have to start leaving the room, despite Leila's protests, or else face sitting there for the next few years. Pregnant with her third child, that was not in Shauna's game plan.

Shauna and Nick still believed in cosleeping but decided to limit it even further with their third child. The plan was to cosleep for four months, and then get the baby into a cot. With each child, they also paid more attention to how often he ate, and whether he was really seeking the breast or expressing some other infant needs and desires. 'I still believe in nursing on demand – but I have to be more aware and recognize what he's demanding, whether he's hungry. I have to be aware when I'm nursing him to sleep,' Shauna said.

She's also seen her own attitudes evolve, and keep evolving with each child. She attributes much of Dylan's warm and affectionate personality to his attachment-parenting infancy and still can't bear to hear him cry. 'If he needs us, we go in.' With Leila it's different. Shauna can tolerate more tears, *and she doesn't feel the need to be as physically close as much of the time. 'With each child, I have more knowledge and experience. I'm still Sears and Sears oriented, I like the attachment-parenting philosophy, but I'm also fascinated by the science of sleep. It's what my heart wants versus what my brain knows I should do about sleep. What feels natural is not the most sleep promoting; what feels natural often gets in the way.'*

13

Helping Twins and Siblings Sleep

M y Sleep Lady guidelines apply whether you have one, two, three, or even more babies, but applying the rules is harder when multiples are involved. Parents need to know how to coordinate two babies' schedules and sleeping styles, to know when the babies should share a room and when they should be apart. In this chapter, I'll pay particularly close attention to families with twins, but I'll also show how families with several children deal with conflicting sleep needs, particularly at bedtime. Be sure to also read the chapter corresponding to your children's ages for specifics on their sleep and schedule needs.

Twins

Taking care of two newborns is an awesome task, and I encourage families with twins to get their babies on a schedule as soon as possible, particularly for feeding. For guidance, read Chapter 5, 'The Right Start for Newborns and Infants,' and Chapter 6, 'Newborn to Five Months.' Begin the gentle first stages of newborn sleep shaping by the time they are six weeks old (if they were premature, use the adjusted age, counting six weeks from due date, not from birth). Start putting them down drowsy but awake at least once a day and watch their sleep windows. Wake them at the same time in the morning, or allow one to wake the other, so you can get them more in sync early on. Some mums tandem feed the babies, one on each breast. Others nurse whichever baby wakes up first, and then wake and feed the other one. That way they should still be waking up within thirty, maybe forty-five minutes, of each other.

Sleep Lady Tip

I urge all parents, *but especially those with twins*, to keep a simple food and sleep log. It's hard to remember everything about one baby's sleep without writing it down; it's impossible with two. The log will also help you see how their sleep windows, sleep cues, and internal clocks differ, and where they overlap.

If your babies were premature, it may take them a *little* longer to sleep through the night. But it shouldn't take much longer if they are healthy, gaining weight, and growing well. Check with your doctor, but it's reasonable for them to sleep about eight to ten hours at a stretch by around four months, and to sleep all night by about six months, age adjusted. Don't convince yourself that their prematurity is an excuse for you not to deal with their sleep needs.

From Womb to Room

These babies have been sharing a womb, and it's usually a good idea to have them share a room. Some families even put them in the same cot for a few months, until they start rolling over. Yes, they may grunt, whimper, and make all sorts of strange baby noises, but they almost always sleep through each other's sounds, and you want to encourage them to do so. Be careful about responding too quickly if one makes a noise. Parents often rush in as soon as they hear a peep, fearing that one will wake up the other one. You may be reinforcing the troubled sleeper while you protect the one who is asleep. You may be teaching her to make noises so you'll come flying in to pick her up all the time. The sleeping twin may be oblivious, or she may stir but then get herself right back to sleep, exactly as you want her to do. Parents of triplets or quadruplets can adapt these techniques for their children, although most don't separate them for naps simply because they don't have enough room! A parent can sit in the middle of the bedroom between the children to soothe them. The children learn quickly to sleep through their sibling's crying and fussing.

Ethan and Nathaniel were both poor sleepers at seven months, waking each other up, demanding to be rocked and held. 'Someone had to hold them until they were asleep. You'd put them down, and they'd wake up, they'd be very upset, and you'd have to rock them again,' Charlotte remembered. It was bad enough at night with two sleepy parents, and it was impossible at naptime when Charlotte was home alone trying to pace and rock two at once.

Working with me, Charlotte and Ed began creating more of a bedtime routine, and learned to put the boys down drowsy but awake. They'd cry, but Charlotte would come in frequently, sitting in the room and helping them calm down. She never let them cry alone for more than ten minutes before she returned to their room. For naps, however, they did separate the boys, and they kept them apart for naptime throughout their toddler and preschool years.

In those cases where one twin sleeps well and the other one wakes up so loudly and frequently that he really does disrupt the other's sleep, I do make exceptions and separate them at night during sleep coaching. Once the poorer sleeper is sleeping through the night (or waking for a single feeding if that's age appropriate and you're satisfied), you can return him to the shared room. It's usually a good idea to leave the poorer sleeper where he is, and move the sounder sleeper to another room, using a travel cot if necessary. Good sleepers tend to be more flexible and can more easily adjust to a temporary new sleeping place, particularly if it's a little noisier or brighter than the babies' bedroom.

Sandy and Jonathan's twins, Marissa and Sasha, had terrible colic and probably some gas pains as well. The couple had plenty of help. Four grandparents lived nearby, but sometimes six adults could not keep up with two colicky infants. When Sandy first called me, I told her to get through the colic as best she could and we'd start sleep shaping when it subsided. At four months, it dissipated swiftly, and we got to work.

At the beginning the girls had slept in a shared cot, in their parents' bed, and finally in a pair of swings. Sandy treated the swing as a temporary colic survival measure; she used it a lot from about eight to twelve weeks and then sensibly began dividing the girls' time between the swings and the cots. Sandy and Jonathan also began trying to get the girls to sleep for longer intervals in the swings, with less frequent feedings, another wise move that laid the foundation for subsequent progress. As the babies got a little older, Sandy and Jonathan began putting them in the cot at bedtime, moving them into the swings only if they had a lot of trouble getting them back to sleep later at night.

When I started working with the family, at about four and a half months, we wanted to complete the transition from swing to cot, and cut back even more on the nighttime feedings, crying, dummy fetching, and assorted other interruptions. I urged them not to run in so quickly, and not to pick the babies up so much when they did run in. Sandy and Jonathan had always had a video monitor on the twins, so they had been rushing to the cots even when they knew nothing was really wrong. They learned to watch the monitor with a more critical eye. 'Even at four months I could see Marissa crying, glancing at the door, and crying some more,' Sandy recalled. 'She was looking to see if anyone was coming in! At four months! That told me that I was the one being trained, and after that, we really picked up the effort to reverse it, to train her.'

Nighttime improved, particularly after the parents decided to stop chasing two sets of dummies all night long, at about five months. Marissa slept better before Sasha. Sasha at one point started throwing all her loveys and toys into Marissa's cot, and then screaming because she didn't have her favorite things anymore, forcing Marissa to rouse herself and hand the blanket back through the cot, so they could both get to sleep. 'They have a lot of empathy for each other. It's really neat to watch,' Sandy said.

Napping was tough at first, because the girls were not on the same schedule, and if one woke the other one up, it would throw the whole day off for both of them and often cascade disastrously into the next day as well. Sandy separated them for about two months during the day, as she worked on lengthening and coordinating their naps.

Napping

Although I normally keep twins together at nighttime, I often recommend separating them for naps, because daytime sleep is so much more of a challenge for most babies. It's even harder if there's a playmate to distract or be distracted by in the next cot. Some parents keep twins apart for naps for days or weeks, others throughout childhood. Do whichever feels best to you and seems to work for your kids.

Nap training duets can be difficult. If you are lucky, one will nap well and you will only have to nap train one, either by using my Sleep Lady Shuffle at naptime or by using the other nap techniques I describe in the age chapters. But if they both need nap training, you'll probably have to calm one, leave him, then go to the other twin and calm him, then after ten minutes or so, go back and check on the first one, and in another ten minutes go back to the second, and so forth. (It's not fun.) If one is napping less than the other, you might have to put him down a little earlier at night, or try to squeeze in an extra short late-afternoon nap if he's under nine or ten months of age.

At seven months, Ryan slept well, but Amber did not. 'Every time Amber got up, the whole house got up,' their mother, Melanie, recalled. 'Ryan was not happy.' Melanie used to rush in as soon as Amber cried, fearing she would wake Ryan. She tried all sorts of things – holding Amber, putting her in her car seat, reluctantly letting her cry once in awhile. Some days the only way Melanie could get Amber to sleep was on her back – on Melanie's back, not Amber's. 'It was killing me; she was getting bigger and bigger and bigger,' her mother said.

When Amber began taking medication for reflux, her nighttime sleeping improved considerably, but naps were still a disaster. Melanie separated them, and concentrated on Amber's napping using the techniques I suggest for a seven-month-old (see Chapter 7, 'Six to Eight Months').

Amber was mad, and didn't even want her mother to stay by her side at naptime. In those first days of nap training, she would cry for the entire hour. But within about ten days, Amber began taking her lovey and falling asleep for a nice, solid nap. Melanie kept the children separate for naps as well as bedtime. The only time they share a room is on vacation – when Ryan enjoys the company but pays a price when his sister wakes him up too early in the morning, no matter how hard he tries to ignore her.

For babies six months or older who are having trouble falling asleep and staying asleep, many families use the Sleep Lady Shuffle, my system of having the parent gradually fade out of bedtime as the child gains sleep confidence. Check out the Shuffle instructions for your children's age. It's obviously easier if only one child needs the Shuffle, and you can temporarily separate the twins while you carry it out. If both need the Shuffle, it's usually easiest if one parent sits in between the two cots, gently moving back and forth to stroke and soothe each child in turn. By the third or fourth night, you will be relying much more on your voice than on your touch to calm and reassure them. For babies under six months of age, follow the sleep-shaping suggestions in Chapter 5, 'The Right Start for Newborns and Infants,' and Chapter 6, 'Newborn to Five Months.'

Bedtime

Bedtime can be quite a juggling act – sometimes ridiculously close to a literal juggling act – with young twins. Melanie, for instance, knew her children needed good, focused attention, and nice, peaceful stories before bed. Easier said than done. 'I can get one sitting in my lap, but not two. I get one down, and the other one climbs away. Bedtime is supposed to be this relaxing, wonderful bonding time, but for us it was very stressful.'

I usually tell parents of twins to close the door, get the pajamas on, and just read. If one gets up, keep reading, try to engage her, but don't force it. When it's time for lights-out, it's into the cot whether they've paid attention to the story or not.

Melanie tried all sorts of variants, depending on their moods and their ages. She usually started out reading and they assumed one of three positions – both on the floor on one side of her, both in her lap, or one on either side of her on the sofa. 'I can't say that any of my three systems worked with complete accuracy, but by mixing up the positions, they seemed to stay in one place for the longest period of reading time.' When they got older, they began to disagree on what books to read, so Melanie would start them off together on a book, but then let Amber pretend to 'read' a book to herself if she turned her nose down at Ryan's choice, and vice versa. 'One twin can 'read' the more interesting book while I read the less appealing story to the other child,' Melanie said.

When work schedules permit, some parents split bedtime responsibilities. For instance, by eighteen months Kayla and Charlie were out of the cot and in separate rooms. Both were waking up at night wanting to drink bottles of milk (when they got older and went through another round of bedtime difficulties, it was juice in a cup) and wanted their parents to lie down with them at night. Each parent led one twin through the Sleep Lady Shuffle, and later the parents divided up bedtime routines. Charles would give Charlie a good-night kiss and then take care of Kayla, while Molly tended to Charlie, who was a little less temperamental at bedtime. After she said good night to Charlie, Molly spent a few minutes with Kayla before she too went to bed. Kayla took longer to fall asleep, and she had more trouble separating, wanting one of her parents, usually Molly, to sit in a chair in the hallway. On nights when Charles had to work late, Molly read to both children in one room, then put the easier-going Charlie to bed, and then Kayla.

Dawn and Clark tried to keep bedtime a whole-family time. Now two and a half, the children take a bath, select three books, and snuggle and read with both parents on a sofa in the children's room. Then Allison turns the night light on. Not to be outdone, Scott then turns it off and back on again. Then they get into their cots. They may happily keep each other company, sparing their parents some of the stalling and curtain calls typical of children this age. But sometimes Allison decides her brother's company isn't quite enough. 'Allison calls; you have to go in, fix her blanket, rub her back. We go through it three or four times, then enough is enough. She may cry until she figures out she isn't going to get her way,' Dawn said. 'Scott is more placid. He goes down, no problem, 85 percent of the time; if she's crying, he'll just lie down and watch her. But once in a while he'll pick up on some of her little traits, and you'll hear him saying, 'I need my nappy changed, too.' He'll see that she can do that and get attention.'

Now three and a half, Nathaniel and Ethan still share a room. Their recent move from cot to bed led to some new bedtime procrastination, asking for a little more of this and a little more of that – in stereo.

Charlotte and Ed responded immediately by enforcing a very consistent bedtime routine, which either parent can carry out. The boys bathe, brush their teeth, read one or two books in the living room, make one last visit to the bathroom, then to the bedroom for a song, a glass of water, and lights-out. 'With two three-year-old boys, you become a limit setter,' Charlotte said, laughing. 'There's no ground to give.'

Nathaniel recently went through a period when he was waking up very early – and the first thing he would do was shout, 'Ethan, Ethan!' until his brother woke up. His parents made a sticker chart for Nathaniel; he had to let Ethan sleep until he could see the sun. If he filled up a whole row of stickers, he could get a toy. (It's always a good idea to get the sibling a treat, too – after all, he was the one so rudely awakened!)

Scheduling Challenges

Twins can have different sleep needs, but they shouldn't be wildly different, not more than an hour off from average. Some researchers have found that identical twins are more likely to need the same amount of sleep than fraternal twins. Either way, you may not get them on precisely the same schedule, but you do want them to be similar.

One trick is to make sure they are awake in the morning within about a half hour of each other. Then coordinate morning naps. For instance, if one twin gets up naturally at 7:00 a.m. and the other gets up at 8:00, wake the sleepyhead at 7:00, too – or maybe let him sleep until 7:30 while you feed the earlier riser. Then they will both be ready to go down for their nap at around 9:00 or 9:30. Similarly, if one tends to take a longer morning nap, start waking him up earlier, so they remain in sync for the afternoon nap. And that afternoon nap is his catch-up opportunity – the one who needs more sleep can take a longer afternoon snooze, and you will still have a long enough gap between the nap and bedtime so that you can put them down together.

You might have to tweak their schedules periodically because at different times, their sleep needs might diverge a bit more, depending on when each child goes through growth spurts or hits developmental milestones.

At five months, Allison and Scott were still in Moses baskets in their parents' room, near Clark's side of the bed. They had wildly different schedules, and no one in the family slept. One baby or the other always seemed to be awake and nursing – or at least demanding that one parent find a dummy.

It was time to get them out of their Moses baskets and their parents' room, and into cots in their own shared room. We introduced loveys, a tiger for Scott, a bunny for Allison. Dawn and Clark cut out the dummies, cold turkey, and sat nearby to soothe the babies when they sought their dummies.

These babies were growing well and doing fine, and no longer needed to be fed all the time. After checking with their pediatrician, we cut back nursing to just once a night. It took several weeks of tinkering and adjusting, but we got them on the same schedule, soothing them without excess nursing as they gradually adapted to new routines. 'If one was asleep and the other cried, that was just the way it was going to be,' Dawn recalled. 'We didn't jump up and pick one up if he or she was crying; we let them learn to go back to sleep.'

Sometimes, even as toddlers, one would wake up too early in the morning and try to entice the other to play, but usually if Clark and Dawn left them alone, both babies would drift back to sleep within five minutes. 'They do amuse themselves,' Dawn said. 'Every once in a while, you'll hear on the monitor Allison saying, 'Scott, look at this. Scott, try this,' and then you'll hear, 'Wheeeeeeeeeeee! Thump-thump-thump,' and you'll know they are having fun at something.'

The biggest scheduling challenge for many families comes at around fifteen or eighteen months, when the twins start moving from two naps to one. That's a strain when you've got one toddler, but it can be really painful when you've got two transitioning at slightly different speeds. (See Chapter 9, 'Thirteen to Eighteen Months,' for more advice on nap consolidation.)

'When one was waking up from a morning nap, we'd wake the other one to make his morning nap short, so they'd both go down together at the afternoon nap. It got kind of complicated, but it was only a few weeks,' said Charlotte.

Dawn recalled a similar experience. 'Allison doesn't like to sleep as much as Scott. She likes to stay up and jibber-jabber, and he learned to just ignore his sister. But when one began switching to a single nap, we dragged the other one along. We had to force it, going by the clock. I could see Scott getting tired; Allison is not as easy to read. But when he went upstairs, she went up too.'

Siblings

For those families who have children very close in age, some of the information I shared about twins in the first part of this chapter may be useful. But here I'll answer some other questions I hear often from families with two or more children, such as:

- How do I put two kids to sleep?
- How should two parents divide responsibilities?
- What about napping?
- Will one crying child wake up or frighten the other sleeping child?
- What if they share a room? And what if one is in a cot and one in a bed?
- What if they have the same bedtime? What if they don't?

Bedtime

The general rule of thumb is to put the youngest one to bed first. Depending on age, personality, and degree of sibling rivalry, the big brother or sister may or may not want to listen to the baby's stories and songs and be part of the baby's good-night rituals before going to bed. If not, make sure the older child keeps busy with a quiet game or activity so she won't keep interrupting the baby's bedtime in a manner that is disruptive or stimulating. You don't want the three year old (or any older child for that matter) running in constantly while you are trying to get the younger one to sleep. That's what I did when my second daughter, Gretchen, was a baby and needed a nice, quiet nursing or bottle before bed and her dad wasn't home to take care of our older daughter, Carleigh. By the time Gretchen was about one and Carleigh three, I could read a 'young' book to the two of them together in Gretchen's room. Then Carleigh would wait for me in her room while I put Gretchen to bed. As soon as Gretchen was down (she knew how to put herself to sleep, so I didn't have to stay there), I'd go to Carleigh and read her an 'older' book and make sure she and I got some just-the-two-of-us Mum-Carleigh time. (I'll talk about shared rooms in a moment.)

If two parents are home in the evening, one may deal with the baby (often the mum if she's nursing), and one takes care of the older child or children. But switch off some of the time, so each child knows how to go through her bedtime routine with each parent. Make sure both children get a few special good-night moments with both parents. It helps if everyone makes the kids' bedtime a priority for an hour or so – take care of other house-hold tasks a little later. Even if you aren't both routinely home by bedtime, see if you can find a time to start coaching when your work schedules will allow both of you to be home for a stretch. If not, see if you can enlist a grandparent, relative, or friend. One adult does the Shuffle with the baby, the other with the toddler. Or it might be easier for you to let the older one stay up for a little while you work on the little one's sleep. Then you can do the coaching for the older one.

> 'We stagger our children's bedtimes,' said Kathleen, whose children, Maude and Sean, are twenty-six months apart. 'That's hard as a working parent, because Maude goes down at 7:00, and I only get an hour and a half with her on the three days that I work. But I know she needs to go to bed then; kids who go to sleep at 9:00 or 10:00 have a lot more temper tantrums.'
>
> While Kathleen is busy with Maude, big brother Sean understands that it's baby sister's special time with Mum. He gets a thirty-minute video, a quiet one suitable for evening, or special playtime with his dad. Then he gets to choose if Dad puts him to bed, or if he wants some Mum time of his own. The other parent comes in for a final message of sweet dreams and a good-night kiss. The family set up this basic system when Maude was an infant and Sean was two, and it was still working with just a few minor tweaks when he was four and a half.
>
> Greta and Matt used to have both boys together for story time. Frederick would happily stand up in his cot and point at trucks while Dad read books to big brother. When that system no longer worked,

when they each needed a more age-specific story, the parents split them up for bedtime.

Some children go through a stage when they only want one parent at bedtime – usually Mummy.

'First I get the baby to sleep, but I often hear Ariella clear across the house; she doesn't want her dad – she wants me. And Peg hears it too, so then I have Ariella stalling and Peg crying. We've tried really hard to let Doyle put the girls to bed, but Ariella really wants me right now, and I have to be with Peg because I'm still nursing,' said Marcy. She and Doyle have gently but persistently continued including Doyle in Ariella's bedtime. He now does baths and dinners and some evening play, although Ariella still insists on Mummy for stories and lights-out. Meanwhile, hoping to avoid a repetition of this pattern with the younger daughter, Doyle has been spending more and more time with Peggy at bedtime, and he's the one who goes in to check on her on those nights when she still wakes up.

Sometimes we worry so much about the younger child's cries waking or upsetting the older one that we rush in too quickly. Try not to fall into this trap, because you are only going to perpetuate the younger child's night wakenings by reinforcing her sleep crutches. If she cries and you come running lickety-split, she isn't going to have a lot of motivation to stop crying! Try going first, briefly, to the older child who has been woken up, rather than the one who is bawling. For instance, if you are sleep shaping with a six month old and the baby is waking up your two year old, go to the two year old first and reassure her. Tell her that the baby is okay and she should go back to sleep. Then go tend to the six month old. If both parents are home, then divide and conquer, one of you with each child. You might also want to try a white-noise machine for the older child. I like the Marpac Sleepmate 980. Some other great new ones have also come on the market, and they aren't expensive. (They are also much smaller and more portable than they used to be, which makes them handy if you want to block out unfamiliar or loud noises when you travel.)

It helps if you tell the older children what sleep training is, and why her baby brother or sister sometimes cries. Most will understand this by around age two and a half. I encourage parents to start with a family meeting, to explain the expectations and find ways of getting the older child (or children) to feel like she's part of the baby's sleep education.

Depending on the age and sleep skills of the older child, you may even help her think of herself as a sleep role model for the baby. Tell her the baby needs to know how to get herself to sleep, just like her big sister does. Explain that when the baby learns, she won't cry as much, but in the meantime you have to be with her or go check on her. The older child will let you go more easily if she understands and you make her an ally. If she gets it, she may not barge in as often with demands on you just as you are finally getting the little one to drift off to sleep. Stickers or other little treats and incentives can help. Your goal, as always, is to prevent the older one from feeling displaced. Instead, you want to make her feel even more needed, more loved, more important. (See Chapter 16, 'Routine Busters,' for advice on the birth of a sibling.)

Sometimes if your children are very far apart in age, with eight or ten years between the oldest and the youngest, it seems that life should get a little easier because the big one can help with the little brother or sister, or at least take care of herself. That's true up to a point, but it's also true that the children have such different needs – logistically, academically, and emotionally – in the evenings that you may feel like you are straddling two parallel parental universes. It's tough to bathe a three year old upstairs while trying to pry a twelve year old away from the kitchen computer, or to get the little one all cozy and drowsy only to have the big one noisily pop into the bedroom every five minutes with questions about maths homework. I know some families who have enlisted the older child to help put the younger one to bed, or even to pretend that he is going to sleep at the same time, although they aren't always willing or able to go along with that gimmick all the time.

Naps

Scheduling conflicts between your children's naps or activities also create sleep barriers. For instance, you may discover that your six month old's natural nap sleep window is wide open precisely when you have to pick up your older child from preschool. See if you can work out a carpool to minimize those disruptions. If you do have to drive and the baby falls asleep in the car seat, either move the car seat inside and let her finish her nap or, better, work on teaching her how to transfer into the cot: if she wakes up while you move her, stroke and soothe her back to sleep. It takes a little while to acquire that skill, but most babies do get it, so don't give up; keep working on it. Then it's lunch and afternoon naps for everyone. Playdates will work best after the p.m. naps, while they are on a two-nap-a-day schedule, or in the morning once the toddler switches to one nap.

Parents often find that no matter how tears-averse they were with their first child, they have little choice once the second one arrives. For instance, if you are nap coaching an eight month old and your three year old is downstairs, it's going to be hard to stay with the baby for a solid hour and leave the preschooler on his own, unless you have a babysitter or a relative who can come over and help at naptime. Even if the preschooler doesn't mind being left on his own (and he probably will mind – an hour is a long time), you are going to be in the baby's room fretting about whether the older child is really quietly assembling that puzzle you left him – or finger painting the living room couch.

Chances are, at some point, you are going to be spending some time with the three year old while you leave the baby to cry for a few minutes. Try to get at least the prenap ritual with the baby done, putting her down drowsy but awake. And check on her every ten or fifteen minutes; you don't want her crying forever. But simply out of necessity, you may have a slightly more Ferber-like approach to naps with a second child.

Marianne and Glenn, whom you met in the chapter on newborns, had three children in four years. Holly was a terrible sleeper, Dean was significantly better, and by the time they got to Ally, it was easy. 'With Ally, I don't know if I got it right, or she got it right,' Marianne said. 'She had some mild reflux and she was on medication, but we did everything differently with her. We let her cry a little more; we didn't pick her up at every whimper. We couldn't! We had two other young kids to take care of. At naptime she would cry, but I wouldn't be able to get up to her room, and I started realizing she was falling right back to sleep. Maybe there were five minutes of tears. When she gets up now, if I know naptime is over, I'll go get her, but if it's not time for it to be over, I'll leave her alone for five more minutes and she'll go back to sleep.'

Occasionally, I've run into families who thought sleep training a younger child would be too stressful on the older child. Ellen, for instance, sent the very sensitive James to his grandparents while she trained Vanessa. Luckily, Ellen had a much easier time with Vanessa than with James, and the sleep coaching took just three days. Usually this isn't a problem; just be attuned to how the older sibling feels about the baby's sleep shaping, or have one parent stay with him and keep reassuring him that the baby won't cry forever, that he'll be sleeping soundly and dreaming sweetly in just a little while.

Sharing a Room

While you focus on getting the baby to sleep, try having the older one play quietly in a nearby room for a little while before coming into her own bed. (If you are all living in a one-bedroom apartment, sleep training is harder but still possible. Check out my advice on page 37 of Chapter 2, 'Getting Started and Tips for Success.')

Parents often ask me for advice on whether children should share rooms, or how old they should be when they are separated, particularly a boy and a girl (assuming the family has enough space for separate bedrooms). I don't think there's a right or wrong answer; do what feels right for you and watch your children for clues to their preferences. They might be old enough to articulate what they want.

It's often helpful to sleep train the baby before you move him into the big sister's or brother's room. You can keep the baby in your room (or another room in the house or apartment) while you train him, and then move him into the shared room once he has it down. Alternatively, if they are already sharing a room, you could move the older child temporarily out of his room into your room or another room in your home. Naturally, this isn't a good idea for a child who may easily start feeling displaced, is having a tough time with sibling rivalry, or who will have a hard time moving out of his makeshift bed in your room if that's where you plan on putting him. But if he is adaptable, explain to him that this is a temporary arrangement while the baby learns to sleep. You might even be able to make it sound fun.

When you do move a baby into the older child's room, teach the bigger child good 'sleep manners.' No talking to, playing with, or waking the baby when he is asleep. Explain that it's so special to share a room and it's important to have good sleep manners.

You can sleep coach two kids or more (I have successfully coached parents of quadruplets) in one room, in cots or beds, even if they are slightly different ages. If it's one parent flying solo at bedtime, sit between the beds or cots and go over to first one child and then the other as needed to comfort them. If one is in a cot and the other in a bed, make sure the older one understands that once he's in bed, he needs to stay there.

Review the tips for good sleep manners in the relevant age chapter. If both parents are available, life is easier if one can sit by each child's bed or cot for the first three nights of the Shuffle. Once you get to night 4, one parent can probably position the chair in a way that works for both children. Some of the details in the 'Twins' section may help.

14

Nightmares, Night Terrors, and Sleepwalking

Nightmares, night terrors, and sleepwalking are distinct phenomena – and none of them is a sign of serious emotional disturbance or disorder.

Nightmares are part of normal development, peaking between the ages of two and three. Children at this age have wondrously rich imaginations and some difficulty distinguishing reality from fantasy. Nightmares occur during REM sleep, and the child wakes up feeling anxious or afraid, but he recognizes his parents and seeks comfort.

Night terrors are less common, occurring in about 5 percent of children, more boys than girls, and can last into the school years. They occur in non–REM sleep, when we do not dream, so the child will not remember the terror. (See Chapter 4, 'Sleep Basics,' if you want to review REM and non–REM sleep.) Night terrors can be disturbing for parents to watch, but they are not a sign of serious emotional disturbance or disorder. You may not be able to eliminate them completely, but you can take steps to minimize them. Usually children outgrow them, and they seldom last past early adolescence.

Like night terrors, *sleepwalking* is a partial-arousal parasomnia disorder, which the child does not remember the next day. As the child can wander around, open doors, and climb stairs, safety is generally the biggest concern with sleepwalking.

Nightmares

Nightmares occur toward the end of a sleep period. The child can recall the dream, or at least know she had a bad one, and it may take her a while to get scary thoughts out of her head and fall asleep again. Nightmares are, of course, common after difficult events or when children are experiencing change or stress or are reliving a trauma. They can also occur when a child is overtired, either because she still hasn't learned to sleep well enough or she's been thrown off her routine for a few days by illness, travel, or a change in the family's schedule. But sometimes they occur for no particular reason, just like we as adults may have a bad dream when nothing particularly unusual or unpleasant is going on in our lives.

Sleep Lady Tip

Children may pick up more than we realize about frightening events, whether it be a distant hurricane, a fire down the block, or the unsettling news of our world. Through snippets of television news or adult conversation, they may get just enough information to be frightened and not enough to truly comprehend how abstract or distant a threat is to them or their loved ones. Keep your antenna up for what they may be hearing or seeing that may cause fear and anxiety. It's often wise to avoid television or radio news when young children are present.

You can't prevent all nightmares – they are part of childhood, just as they are an occasional part of adulthood. But you can try to minimize them and make them less frequent. Avoid scary videos, books, games, and stories prior to bed. Don't play scary games, not even during the day if your child is fearful, unless you can turn them into empowering games where your child transforms the scary monsters into giggly monsters or something like that.

When a child does have a bad dream, respond very quickly and assure her that she is safe. Hug her and hold her if she needs it, even if you are in the middle of a sleep-shaping program, or the Sleep Lady Shuffle, that asks you to minimize your nighttime physical engagement. Stay in her room until she falls asleep again. It's tempting to lie down in her bed with her, but try to avoid it, or to keep it brief, particularly if you are trying to break a cosleeping pattern, or you have been cosleeping until recently.

The same rich imagination that contributes to the nightmares may also help combat them. For instance, many three and four year olds have imaginary friends, and you can help the child enlist those friends to ward off bad dreams or monsters. Draw on the lovey, too; remind her that the lovey is by her side all night and will make her feel safe and sound. Children also like applying their imaginations to a dream agenda. 'Tonight I'll dream about playing football.' Or 'Tonight I will dream about building a sand castle.' Or 'Tonight I will dream about being a beautiful ballerina.' It helps them feel more in control of what happens to them after they fall asleep, particularly if they are worried about nightmares. My 'Dream Cards' (also on my Web site) might help children feel in control of their dreams. Based on my experiences in 'creating' dreams with my own daughters, the cards guide children through a progressive relaxation exercise and have images for dream ideas such as a tree house, a beach scene, a field of flowers, and a rainbow.

By the age of five, many children understand the difference between dreams and reality. Despite that cognitive leap, they still need TLC and reassurance, just as we adults still want an extra hug when we have a bad dream.

Sometimes kids become fearful of their own room because of the nightmares, or just start stalling more at bedtime or running out of bed more at night. Spend more time playing with her in her own room during daylight so that she feels safer and more comfortable there. At night, allow a little extra time for the bedtime rituals and relaxation. Include bedtime stories about children conquering their fears. (I suggest some good bedtime stories, as well as relaxation guides, in the 'Resource Directory' at the back of this book.)

Review her sleep chart, if she has one, to remind her of good sleep manners, and then reward her liberally for following them. If she wakes with a nightmare and comes to your room, take her back to her own bed and stay near her until she feels better.

Sometimes parents sleep in a child's bedroom after bad dreams, but be careful about doing this too long or too often. It can become a negative association, or a sleep crutch, and she will need you to be there all the time. (You may decide lying down with her is worth it if you feel you will be able to retrain her out of that habit fairly quickly, when the fear of nightmares subsides.)

At bedtime, if she's apprehensive about bad dreams, tell her you will be nearby, and be very specific. 'Mummy will be in her room reading,' or 'Daddy will be right down the hall hanging up his suits.' Promise to check on her frequently and then live up to that promise. Not only will those checks make her feel safer, but they will also help keep her in her own room instead of scrambling out every five minutes in search of you. Leave the door open a little if that makes her feel better, and keep a night light on, or even a little more hall light than usual. Discuss bad dreams if your child brings them up, but don't 'lead the witness.' In other words, you shouldn't be the one to remind her about last night's scary dream, and if she runs into your bedroom at night, your first words should not be, 'Did you have a nightmare?' Be sympathetic – don't yell at her for getting out of bed when she may be frightened, but don't plant the idea of bad dreams if it isn't already there.

A few other suggestions follow. Not every idea will help with every child, but experiment to see which works for you, or which leads you and your child to your own helpful variants:

1. Allow a pet to sleep in the child's room.
2. Try letting your children share a room as long as they both have good sleep manners and won't keep each other up.
3. Use some kind of 'monster-away spray' or, if it seems too confusing to be chasing away monsters at the same time you

are trying to teach your child that monsters don't exist, use a 'bad-thought spray.'

4. Let your child create his own bad-dream defenses. One slightly older girl I worked with, about eight, made a shield with pictures and images that she felt protected her, and kept it by her bed. Another one put up a dream catcher. Several kids I know have arranged their stuffed animals or action figures around their bed in a way that makes them feel protected. I heard about one insightful preschool teacher who had families make a 'monster box' – with a lid to capture monsters and keep them confined.

5. Include in your bedtime preparations some kind of prayer for safety if that fits your beliefs, or create a more secular anti-nightmare ritual or mantra. Your child might imagine a guardian angel watching over him, or recite a prayer with you that surrounds him with love, light, and protection.

6. Help your child act out throwing away his bad thoughts in a concrete way that can make him feel they are really gone. Throw them out the window (you don't really have to open the window) or dump them in the trash or flush them down the toilet (just make sure he knows that they are flushed far away, so he doesn't get afraid of the toilet in the morning!). One mom I know made a 'worry tree' with her kindergartner. She made the trunk and branches out of brown construction paper and formed leaves out of green stick 'em notes. Each night the child plucked a leaf off the tree, and ripped it up, eliminating a worry.

7. If your child has adequate verbal skills, teach him progressive relaxation techniques, tightening and releasing muscles starting at the toes, then the feet, and all the way up to the top of the head. If you don't want to do this yourself, you can play a relaxation CD (see my suggestions at the back of the book or try the Sleep Lady CD, *The Sweetest Dreams*). You can also try creative visualization, helping your child imagine playing on the beach with his cousins or walking in the park as the leaves change color, any image that will make him feel happy and calm. Children sometimes like to pretend they are a character in a favorite (nonscary) book or like making up stories where they are a prince or princess or magic fairy in a beautiful garden. (I

have some resources at the back of this book and on my Web site, www.sleeplady.com.)

8.   It is also wise to avoid high-dose vitamins close to bedtime, and if your child takes any medication, talk to your doctor about whether it might interfere with sleep and whether you can find an alternative or at least change the dosing times.

Night Terrors

Night terrors are not bad dreams, and although they are distressing to witness, they are not a sign of psychological problems. They are different from nightmares, although the first time your child experiences one you may not immediately recognize that it's a terror.

A child experiencing a terror may scream, shout, sweat, have a racing heart, appear anxious, and seem inconsolable. His eyes may be wide open and he will look awake, but this is a partial-arousal disorder and he is actually still asleep and probably won't recognize you. He may even push you away, or flail at you, even while he is calling out for you. The terror usually lasts five to fifteen minutes and then subsides. It is often more upsetting for the parent to endure than for the child to experience, since the child usually won't remember it – and the parent will.

Night terrors occur during non–REM sleep (when they are coming out of deep sleep) and usually within two hours of falling asleep. The single biggest risk factor is probably being overtired – terrors may stop when your child starts getting more sleep. Sleep apnea can be a factor, so discuss that possibility with your doctor. Stress that disturbs sleep, such as a major change in the child's sleep schedule or a new place to sleep, can also be a factor. A child who has an erratic sleep schedule is also at higher risk. Terrors may also occur during developmental milestones, or when a child is sick or running a fever.

'My child didn't have too many bad dreams, and I don't think he had any full-fledged monstery nightmares that I was aware of. Then one night when he was sick and had a slight fever, just before his third birthday, I heard this earsplitting, terrorized screech at about

10:30 or 11:00,' the mother of that three year old said. 'He was screaming, 'Mummy, Mummy!' and when I ran to him and told him I was there, he kept alternating between screaming for me and hitting me, like he didn't recognize me and I was scaring him. I picked him up and held him, which I later realized I probably shouldn't have done, and he kept screaming for me, and I kept telling him I was there, and he seemed to go back and forth between recognition and terror.

'Then all of a sudden, it was over. The tension went out of his body, and he went right back into a peaceful sleep, looking perfectly calm and content. I was so shaken that I slept in his room the rest of the night, but he was fine and never said a word about it in the morning. He didn't have any problems again, including the next time he had a cold and tummyache, but then a few months later it happened again when he was running a fever. It still took me a few minutes to realize what was going on, but at least I was a little better prepared. It still felt horrible to watch and I felt helpless, but at least I knew it was only the fever and that he would be okay in just a few minutes.'

Children are more likely to experience night terrors if either parent had them as a child or if a parent had a partial-arousal sleep disorder such as sleepwalking. If your child gets up and walks around while having a terror, which can happen occasionally even with children who do not otherwise sleepwalk, make sure she is safe. Think about placing a gate at the top of any nearby stairs.

During a terror, monitor the child to make sure he is physically safe and not thrashing around in a dangerous way during the episode. But don't interfere, as this could intensify it. Try not to touch your child or pick him up, since this can actually prolong the terror. Go to him, stay in his room, and calmly reassure him. Don't talk to him about the terror in the morning. Since sleep deprivation plays a major role in night terrors, put him to bed earlier, even if only by thirty minutes. Be extra vigilant about keeping him on a consistent sleep schedule.

If night terrors seem to be regular events, not an occasional side effect of a fever or temporary schedule disruption, keep a sleep log to monitor the timing and frequency. If they are occurring two to three times a week at set times (e.g., two hours after going to sleep), try waking him fifteen minutes before the typical onset of the terror. Don't get him completely wide awake, rouse him just enough for him to mumble, move, or roll over. Then let him fall asleep again and see if you can disrupt the sleep cycle that leads to the terrors. Do this every night for seven to ten days. If the terrors return, do the waking again, but this time do it for two full weeks to see if you can extinguish the problem.

Sleep Lady Tip

Although this may not be a psychological problem or an illness, you might want to discuss frequent ongoing terrors with your doctor to make sure there is no underlying trauma, illness, or apnea that must be addressed. Check to see if any medications he is taking, including any over-the-counter drugs, could be interfering with his sleep and contributing to the terrors.

Sleepwalking

Like night terrors, sleepwalking is a partial-arousal disorder that occurs during non–REM sleep, when the child is not dreaming. Episodes usually occur within two hours of falling asleep, and the child doesn't remember sleepwalking later. A sleepwalking child looks awake but usually appears confused, and may be clumsy and do strange things. He may not want comfort from a parent, although he probably won't scream and act afraid as he would if he were having a terror. Sleepwalking, as with terrors, often runs in families.

You may be surprised to find that sleepwalking is actually quite common, although chronic or frequent sleepwalking is relatively rare. In *A Clinical Guide to Pediatric Sleep: Diagnosis and Management of Sleep Problems*, Jodi Mindell and Judith Owens write that between 15 and 40 percent of children sleepwalk at least once, and 3 to 4 percent have frequent episodes. The peak ages for weekly or monthly episodes are from four to eight years of age, but about one-third of sleepwalkers will experience episodes over a five-year span, and about one in ten will sleepwalk for ten years.

The most important concern is, of course, safety. You don't want a sleepwalking child to fall down the stairs, climb anywhere he shouldn't be, stumble into the basement, or go outside. You should put gates on the stairs and lock doors. If you hear him walking around, don't wake him, but try to gently guide him back to bed. If you are afraid you won't hear him, think about installing an alarm, or even some kind of makeshift system like a bell that will ring if he opens his bedroom door. Sleep deprivation is a risk factor for sleepwalking, so make sure he gets plenty of sleep and is on a consistent schedule. With sleepwalking, I do recommend you contact your doctor. Depending on the frequency of the episodes and his risk of injury, she may want to prescribe a short-term sleep medication.

15

Medical Problems

Coughs, colds, ear infections, and tummyaches, those routine childhood illnesses, can temporarily disturb sleep, and my next chapter, 'Routine Busters,' will help you through those rough spots. Here I will talk about some of the more complex and persistent medical problems. As I'm not a medical doctor, I called on my own family pediatrician, Dr Faith Hackett, to review this chapter. If you have consistently applied a behavioral modification program – whether it's my Sleep Lady approach or one of the crying-it-out alternatives – and your child is still not sleeping well, please consult your doctor to determine if her sleep problems have medical roots and to refer you to a specialist if necessary.

When you do talk to your doctor, including at routine checkups, make sure you mention your child's sleep patterns, even if the doctor doesn't bring it up herself. Provide her with enough information to evaluate the problem. Keep a sleep log, or at least jot down some notes, and be prepared to explain the behavioral approach you have adopted. If your child throws up regularly and you wonder if it may be a symptom of reflux, try to keep track of how often and when. For example, telling your doctor that your baby throws up five to seven times a day, ten minutes after eating, is more helpful than telling the doctor that the baby throws up 'a lot.' Similarly, if you think your child may have allergies, note the circumstances of the reactions. If you suspect apnea, make a five-minute tape of the snoring, snorts, or those other loud and strange nighttime noises so the doctor can hear for herself.

Sleep Lady Tip

Even children with medical components to sleep difficulties can benefit from behavioral modification techniques. For instance, your child might have health concerns that require night feedings past the age where most other infants are learning to sleep longer intervals. But you can still work on teaching good sleep habits at bedtime and naptime, even if you can't grapple with those night wakenings yet.

Reflux and Colic

Spitting up is a normal part of infancy. It may create a laundry problem, but it's not a health problem. However, when babies spit up or throw up excessively, numerous times a day, they may have gastroesophageal reflux disease.

Reflux is very common, affecting as many as one in ten babies. It can be caused by a host of factors, often related to the fact that in many babies the gastroesophageal valve (in layman's language, the valve at the top of the stomach) has not yet fully developed and needs more time to grow. In mild cases, it's akin to baby heartburn. In more severe cases, the stomach acid as well as food, breast milk, or formula get pushed back up out of the stomach, up the esophagus, and out the mouth, or even sometimes the nose. In addition to the vomiting, many babies develop related respiratory symptoms and may face a risk of aspiration. Luckily, reflux can usually be managed, and your doctor can suggest many techniques, possibly including medication. Most babies will outgrow the condition in six to ten months.

Reflux babies can develop sleep problems that can persist even after the reflux symptoms are controlled. More than a third of the children I work with have, or have had, reflux past the age of three to four months. (If they get over it very early, you should be able to follow the sleep-shaping ideas in the age-by-age section of this book without having to worry too much about longer-term sleep disruption.) My own second child, Gretchen, had reflux, and her first few weeks were not easy. But with our doctor's help, we were able to manage her condition with medication and have a happy, healthy baby who slept eight hours at a stretch pretty consistently by the time she was ten weeks old.

Parents often confuse reflux with colic, but they are not the same. Reflux is a structural, though not permanent, problem with the digestive system. *Colic* is a catchall term that basically means a baby cries a lot, mostly in the late afternoon and early evening. Up to one in four babies under age three months experience these crying jags. But it doesn't mean you are a bad or incompetent parent, or that your baby is in pain, or that he will be a fussy or unhappy child. Some people believe that colic may be a sign of overstimulation, and that your attempt to calm the baby will only add to the problem. Dr Ferber, for instance, says that if the colicky baby doesn't respond to our soothing, then soothing isn't what he is seeking. He recommends that you let the colicky baby cry for fifteen to thirty minutes and see if he can calm himself down. My own preference is for you to review the soothing techniques, such as swaddling and swinging, that I outline in Chapter 5, 'The Right Start for Newborns and Infants.' *Remember – don't get in the habit of nursing him every time he cries.* Since the crying might make it harder to read his sleep-window cues, keep an eye on the clock so you know how long he's been awake. Try taking him into a quiet, dimly lit room where he may start showing signs of tiring.

How to Recognize Reflux

Reflux symptoms can emerge in very young infants. They can include:

- Frequent vomiting – sometimes and quite unpleasantly through the nose. (Some babies have *silent reflux*, meaning they have the pain and surges of acid without spitting up.)
- Slow weight gain or even weight loss. However, not all reflux babies are underweight.
- Reluctance to eat or signs of pain when eating, such as stiffening up, arching his back, or pushing away from the breast or bottle.
- Wanting to eat, but just a little at a time.
- Frequent coughs (this can have other causes; check with your doctor).
- Aspiration causing chronic nasal or sinus congestion.
- Choking or gagging.
- Sour breath.
- Excessive crying – more than a few hours a day.
- Baby wakes up frequently, often showing signs of pain in his stomach or chest.

Don't panic if your child displays a few of these signs once in a while. You are looking for a pattern, not a single episode. But if you do suspect a problem, call your doctor. It's important to get an accurate diagnosis. You might think the baby has reflux when he is lactose intolerant or just gassy. In severe or stubborn cases, your doctor may suggest you consult a pediatric gastroenterologist.

Managing Reflux

Sometimes we can control reflux with a few simple positioning and feeding tricks, which I'll address in a moment. But sometimes we face slightly more complicated choices, and the solutions you choose will be a blend of your values and parenting style and your doctor's advice. For instance, if you are completely committed to breast milk and don't want formula, you may opt for medication and modify your own diet by reducing or eliminating dairy. Conversely, if you don't want to put your infant on medication, you might prefer to cut back on breast milk and try to find a formula that works for her instead of or in addition to nursing. Sometimes you won't have a choice. Your baby will clearly need medication, and your doctor will explain why.

The following suggestions are widely accepted by pediatricians, but check with your own doctor anyway. Not every doctor agrees with every element on this list, and your doctor may feel that some aspect of reflux management is inappropriate, unwise, or even unsafe for your unique child. Keep in mind too that some of these tools will tame the spitting up but will not necessarily stop all the surges of pain.

Sleep Lady Tip

Babies tend to like bouncy chairs even if they don't have reflux, and not just after eating. Bouncy seats hold babies at an angle that 'folds' them less than a car seat. You don't need all the bells, whistles, and elaborate sound and light effects; a simple seat is fine.

Gravity is your baby's friend. Keep your baby upright, but not slumped over, for twenty to thirty minutes after all daytime and bedtime feedings to help digestion. You can seat her in a bouncy chair or hold her in your arms – *but don't get into the habit of holding her until she falls asleep in your arms.* Time the feeding early enough so that you can feed her, hold or sit her down for a half hour, and then put her to sleep drowsy but awake.

- Offer frequent, small meals.
- When possible feed the baby upon waking, not before sleep, which allows time to digest before lying down again.
- Burp your baby several times during the feeding, not just once after feeding.
- Experiment with different formulas. Some babies do better with soya formula or a hypoallergenic formula or a thickened formula made for babies with reflux, making it more viscous and easier for the baby to keep down. (Some doctors recommend that you thicken your own formula, adding one tablespoon of dry cereal

to two ounces of formula, but ask your pediatrician before you try this on your own, particularly with very young infants.) You might even find that your baby does better with one brand of formula than another, or that he still throws up the powdered version but does better with the thicker (and alas usually costlier) premixed canned variety.

- Elevate his cot or Moses basket under the head. You can buy a simple, inexpensive wedge at a baby store that goes under the mattress cover or the fitted bottom sheet (and is also helpful when he has a cold). One family I worked with, following their doctor's advice, rolled up a baby blanket in a U shape to make a nest in the elevated cot so the baby wouldn't roll down to the bottom of the cot. For safety's sake, they stuck the U-shaped blanket under the fitted sheet, and placed the baby with his feet at the bottom curve of the U. The sides of the U shouldn't reach past his chest. Some families use a Tucker Sling, which keeps the baby elevated, or an Amby bed, which is like a baby hammock. Both are available online. Of course, review the safety precautions.
- Dress him in outfits that are loose at the waist.
- Try having him sleep on his left side, once he is old enough to do so safely. Talk to your doctor and familiarize yourself with safety precautions to avoid SIDS ('cot death').
- Encourage him to sleep on his tummy, once he learns to roll over in both directions and the SIDS risk lessens (usually around six months; check with your doctor). Citing a few small studies showing that even younger infants with reflux do better on their tummies, some websites urge this sleeping position for reflux. However, the North American Society for Pediatric Gastroenterology and Nutrition does *not* endorse sleeping on the stomach for young infants, except in extremely rare cases where the reflux disease is so severe that the risk of death from reflux outweighs the risk of SIDS.
- It also helps to have a sense of humor and a Mummy or Daddy wardrobe that does not require dry cleaning! Carry around a lot of spare clothes in your car, stroller, or nappy bag – for your baby and for you!

How to Help Reflux Babies Sleep

As parents, our natural instinct is to soothe a baby who hurts. That's exactly what we should do. But we need to pay attention to how we soothe a reflux baby. While a baby without tummy problems is learning to rock himself to sleep, a reflux baby dealing with projectile vomiting may miss out on the chance to learn how to self-soothe and fall asleep on his own! As we comfort our babies, we may inadvertently reinforce poor sleep habits. Then, even after the reflux (or colic) has passed or been controlled, our babies still don't sleep well. They must then learn, or relearn, how to put themselves to sleep without being walked, rocked, fed, put in the swing, the car seat, or ridden around the block – you know the drill.

I will give you two related sets of suggestions – one on how to deal with sleep while you and your child are still handling the worst of the reflux, and a second one on how to get him on a better sleep path once the medical part is under control or he has outgrown it. In both cases he'll do better if you tackle bedtime first, then naps. Before the nap piece falls into place, do whatever you need to do to get him some sleep during the day, even if it means breaking my usual rules of not using the car to get him to sleep. If you are feeding him at night for medical reasons, don't worry about changing that right away, although the night wakenings might diminish on their own as other aspects of his sleep improve. Work with the information here as well as the relevant age chapter earlier in this book.

As with a colicky baby, reading reflux babies' sleep cues can be difficult. I suspect this is because they don't learn to differentiate their cries because pain, vomiting, hunger, and tiredness all sort of blur together for them. We then have more trouble figuring out what they're crying about and may not respond as consistently to whatever it is they're trying to tell us. So you have to be more diligent about watching the clock, not just your baby. Keep track of when he ate. As he gets older, you'll want to stretch out the time between feedings as long as you can without provoking more vomiting, particularly overnight. Also pay attention to how long he has been awake. Make sure he naps on time. The last thing he needs is an overlay of exhaustion on top of his burning esophagus. Taking him into a quiet, dim room for a while before nap or bed often helps. He may show his sleepy signals more clearly in such a setting. Also, the quiet environment may cue him that it's time for bed.

As I mentioned, your doctor will probably recommend that you hold or seat your baby upright for about twenty to thirty minutes after he eats. Don't hold him until he falls asleep. You don't want him to develop an association between sleeping and being in your arms, or otherwise you'll have to hold him to sleep all the time, including overnight, for months to come. Don't worry if he falls asleep in your arms occasionally. Just don't teach him that your arms are his bed. Allow enough time between feeding and bedtime for another activity in between. Feed him, hold him upright, and then read him a book, give him a bath, and let him get some tummy time on a play mat. When it's time for him to sleep, put him down drowsy but awake. Try to arrange his daytime schedule so that you are feeding him when he wakes up in the morning and when he gets up from naps, instead of before he takes naps, to avoid that holding-sleeping association. That gives him time to digest before he lies down, a position that increases the reflux.

Some reflux babies fare better if they eat small, frequent meals. That might mean you will have to feed him overnight to an older age than you would a baby without reflux. But the night feedings can also add to his discomfort, so talk to your doctor about when you can stop them. At some point, the nighttime nursing (or bottle-feeding) ceases to be a physical requirement and starts being a sleep-disrupting habit. When that happens, you need to stop those nighttime feedings. Please don't let this go on too long – address it before his first birthday. If not, you may well have a child who wakes you up demanding a drink every few hours well into his second or third year.

Babies who feed at night also tend to get emotionally attached to the cup or bottle, as though it were a dummy or a teddy bear. Some babies give up the night feeding much more easily than you might guess, in a night or two. Some resist longer. In each age chapter, I give detailed advice on nighttime weaning. For older babies who did not have reflux but still have a nighttime eating pattern, I usually recommend a pretty quick end – maybe not quite cold turkey but something close. However, with children who had reflux, you might want a more gradual and gentler approach. I give many suggestions about night weaning in the age chapters (with the most details in Chapter 7, 'Six to Eight Months').

In my own sleep practice, I have found that postreflux babies often remain very sensitive to their environments. They react more to such stimuli as bright lights, crowds, food, and textures. You then need to be sensitive to their sensitivities! (I talk a little more about sensory processing issues and give some resources in the section on attention deficit disorder and attention deficit/hyperactivity disorder later in this chapter.) Continue to be very careful about his schedule. Watch the clock, and keep using that quiet, dimly lit room to help him calm down.

Tracy and Drew's son, Lucas, had been diagnosed with reflux shortly after his birth. His pediatrician prescribed Zantac. It took a while to get the dosing and timing right for Lucas, but by four months, the medication and reflux management techniques had brought the problem under control. But they didn't do anything for his sleep. If anything, his sleep was getting worse. While other babies had been learning rudimentary self-soothing techniques, Lucas had his mind on his hurting tummy. Now he was getting up every three or four hours – more on a bad night. Naps were also problematic, and sometimes he woke well before dawn.

Tracy started paying a lot more attention to his schedule and the timing of his meals. She shortened his feedings, sometimes letting him nurse only two or three minutes. 'I shaved minutes off nursing to convince myself it was about soothing, not feeding. He was doing it for fun!' she said. 'I knew he really didn't need to eat that often. And it wasn't the reflux cry anymore – it was the unhappy cry.' At four months, the pediatrician said they should try to get Lucas to sleep, without food, for about seven hours a night. Seven hours seemed beyond comprehension to the sleep-deprived couple. They called me.

Tracy still breastfed Lucas before he went to bed, at about 7:00 p.m. But for the next feeding, at about 10:00 or 11:00, I suggested they give him a bottle of formula or expressed breastmilk (I talk a lot about these 'dreamfeeds' in Chapter 6, 'Newborn to Five Months'). They also gave him his medicine then. Then they would not feed him again until at least 6:00 a.m., or even 6:30 if he slept that late. They would stay with him and comfort him if he cried and protested, but they did not feed him or lie down with him. (I gave them the option of picking him up briefly if they needed to calm him down, although they chose to soothe him without lifting him out of the cot, a decision that might have made their first few nights a little more teary than they had to be.)

'The first night, he cried for a long time. Then he collapsed. We soothed him, but we didn't pick him up. It took about two weeks before he wouldn't cry at all, but other nights he didn't cry as long,' Tracy said. By the end of the two weeks, he was getting up once for ten minutes or less in the middle of the night, but they wouldn't feed him and he woke up less and less. At about six months, they took the next step and gave up that dreamfeed. 'It was pretty easy,' she said. 'He woke up and fussed, and we went in and said, "Sorry, buddy!"' So then he went to bed at 7:00 at night and slept all the way through until 7:00 in the morning.

Although those first two weeks of transition were unpleasant, Tracy and Drew's wholehearted belief that Lucas needed to learn to sleep better made it a lot easier for them to be consistent. And with Tracy having to go back to her job at five months, they knew they needed to deal with his sleep problems now. 'We couldn't have done it if we had to leave him alone crying. Being in the room made it easier. But we really believed he would be better off if he could sleep. He had to learn how to do it.'

Tracy was also motivated by the secret confessions of her girlfriends that some of their kids were still waking multiple times at night at ages two and three. She was also clear-sighted enough about herself to know that she needed more sleep to be the mother she wanted to be. 'I was so tired, I couldn't function, and I wasn't enjoying him as much as I wanted to,' she said.

Those first few nights, she let Drew give Lucas a bottle and deal with his protests. That was partly to avoid getting Lucas even more upset by letting him see his mother but not letting him nurse. But it was also because by then Tracy really needed a break. She went *downstairs, put in some earplugs, and slept for three nights. 'I felt I'd been reborn.'*

Allergies and Asthma

Milk sensitivities, eczema, and environmental allergies can all hamper a baby's ability to learn how to sleep, and they can disrupt sleep at any time from infancy through childhood.

Food and Milk Allergies

If you are nursing and suspect your child is allergic or intolerant to milk, you can try eliminating all dairy products (check labels, as dairy ingredients can be hidden) from your diet for three or four weeks. Make sure you get alternative sources of calcium for your sake and your baby's. Some mothers mistakenly expect to see a difference in a few days, so they don't stick to it. Milk sensitivities can contribute to mild reflux and may also cause nasal congestion that can contribute to apnea.

Talk to your pediatrician about giving your baby a milk test. You might also, with your doctor's guidance, try hypoallergenic, lactose-free, or soya formulas. Think about eliminating or cutting out caffeine and alcohol if you are nursing. Because peanut and other nut allergies are becoming more common and can be dangerous, some pediatricians advise nursing mothers to eliminate peanuts, peanut butter, or other nuts from their diet. Also, if you or your husband had childhood food allergies, tell your pediatrician. She may want you to delay introduction of certain solid foods – like wheat, eggs, citrus, shellfish, berries, chocolate, or corn – or modify the timetable. For instance, she might want you to introduce one food a week, instead of trying a new one every few days, so you can more easily monitor reactions.

Eczema and Dermatitis

Numerous allergies can cause hives, rashes, and itchy skin – and it's hard to sleep if you itch like crazy. According to *Guide to Your Child's*

Sleep: Birth Through Adolescence, from the American Academy of Pediatrics, allergic children can have trouble sleeping even at those times when they are symptom free. Some research suggests that children with skin allergies may be at higher risk for developing asthma. There are a lot of treatments, some over-the-counter, some by prescription, for eczema and related conditions, so you and your pediatrician should be able to get this problem under control with relative ease.

Stuffy Noses, Coughing, and Other Allergy Symptoms

Your child might have seasonal allergies, or a sensitivity to dust, pollutants, mold, or a household pet. You know how poorly you sleep when you have a cold. Children with these allergy symptoms feel like that all the time. Seasonal allergies can also inflame adenoids and tonsils, which in turn can cause sleep disturbances or sleep apnea.

Allergic or asthmatic children often have disrupted or poor-quality sleep. They may then struggle to stay awake during the day and perform poorly in school. Sometimes they are judged to be hyperactive or to have behavioral problems when in fact all that fidgeting is just their attempt to stay awake. Good diagnosis and treatment lead to better sleep – and to a better-behaved, higher-functioning daytime child.

Depending on your child's age and the severity of symptoms, your doctor may recommend a saline spray, decongestant, bedroom humidifier, or allergy medicine. A lot of over-the-counter cold and allergy medicines are no longer recommended for children under the age of six and many products for the under twos have been taken off the market, so be careful and talk to your doctor.

Unfortunately, some asthma medications themselves disrupt sleep. Watch out for changes in sleep patterns if your child takes asthma or allergy drugs. You might need to try a slightly different drug, or a different dose. Ask your doctor if the child can take the medication a little earlier in the day, rather than just before bed, to see if that helps.

Sleep Apnea

A child with sleep apnea stops breathing briefly during sleep because of obstruction of the upper airways, in the back of the throat. Swollen or overly large tonsils or adenoids cause the obstruction. (But not all large tonsils or adenoids cause apnea – many kids will 'grow into' them in time.) Lax neck muscles during a child's sleep can also contribute to apnea.

Even mild cases of apnea can disrupt sleep and may warrant surgical removal of the adenoids or tonsils or both. When the child can get some air despite the obstruction, you might hear loud snoring. When he can't get any air, his brain will tell him to get up and breathe ASAP! He will get up to move the muscles in the tongue and throat to open the air passage. But he won't necessarily be able to get himself back to sleep again without calling for you.

Loud breathing and persistent snorting and snoring are often key symptoms of apnea, and it's a good idea to make a five-minute tape of those strange nighttime noises so your doctor can evaluate them. Also, while it's worth getting a good evaluation, first from your doctor and then from a pediatric ear, nose, and throat specialist, don't be in too much of a rush to get those tonsils or adenoids removed surgically. Sometimes it's necessary, but you don't want your child to go through unnecessary surgery if it's not. It's a myth that removing tonsils or adenoids will reduce the number of colds and sore throats he catches or will 'cure' allergies. It doesn't even help recurrent ear infections except, according to Dr Barton Schmitt's book *Your Child's Health* (2005), in those children whose large adenoids are causing the nasal obstruction that leads to the ear problems.

How to Recognize Apnea

Apnea has one set of symptoms by day and another by night. Day symptoms include:

• Breathing through the mouth
• Nasal congestion

- Nasally voice
- Difficulty swallowing
- Frequent infections (ears and sinuses)
- Poor appetite
- Morning headaches (if they are old enough to tell you)
- Waking up tired and being very sleepy during the day
- Behavioral problems

Nighttime symptoms include:

- Snoring – often loud ('grandpa' snoring, as one specialist puts it)
- Loud breathing
- Pauses in breathing while sleeping
- Frequent nighttime wakenings – particularly if they don't have any other sleep crutches
- Waking up thirsty during the night
- Very restless sleep
- Sweating during sleep (body is working harder to breathe) particularly on the head
- Unusual sleep positions such as sleeping on their knees, propping themselves up on pillows or stuffed animals, hyperextending their neck, sitting up, and so on; these positions reflect an effort to keep the airways open
- Bedwetting if the child is trained during the day and had been trained at night
- Mouth breathing
- Sleeping fewer hours than the average

If you cosleep and your toddler or preschooler wakes up frequently, you might want to think about apnea. This isn't true if she is nursing on demand and still wakes up to nurse frequently, but it is a possible indicator for a child who may wake up, sit up and reposition herself, and then go back to sleep.

I worked with a two year old who slept with his parents and would sit up, cry out, and plop back down in the middle of the night. He didn't need them to do anything else for him to get back to sleep. We worked on bedtime, and naptime, and we did a lot of sleep coaching to reduce night wakenings. But we didn't eliminate them completely. He didn't snore, but he was a mouth breather and he had milk allergies. His doctor finally ordered an X-ray of his adenoids, and sure enough, they were quite enlarged. He had them removed, and started sleeping all night almost immediately.

How to Help a Child with Apnea Sleep Better

If your child has even mild sleep apnea, behavioral modification will get you only so far. You can teach him to get himself to bed at night and at naptime, but you will have a very hard time stopping the night wakenings since it is a physical condition that is getting him up. So you need a double-pronged approach. Get him evaluated, by a pediatrician and by an ear, nose, and throat specialist if necessary. You may need to take him to a special clinic for an overnight sleep study. Few clinics deal with pediatric behavioral sleep problems, but many do evaluations for apnea or other breathing disorders. Your doctor can refer you. Sometimes treatment, which can include surgery or allergy medication, solves all the sleep problems. In many cases, however, you will still have some behavioral problems to address. Follow the advice in this book for your child's age. You should find that improvement comes quickly.

> *Amanda and Tony, whom you met in Chapter 11, 'Two and a Half to Five Years Old,' went through my whole Sleep Lady Shuffle with Wes. He quickly learned to fall asleep on his own without protest and to go back to sleep with less parental intervention. But while Wes woke up a lot less frequently at night, no matter what behavioral approaches Amanda, Tony, and I tried, we never got him to stop waking up at least once or twice a night, often around the same time.*
>
> *Approaching his fourth birthday, he often seemed very tired during the day, as though he were fighting to stay awake. During one of our follow-up conversations, Amanda mentioned that Wes breathed very, very loudly at night. I urged them to call their pediatrician.*
>
> *It turned out that Wes had severe allergies. Not quite full-fledged asthma, but enough difficulties to keep some emergency medicines on*

hand if the wheezing got too bad. The doctor also suspected apnea. Amanda and Tony tried to get Wes a thorough overnight sleep study at an established clinic — but he got so distraught each time that they always had to give up and go home. But the ear, nose, and throat specialist and the pediatrician agreed that his extremely large adenoids and tonsils should come out. Unfortunately, the operation took place on his fourth birthday, and he had a pretty miserable few days. When he began to feel better, his parents revived his old sticker chart and started talking to him again about the Sleep Lady and sleep manners. This time, lo and behold, Wes started to sleep all night.

'He was always a happy and loving child, but he's even happier now,' his mum said. 'He needed so many naps, he struggled so much, it has made such a difference for the whole family. Back then, I would look at myself in the mirror and I looked all fuzzy — I was so exhausted. I feel much more patient now.'

Attention Deficit Disorder and Attention Deficit/Hyperactivity Disorder

The conditions ADD and ADHD are not usually diagnosed in very young children, but they sometimes do become an issue in preschool years. Children with other behavioral or attention problems, including sensory processing issues, may be mislabeled as ADD/ADHD, particularly in these early years.

Whatever the cause, hyperactive children often have trouble falling asleep. These children, even more than others, need a lot of consistency and a steady parental hand. Set bedtime rules, and make sure your child understands that they are rules, not suggestions! Give your child an extralong wind-down period before bed — maybe forty-five minutes will do the trick.

Try to get tension-producing activities out of the way in the afternoon or early evening, leaving plenty of time for the child to switch into a calmer gear before bed. Stimulating games (including computer games and DVDs) should also be over and done with well before bedtime — and keep them out of his bedroom. Bedtime activities should be quiet, gentle, borderline boring. ADD/ADHD kids, even more than other children, may stall, engage, delay, provoke – they do whatever it takes to keep themselves up and you at their side before bed. Be patient but firm.

If your child takes medication for ADD/ADHD, it may make it harder for him to fall asleep. Work closely with your doctor on timing and dosage. You want to time the medication so it helps the child during the day, but wears off early enough that it does not interfere with bed. If you think medications are keeping your child up, or making him have trouble falling asleep, talk to your doctor about alternatives. There are several medications on the market now for ADD/ADHD, and if one is creating sleep difficulties, it might be worth trying another.

There are many good books on ADD/ADHD. My favorites include *Healing ADD* (2002) by Daniel Amen, and *Taking Charge of ADHD* (2000) by Russell Barkley. You may also want to explore whether your child has sensory processing difficulties, which I find often play a role in sleep problems. These sensory problems can include a lack of focus and an oversensitivity or an undersensitivity to stimuli such as light, food, textures, water temperatures, loud noises, and being touched. By far the best book on sensory processing is *The Out-of-Sync Child* (2006) by Carol Stock Kranowitz. It's a superb, easy-to-understand resource. I also like *Sensational Kids* (2007) by Lucy Jane Miller and Doris Fuller. You may also want to consult an occupational therapist certified in sensory processing (sometimes also called sensory integration). If you do, share your observations and concerns about your child's sleep patterns.

Bedwetting

Most children are potty trained by day sometime between the ages of two and three, some earlier, some later. Girls are usually, but not always, earlier than boys. Listen to your child's signals regarding potty training – if he isn't ready, it won't go smoothly. I don't see any problem in working on daytime potty training, with a receptive and enthusiastic child, at the same time that you are doing Sleep Lady coaching. But I would not make a big push about using the potty at night in the midst of sleep coaching. Think of how confusing it would be for him to go through this behavioral modification program to learn to go to bed and stay in bed – and then be told he'd better get up and pee!

It often takes until the age of four or five for a child's bladder to grow big enough to contain the night's urine production, or for his sleepy brain to learn how to respond when his bladder shouts, 'Full!' Do get in the habit of having him go to the bathroom before bed, but just keep him in a nappy or pull-up at night until the age of four or five. If he stays dry, fine. It will make it easier for you to help him start using the potty at night when he's a little older. You may notice that he's always dry, that he's learned this on his own, so you can get rid of nappies or pull-ups.

After the age of five, bedwetting still affects about one in ten children. It's twice as common in boys as girls. The reasons for bedwetting are not well understood, but there is often a family history. Many doctors now regard it as a *parasomnia*, a sleep disorder found in deep sleepers. Sometimes bedwetting – particularly if the child was trained at night but then starting wetting the bed again – can be a sign of sleep apnea, so discuss that possibility with your doctor.

In *Waking Up Dry: A Guide to Help Children Overcome Bedwetting* (2005), Dr Howard Bennett says the main factors in bedwetting include:

- family history – 75 percent of bedwetters have at least one parent or a first-degree relative who wet the bed as a child
- small bladder, which limits nighttime urine storage
- deep sleep so that the child does not respond to the bladder's signals
- constipation, which can create pushing on the bladder and confusing signals
- minor illness and fatigue

Some families report success when they wake up the child an hour or two after he goes to bed, or right before the parents go to bed, to use the bathroom. But it isn't a surefire solution.

Other Medical Problems

A host of serious diseases and syndromes can disrupt children's sleep – autism spectrum disorders, rheumatoid arthritis, neuromuscular disorders, sickle cell disease, and brain injuries, to name a few. (Narcolepsy and restless leg syndrome are extremely rare in young children.) These diseases require medical expertise well beyond the scope of this book. However, even children coping with severe physical challenges and the accompanying emotional trauma can benefit if they learn to sleep better – maybe not perfectly, but better. As Ayanna's experience illustrates, these children usually make the most improvement when their physical symptoms are under control, or at least reasonably contained, and they can begin to shake off some of the bad sleep habits they developed while they were sick.

Ayanna

For the first ten months of her life, it seemed that Ayanna never slept. She coughed, choked, and gagged. She cried. Her frantic parents, Lakeisha and Al, never left her alone. They slept beside her, watching her breathe and hoping for the best. At ten months, she was diagnosed with cystic fibrosis (CF), a very serious lung disease. Although there is no cure yet for CF, Ayanna benefited from the recent advances in treating and controlling it. Within a month of her diagnosis, she was on medication that made her breathing less labored. Her overall health improved. She was happier. But she still didn't sleep.

'Once she got diagnosed and everything got better, we thought, 'Well, she'll sleep better.' But she didn't,' her mother, Lakeisha, said. Although Ayanna was doing better physically, she was used to being near her parents at night. And since her health was better but still fragile, they were understandably reluctant to be very far from her, despite their doctor's reassurances that she could and should be in her own room.

Lakeisha and Al did get her out of their bed, but she moved into a toddler bed, right alongside theirs. 'Too convenient,' her mother laughed. 'We spent all night putting her back in her bed.' In addition, one of the medications she took often made it hard for her to fall asleep – and her parents aggravated that by letting her stay up too late, until 9:30 p.m., meaning she was both pumped up by the drugs and overstimulated by the late hour. It was often 10:00 or 10:30 before she would finally fall asleep, and then she'd be up many times, all night long, tossing, turning, screaming, and yelling.

This went on for a very long time, until one of Lakeisha's coworkers commented on how tired she seemed. That coworker happened to be my brother Glenn. He gave her my number, and she waited about one whole minute before she called me. Ayanna by this time was two and a half, and Lakeisha was beyond exhausted.

'I had wanted to get her into her own room; I knew it would be healthier for her. But I didn't know how. I didn't want to go through the whole crying-it-out thing,' Lakeisha said. 'My kid had gone through enough crying in her life. I just wasn't going to do that to her.'

I knew that Lakeisha had very low expectations. She kept telling me that this case was going to be my first failure. I surprised her — or rather I helped Ayanna surprise her. Lakeisha and Al did my Sleep Lady Shuffle, and Ayanna responded immediately. In fact, they didn't even have to go through the whole program; within a week she was going to sleep on her own. 'We had to remind her, 'No talking, lie quietly, sh-sh, night-night,' but that's all it took,' her mother said. 'In the morning, she would tell us she slept in her 'big girl' bed. She was so proud — she'd get her stickers.'

Sleeping through the whole night took longer, about two or three weeks. It wasn't completely consistent. Some nights she slept, and some nights she woke up and wanted her parents to sit by her. 'We'd sit, and she'd fall right back to sleep. It wasn't an hour — it was five, ten minutes, and then she'd be out again. I'm still in awe.'

Ayanna is lucky in that her CF is relatively mild, and the worse of it can be controlled. But she still gets sick a lot, which causes sleep disruption and much more anxiety than in other households where the worst thing is an occasional earache. When she's sick, Lakeisha and Al still stay with her, but they don't take her into their bed, and they try not to climb into hers too much, either. Instead, they try to restrict themselves to sleeping on a mattress on the floor beside her. When the episodes are over, they quickly go back to their own room, and she can deal with the transitions. At the age of three, she was usually sleeping from 8:30 p.m. to 7:00 a.m. without interruption. 'I couldn't believe it,' her mother said. 'Oh, my goodness, I absolutely have a life back. I have time with my husband now. Our life does not revolve around getting our baby to sleep. We talk about things other than what an awful night it was.'

They go out sometimes now and leave Ayanna with a babysitter. She goes to 'cousin slumber parties' at her aunts' homes, and Lakeisha and Al get a night off, which is great for all couples and absolutely invaluable for a couple dealing with this kind of stress. When they gave away the cot, though, they had to blow the dust off it first. Ayanna had never spent a night in it.

16

Routine Busters:
Dealing with Travel, Illness, and
Life's Other Disruptions

No matter how hard you try to keep your child on a predictable and comforting routine, disruptions are inevitable. Some routine busters, like a vacation or a weekend visit to the grandparents, are planned and welcome. Others, like illnesses, strike without warning and can turn a child's sleep upside down.

In this chapter, I explore ways to get through such common disruptions as travel, illness, teething, the birth of a sibling, and moving to a new home. I also offer some advice in the event of big life changes, like Mum returning to work, or a divorce. I offer guidelines but not rigid rules. Some children are more adaptable than others, and get back into their normal routine without missing a beat. Parents also react differently. Some families strive to keep the schedule in place at all costs. Others consciously decide that the circumstances warrant breaking the sleep rules temporarily, knowing they may have to pay a price later.

During the autumn when Ilan turned three, Joanne's normal three-day workweek became a grueling marathon of fifteen-hour workdays – sometimes even longer – five or six days a week. Ilan didn't see her before bedtime, and woke up frequently wanting to see her at night. She was exhausted, he was miserable, and she decided to cosleep temporarily. After the work crisis ended, she took several days off and spent a lot of time with him and explained he was going to sleep alone in his fire-truck bed again. She cuddled him a lot right before bedtime and sat in the hallway while he fell asleep. He began sleeping through the night again within a week.

As a rule, if you have deviated, it's a good idea to return to your normal routine as soon as possible. Most kids adapt quickly, particularly if they have already developed fairly good sleep skills. Sometimes you'll have to do another round of sleep coaching (often accompanied by some intense crying or, as I like to call it, the inter-mittent-reinforcement shriek), but it usually goes faster than the initial go-round because you are reminding them of a learned skill, not introducing it from scratch. At the end of this chapter I give some help on how to do a refresher version of training, and, as always, you can comfort your child as you ease him back into his routine.

I like reminding children of sleep rules even while we're bending them. 'You are sleeping in the same room as Mummy and Daddy while we are at the lake, but as soon as we get home, you and Teddy Bear will be back in your princess bed and Mummy and Daddy will be in our bed, but we'll come check on you every night.' Or 'I'm going to pick you up and hold you until you fall back asleep to make you feel better, but as soon as your tummyache goes away, you won't need Mummy to do this. You are going to sleep great again, and I'll give you so many stars and stickers because I will be so proud.' Even very young toddlers understand some of this, and older ones get it quite well. It helps to make the rule breaking less confusing to them and makes the intermittent reinforcement less powerful. By understanding your expectations, they may have an easier time readapting to their old routine once the disruption has passed.

Developmental Milestones

Cognitive, emotional, or motor developmental milestones often affect sleep. In fact, Dr T. Berry Brazelton in his book *Touchpoints: Your Child's Emotional and Behavioral Development, Birth to 3* reminds us that we may see regression or a period of disorganization not just in sleep, but in social, emotional, and feeding patterns as well.

I find that the most pronounced, although temporary, sleep problems occur as a child is learning to walk. You may also see problems right before your child sits up, crawls, stands, and is potty trained. I address many of these leaps in the relevant age chapters, but the key is remembering that these new skills excite children and change their view of their world, sometimes quite literally. For instance, when your child stands up in her cot for the first time, she may discover everything looks different from up there!

Of course, it's hard to know that a child is about to reach a milestone. We see the disorganization, the regression, and we may think something is wrong. We might even rush to the doctor. Only in hindsight do we realize that she was about to take her first step. Be flexible, but stay consistent during these periods. When a child is sick, or when we travel, we do have to deviate from normal sleep rules, but with the developmental milestones, if you stay the course, the child will quickly adapt.

'I don't know if this is true for all babies, but for both of mine, sleep got worse before they reached a new milestone. Both kids would have two or three fussy nights – it usually didn't require any intervention from me, but I could hear their disrupted sleep,' said Lisa, mother of Teddy and Brittany and a champion keeper of sleep logs. 'Then they would roll over, or stand up, or sit for the first time.'

Sleep Lady Tip

If your child has only recently started sleeping through the night or going to bed without a great deal of fussing, try to postpone any discretionary travel for at least three weeks.

Travel

The better a child sleeps at home, the better the odds are that he will sleep well when you travel. Even if he does get out of kilter while you are away, if he's a good sleeper, he'll probably return to good patterns when he gets home. Conversely, if your child has only recently started sleeping through the night or going to bed without a great deal of fussing, try to postpone any discretionary travel for at least three weeks.

When you travel, your child will probably backslide a little bit, but try not to throw out all your gains and try not to rely on whatever sleep crutch you've just eliminated. For instance, if you stopped nursing during the night, don't start again. Go ahead and do a lot more soothing and comforting on the road than you would at home, but find some way of soothing that won't lead you back to where you started, that won't let you get caught in the intermittent-reinforcement trap. You don't want him thinking, 'You got me up to nurse when we were in that strange place; maybe you will still get me up to nurse now that we are home!' You can't blame him for trying.

Always bring along the lovey and pack a night light, and, since there's no such thing as traveling light with a small child anyway, go ahead and take along favorite books and toys. Many families bring cot sheets or blankets, too. (Some hotels don't provide much in the way of bedding with a cot or travel cot, so check in advance or pack linens just in case.) You want the child to have items that feel and smell comforting and familiar. If you are one of those parents who always keeps a small bag stocked with first-aid supplies, travel-size medications, and baby toiletries, stick the spare night light and bulb in there as well, so you don't have to worry about forgetting them. If you are staying at a relative's home or in self-catering accomodation, you may want to take your baby monitor with you, too, so you don't feel like you have to stay by his side in a dark room from 7:00 p.m. on!

'We visit my parents, just about an hour away, pretty frequently. I used to bring the whole sheet set — including the bumper and the mobile! But I don't do all that anymore,' said Jayne, who worked

with me when Cynthia was four months old. 'She sleeps in a cot there, and although she usually doesn't sleep well the first night, she's okay the second night. I try to be consistent with her routine there. I don't skip naps, and I put her down at her usual bedtime. She's fine as soon as she gets home.'

One obvious drawback to staying in a hotel or motel is that young children go to bed early, and you may not want to sit in the dark all night. (Some couples take turns reading in the lobby or even in the hall. A balcony can be a good alternative, weather permitting. If you have older children, one of you might want to put the baby to bed in the hotel room while the other keeps the big kids occupied – ice cream, minigolf, or something like that – but then try to have them tiptoe into the hotel room and get into bed as quietly as possible.)

Think about how to position the child's cot or bed so that you may be able to turn on a small lamp later without having it shine in his eyes, or maybe take one of those little travel book lights along. Some all-suite hotels oriented toward long-term business travelers have good deals for families on weekends and holidays. Even in a suite, you may have to turn off all or most of the lights for a few minutes when you put the baby to bed, but then you have some adult space to talk or read or watch a movie with the volume on low (and the kitchenettes are great when traveling with children). One creative mum I know packed an extra sheet and thumbtacks with her every time she stayed in a hotel with her child. She could make a curtained 'wall' between the cot and the bed à la *It Happened One Night* so the child wouldn't think she was going to get to sleep in Mum and Dad's room from now on.

'Randy travels for work, and since I'm not working right now, we try to travel together. I bring everything – the blanket, pillow, more than one teddy bear, toys, and food,' said Suzanna's mother, Sheila. 'We try to get a suite – if she's in our room, it doesn't work as well.' Initially, Sheila would 'do anything' to get Suzanna to sleep away from home, including cosleeping, and that set up problems when they got home. Over time, Suzanna became more adaptable, and Sheila

got better at figuring out how to backslide on the road without creating
longer-term disruptions at home.

Before you go, talk to the hotel about whether it has cots, travel
cots, or Pack-'n-Plays. Or if you are visiting relatives, think about
whether enough grandchildren will visit over the years to make it
worth investing in an inexpensive cot, even one of the smaller fold-
up varieties. Some babies don't really like sleeping in those travel
cots with thin mattresses. You'll learn quickly what your child can
adjust to, and you'll then be able to pack and plan accordingly on
subsequent travel.

With older children who are no longer in a cot, you may request
a rollaway bed, or if the child will be in a regular hotel bed in your
room, you may see if you can move it closer to the wall for safety.
Put an extra pillow on the floor in case he falls out, or place the
mattress on the floor so it doesn't matter if he rolls off. You may
want to place the mattress next to your bed, or between your bed
and another bed holding older siblings, so that the little one is reassured by being close to you.

There's a good chance he will get out of his bed and sneak into
yours. Some parents return the child to his own bed; others figure
it's a losing battle in the hotel. If he does end up with you, carefully explain that he can sleep with you in the hotel (or at Granny's
house or wherever) but will have to go right back into his own
bed when you get back home. Ilan understood this immediately,
and even if he didn't sleep through the night right after a schedule
disruption, he did understand that he could sleep with Mummy in
a hotel or at Granny and Grandpa's house, but at his own house
he'd be in his fire-truck bed with his stuffed animal friends, and
Mummy would be in her room with Daddy.

If possible, try to have your child sleep in one place throughout
the whole vacation. You may be better off with a week at the beach
than on a road trip with a different hotel (and possibly a different
cot) every night. If you are visiting several relatives, it may be worth
sleeping in one home for the entire trip and visiting with other
family members during the day or over early dinners. For instance,
one couple with a nine month old originally planned a five-day

vacation – two nights with one set of grandparents, two with the other, and one night at an aunt's. I gently suggested they might want to reconsider, so they chose one set of grandparents as a 'base camp' and arranged to have relatives visit them there or to spend part of the day at other family members' homes. They carefully explained to all concerned why their baby needed this, and to avoid bruised feelings or rivalries, they immediately let all concerned know that the other grandparents would be the 'base' for the next visit.

Try very hard to make sure your children get enough rest on vacation. With all the change and stimulation, they may not nap while traveling. It's up to you how hard you press the nap; you may get a sense that if you insist and make the effort, he will nap. Alternatively, you may figure that you can spend the whole afternoon in your hotel room and he still won't sleep a wink, so you might as well go out and enjoy yourself; maybe he'll doze in the stroller. It depends on how old the child is, and how long you are away. An infant absolutely still needs naps. A three year old can probably skip naps for a few days as long as you get him to bed at night earlier than usual.

You might also want to plan some of your travel to overlap with naptime. As you know, I normally want children to sleep in their beds, not in cars, but on vacation, a car nap might be the best you can do. Plus, if you are going to be in the car for a few hours anyway, it may be easier on everyone if he sleeps through it. Try to get back to your hotel (or relatives' home) on the early side, to have an early bedtime. A vacation isn't much of a vacation when the kids are melting down all day.

'We had trouble with naps on vacation,' said Lucas's mother, Tracy, whom you met in Chapter 6, 'Newborn to Five Months.' 'But we found that if we had to disrupt his day, we were better off disrupting it in the morning. He'd often fall asleep and catch up later.'

When you get home, make it a top priority to return to your normal routine as quickly as possible. Some families keep their activities very light for a day or two when returning home to really focus on getting napping and bedtime back in place.

Traveling Across Time Zones

If you are traveling across time zones, get your child up at his usual wake-up time, both when you start your vacation and when you get back home. In other words, if he wakes up at 7:00 a.m. at home in Miami, wake him up at 7:00 a.m. Pacific time in Seattle, and then when you get back home to Miami, wake him at 7:00 a.m. eastern time. Do this the day you arrive on vacation, or if you all need to recover from a long trip or a red-eye, do it the next day.

Switch naps and sleep times to local time the first full day after your arrival. So if you got in late and everyone goes to bed later than usual and then sleeps in, naps will obviously be off that first day. But don't let him nap late. Wake him from his last nap (or his only nap) early enough so you can get him to bed at his regular bedtime. In other words, if you arrived in Seattle at midnight, everyone will sleep late in the morning (you hope!). Then instead of napping from 1:00 to 3:00 p.m., he might not begin his nap until 4:00. Don't let him nap too late, though, even if he's a little cranky when you rouse him, so you can get him to bed that night at his regular bedtime, at 7:00 or 8:00 (Seattle time). Don't fret if you can't follow this exactly. A few car or stroller naps aren't a big deal on a vacation; you'll get everyone back to normal when you get home.

Sleep Lady Tip

Use the naps to help your child reset his clock to his new location. Exposure to sunlight, especially in the morning, helps the body adjust. And there's nothing like a hotel swimming pool to tire kids out and help them get ready to sleep.

'We went to Hawaii with two young kids, and we had to lie down with them. We knew it was a no-no, but we had to do it. They were getting up so early — 1:30 a.m.,' said Kathleen. 'Sean had an easier adjustment than Maude, although he did want dinner at midnight.

But when we got home, they readjusted in four nights. They both cried a little on the third night, but just for a couple of minutes, that's all.'

Enjoy Life!

Although I stress routines and consistency, I don't want you to take it to such an extreme that you can't enjoy your life! I'm not sure I would have been as courageous as Kathleen, flying to Hawaii with two children under the age of four. But don't let yourself get caught in the trap Linda and Miguel experienced, either. Four months after they got Amy sleeping well, they were still too petrified even to visit out-of-town relatives for a weekend, never mind try a vacation.

'I'm afraid to get her out of her routine. I'm afraid she'd get out of whack. She would probably adapt better than I think, but I would dread going back to the way things were – it was just so awful,' Linda told me when Amy was fifteen months old. Finally, after a few more months, they did venture away for a weekend with great trepidation. 'She did great!' Linda said. 'Naptime the first day was nearly nonexistent because of the strange environment and a new travel cot but beyond that she did wonderfully!'

Daylight Savings Time Changes

When we change clocks in the spring and autumn, switch immediately to the new time. In other words, if her bedtime was 7:00 p.m. and you moved the clock to 8:00 p.m., keep putting her to bed at 7:00 p.m. according to the new time. Make sure your child has taken a good nap so she can make it to the new time. She may wake up a little early or a little late for a few days, but then she'll adjust. Stay consistent, and don't let her start her day before 6:00 a.m. (new time). Schedule your next day's meals and activities according to the new clock time. The adjustment seldom takes even a week.

If you think your child can't make a one-hour adaptation that easily, split the difference. Using the example above, put her to bed at 7:30 p.m. (new time) for a few days, and then shift it to 7:00 p.m.

Routine Childhood Illnesses

You have some control over when your child travels, but you don't get to choose when he gets an ear infection, a tummyache, or bronchitis. If he gets sick during a sleep-training program, pause until he's feeling better. Don't abandon the program. If you can, 'freeze' or maintain your Shuffle position until he feels better. If you feel he absolutely needs you closer, go back to sitting near the cot as you did on the first three nights of the Shuffle, and then move halfway across the room when he feels better. Don't draw this out; you will just make it harder for him. If he gets sick shortly after you complete his 'coaching,' he'll probably backslide a bit, and you may have to do an abbreviated version of training to get him sleeping all night again.

When your child is sick, respond immediately to his cries at night. Do whatever you need to do – give him medicine, aspirate his nose, clean him up after a tummy attack. Go ahead and hold him and comfort him as much as you think he needs, even if it sets back sleep training a few days. My advice about not picking up crying children during sleep shaping does not apply when they are sick.

Don't totally overdo it, though. You want to take care of your child, you want to soothe your child, but there's a difference between a little backsliding and total regression. In other words, if you've recently ended cosleeping, don't put your child back in your bed at the first sniffle. Sit by his side, hold his hand, stroke him, snuggle him, but try not to take him back into your bed. I would even rather have you sleep on a makeshift bed in his room than have him back in your bed.

But obviously, if you have been trying to get rid of his water bottle at night but he's now got a tummyache, give him whatever fluid he needs to stay hydrated until his stomach calms down. Once you make a health-based decision to give him a drink, do it as soon as he needs it; don't make him cry for it. If age appropriate, feed him in a slightly different way during illness. In other words, if you just weaned him from nighttime nursing but he needs liquids because he's sick, try a cup or a bottle instead of nursing. If he was emotionally attached to a specific sippy cup, try letting him having a few sips out of a 'big boy' cup.

Occasionally, we find a silver lining to an illness. I know one six month old who was very dummy dependent, but he got so congested by a bad cold that he couldn't suck on it and breathe simultaneously. When he didn't use it for three nights, his parents seized the opportunity to make it disappear for good.

During and immediately after an illness, expect your child to wake up more at night and to take longer to get back to sleep. Don't assume over-the-counter cold, allergy, or pain-relief medications will help your child sleep (and don't give them without checking with your doctor as many are not recommended for children under age six and recently, many cold and cough mixtures for children under two have been taken off the market). These medicines do make some children sleepy, but they stimulate others, and they can get so wired that they stay awake for hours. Some mums have found dye-free medicines reduce this problem, but it's not always a solution. And even if they do induce sleep, most medications wear off in a few hours.

Vaccinations throw some children off for a night or two. Ask your doctor whether you should give him Calpol or a similar analgesic before the shot, and offer the baby more reassurance at bedtime and when he gets up at night because he might not be feeling completely himself. He will usually feel better and be sleeping normally within a few days.

Ear infections are particularly brutal on sleep, because the pain intensifies when a child lies down. In fact, frequent and distraught awakenings may be one telltale sign that your child has an ear infection. If your child has chronic infections, talk to your doctor about consulting an ear, nose, and throat specialist on the wisdom of using a longer or different course of antibiotics, or whether he's a good candidate for surgery to insert grommets. If he gets an ear infection while you are doing the Sleep Lady Shuffle, pause where you are, and start moving ahead again after he's been on antibiotics for two or three days (faster if he feels better after only one day).

Teething

Teething can interfere with sleep, but far less than many parents anticipate or believe. Usually, children who sleep well will experience minor disruptions when they begin to teethe (except for the molars, which come in between ages one and two and can cause more pain). But children who are overtired, or who don't know how to put themselves to sleep, may have more trouble when teething. It's like she is saying, 'I'm already tired, I'm not sure how to go to sleep, and now I have this pain in my mouth. That's going to put me over the edge, so I'm going to stay up and yell.'

To sort out how much of the sleep disruption stems from those new little teeth, compare day with night behavior. If she's her usual self all day but extra cranky or difficult at night, it is probably not the teeth. If a usually cheerful child is miserable around the clock, the trouble may well be a particularly painful tooth. The pain usually subsides as soon as the tooth comes through the gum. Ask your pediatrician about using Calpol or a similar painkiller. I also found that letting my daughters chew on cold objects during the day, like a washcloth that I had put in the freezer for a few hours, was very soothing. They also liked chomping on a toothbrush. Occasionally, I've worked with children who have a slew of symptoms – nappy rash, low-grade fever, diarrhea, disturbed sleep, excessive drooling, poor appetite, and crankiness – but they are a minority, and the problems usually pass as soon as the tooth pops out.

If teething problems crop up while you are in the middle of Sleep Lady behavioral modification techniques, progress may slow down for a few days while the tooth comes through, but stick with it. You might want to be a little more soothing, do a little more holding or patting, but don't regress to all the patterns you are trying to change. If you are just about to embark on the Sleep Lady Shuffle or are introducing new sleep manners and you suspect a tooth is about to erupt, consider delaying any changes for a day or two.

Moving to a New Home

A lot of families regard the move to a new home as a time to make sleep changes, but I'd be careful about this. Moving means change and stress, and you don't necessarily want to add to it if your child doesn't do well with change in the first place.

Make sure you give your children plenty of time and attention because it's an enormous change for them. Play in their new bedrooms, to promote comfort and familiarity. At night, babies, preschoolers, and even school-age children might want some extra reassurance as they acclimate to new surroundings, so sit in her room or by the door at bedtime. Don't forget a night light and a few practice runs at finding the bathroom!

With older children, even around the age of three, you might want to let the child help arrange her room. Choosing colors or decorations will help her feel in control and make the move feel more fun. Be sure to let children talk out their concerns, including questions about their new routines, babysitters, preschools, or schools.

After Reid lost his job, he and Julia traveled by car with three young children while they tried to figure out where they wanted to resettle. They spent a lot of time in cars and hotels, and did a lot of backsliding regarding sleep. 'We gave Todd back his dummy,' said Reid. 'I'm not sure whether it helped him, but I think it helped the real estate agents.'

When they finally did settle in a lovely southern coastal city and Reid opened his own business, the kids manifested pretty typical behavior. That's when the oldest daughter became a champion bedtime negotiator, earning that 'Captain Loophole' sobriquet. The second daughter, who was moving to a new area and starting kindergarten simultaneously, started showing up in her parents' bed at night. And Todd needed that dummy again – but he would get furious at bedtime, hurling it across the room. 'It's an interesting ritual, if you stop to think about it,' Reid said. 'He was throwing the one thing he really needed to get himself to sleep.' Naturally, as the parents gave their

children reassurance and everyone adapted, life calmed down, or got
as close to calm as any home with three children age seven and under
can be.

With a very young baby, a move to a new house or apartment
is a good time to move the cot out of your room and into her
own room. If she's more than six months old, you might want to
start the Sleep Lady Shuffle as you make this switch (although you
may not want to tackle everything at once; for example, if you
move her to her own room, you might not want to try to wean
her off of her dummy that same night).

If she's less than six months old and too young for the Shuffle,
sit in her room and give her some extra soothing and reassurance
as she acclimates. For an older child, a move is not usually a good
time to switch from a cot to a bed. Let her get accustomed to the
new space first, or you will be inviting more bedtime conflict. If the
room configuration allows it, I like putting the cot in the same place
in relation to the door as it was in your old house or apartment.

As with all changes, the better your child sleeps, and the longer
she's been sleeping well, the less disruptive a move is likely to be.
If your child doesn't sleep well and you want to do some concerted
sleep coaching, wait a few weeks after the move until she's adapted.
You as a parent will also cope better with her sleep training if
you've got the first wave of moving chaos under control.

We moved when Carleigh was two and half and Gretchen was
minus three weeks (I was pregnant!). Being a little hyperfocused on
sleep, I had the estate agent help me figure out which of the four
bedrooms got the earliest sunlight. I then put the girls in the rooms
with the least morning sun. Some people move into a new home
and get the kitchen set up first, or maybe the big-screen TV. The
first thing I did was put up room-darkening shades in the kids'
rooms and get their furniture in place.

Child-Care Nap Obstacles

Child-care centers have their own approach to naps, and they aren't
always the approaches that are right for your individual child, even

if the overall care is excellent. For instance, many child-care centers will not allow a baby to cry in the cot at naptime for fear of waking all those other babies. So the caregivers often rock or hold the babies to sleep.

You should work on nighttime sleep and weekend naps, and when you are fairly confident of your child's ability to get herself to sleep, talk to the child-care providers. Explain what you have accomplished and ask them to work with you on getting her down drowsy but awake. Perhaps they can put your child in the sleep room or nap area a few minutes before they bring in the other babies, to give her a chance to get used to falling asleep on her own there. Maybe they can just rock or hold her for a shorter period of time and then pat and 'sh-sh' her to sleep, instead of rocking her until she's totally out. Talk to them about meshing their nap schedule with your child's sleep windows. Share your knowledge of sleep science to see if you can get them to work with you. Talk to them about keeping a special lovey, blanket, or pillow at child care or preschool. At the very least, ask that they work on 'filling her sleep tank' any way they can so that she is not totally nap deprived when you pick her up.

One family I worked with had a very active, alert six month old who had difficulty napping in a bright, somewhat noisy room with other children. Her child-care center would not tolerate any naptime crying, so the staff held her to sleep. Even that stopped working; as soon as they put her in her cot, she would wake up and cry. The baby would end up taking several short half-hour naps and be a wreck by the time her parents arrived. They then had trouble with her at dinnertime and bedtime, and she started waking up more frequently at night because she was overtired. The otherwise excellent child-care center would not bend on their sleep rules, so the parents withdrew her and hired a nanny. It was much more expensive, but they felt they had no choice, given their daughter's temperament and sleep patterns. The child-care center did agree to reserve a slot for the little girl, and she happily returned at age two.

Some child-care centers transfer babies on their first birthdays to a new care group where all children nap once a day. Unfortunately, this is premature; most children don't transition to one nap until about fifteen to eighteen months. Talk to the center about leaving your one year old in the baby room for a few more months until he's ready to give up his morning nap.

In toddler classrooms, children usually nap on mats or camp beds (not cots) in a darkened room with a lot of other children. If it works, leave it alone! You can work on bedtime and weekend naps, and many children can separate what happens at child care from home patterns.

With a three and a half or four year old, your challenge might be convincing the child-care staff that he no longer needs to nap, that he stays up way too late if he sleeps for two hours each afternoon. Most providers give sleep reports; if yours doesn't, ask them to fill you in.

Family Trauma

Obviously, going through a divorce, illness, or a death in the family is an upsetting time for everyone, and your goal should be to provide your child with maximum comfort and security. You will almost certainly see some sleep disruption – more clinginess at bedtime, more night wakenings, maybe more bad dreams.

I wouldn't attempt to embark on any major new sleep training until the trauma (your child's and yours) has diminished and new routines have been established. You can, however, try to avoid creating any new sleep crutches during a time of stress. For instance, you might be tempted to start cosleeping to comfort your child (or yourself), but I would recommend that you do a lot of snuggling before bedtime and a lot of comforting from a chair or the doorway rather than getting into a new habit that may be difficult to break later.

Separation and Divorce

With separation and divorce, as always, maintaining a routine will provide your child with a great deal of security and comfort. Children may adapt better than you expect to two different sets of sleep rules and expectations. They understand, for instance, that

Mummy will lie down with them until they fall asleep at Mummy's house, but Daddy won't lie down with them at Daddy's house (or vice versa). What counts is consistency from each parent. In other words, if you lie down with her on Tuesday, she has every reason to expect you to lie down with her again on Friday, no matter what happened at the other parent's house on Wednesday and Thursday.

Similarly, it's fine if your kids share a room at Dad's house but have separate rooms at Mum's. If you have to sleep coach them, you may have to separate them temporarily. It's generally better to move the better sleeper to a temporary bedroom, and leave the one being coached where he is. (Chapter 13, 'Helping Twins and Siblings Sleep,' has more advice on sleep training more than one child.)

A parent with shared custody can do the Sleep Lady Shuffle on his or her own, no matter what the other parent is doing. It may take longer and not be perfect, but you will see improvement. For instance, if you're now a single father and don't want to cosleep with your three-year-old daughter, you can start the Shuffle by having her sleep on a mattress on the floor of your room for a weekend or a week. Then, the next time she's at your house, you can sleep on the floor of her room while she gets into her bed. Continue the Shuffle, step by step, as best you can within the confines of your custody arrangement. Obviously, the ideal is for both parents to work this out together, but that's a tall order amid a divorce. Don't despair of sleep improvements even without cooperation from your former spouse or partner.

Sleep Lady Tip

Some parents have tremendous trouble setting any limits during the first year of divorce. They feel sad and guilty and don't want to 'ruin' their time with their children by setting limits, enforcing rules, or risking arguments. Again, I must emphasize that children find routine, structure, and boundaries comforting, especially in times of stress.

Loss of a Family Member

In the sad event that your family experiences a death, follow the same advice mentioned above: Be gentle and offer extra reassurance, ideally without creating new sleep crutches. Make sure you don't tell your child that Grandpa went to sleep and won't wake up again. That only exacerbates children's evening fears. Incorporate your own beliefs in explaining death to your child. If your spouse has died, then you may want to seek grief counseling and discuss further strategies with the therapist on how to help your child. Some parents may decide to do whatever works and deal with the sleep fallout when they are feeling better themselves.

School and Work Changes

All sorts of disruptions unsettle our children's lives – new childcare providers, Mum's going back to work, a parent's traveling on business. Basically, you need to give extra reassurance and comfort without throwing your whole routine out the window. Keep bedtime and bedtime rules consistent, but make sure you are providing the sense of security your child needs.

> 'When Vince travels, I stick to the plan. If I vary it for even one second, it's all over,' said Beth, whose daughter, Madison, was then two and a half.

Be extra diligent about making sure your child gets enough sleep because she will be able to handle stress and change better if she's well rested. Some parents who travel like to leave a tape or video recording of themselves singing a lullaby or reading a favorite bedtime book. Children sometimes like to mark off the days on a calendar until Mum or Dad comes home. It's very concrete, and they can actually see that the parent's homecoming is approaching. It's nice to include the missing parent in bedtime songs or prayers. Be careful, though, about talking to Mum or Dad on the phone just before bedtime. This can be upsetting to a child who doesn't understand where his parent is. If your child reacts badly, try scheduling the phone calls earlier in the day.

Baby Brothers and Sisters

Most children experience some understandable regression when a new baby comes along. They may have temper tantrums, or ask for a thing they've outgrown, such as a nappy, bottle, or dummy, or need your attention urgently every time you start to nurse the new baby.

Sleep is also affected. If the older child starts waking up more frequently at night, walk him quietly back to bed. If he's waking up because he hears the baby, explain that everything is okay, that new babies need to wake up and eat, but that soon the baby is going to sleep all night just like his big brother or sister. Remind him during the daytime, too, if he's old enough to understand.

Sleep Lady Tip

No matter how busy you get with the baby, it's essential that you spend special one-on-one time with the older child every day.

If he starts demanding more of your attention at bedtime, start bedtime earlier so he has longer to unwind with you. (Depending on everyone's nursing and sleeping schedules, this might only work if both parents are at home.) Or involve him in the baby's bedtime. He could 'help' you read the baby a simple story, or you could read to him while nursing. (See Chapter 13, 'Helping Twins and Siblings Sleep,' for more advice on how to coordinate two bedtimes.)

If the baby is sleeping in your room and your child knows that he used to be there, explain that the arrangement is temporary, that the baby will go to her own room (or their shared room) in a few months. If your older child is cosleeping with you, please don't kick him out of bed to make room for the new one! Keep the baby in a Moses basket or cosleeper, but don't add to the older

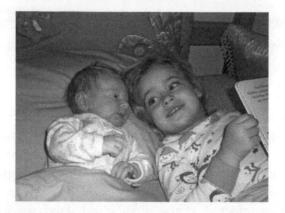

child's feelings of dislocation. Sometimes the father sleeps with the older child in the child's room, while nursing Mum sleeps with the baby in the parents' room.

If you are going to transition a child to a bed before the birth of a sibling, do it at least two and up to six months before the birth. If you wait until after the baby is born, give it at least four months. Please don't rush this transition because you need a cot, particularly if your older child is under two. If your older child is still happy in his cot, leave him there and buy or borrow another cot or Moses basket for the baby.

Occasionally, an older child who is already in a bed will want his cot back. He may say it, or he may show you, for instance, by climbing into his baby brother's cot. Highlight the advantages of a 'big boy' bed. Point out things that he gets to do with you that the baby doesn't – like going to the playground or eating cookies! Cot envy is usually his way of voicing a fear that he is being replaced, so just keep giving him all the reassurance he needs. But if he's under age two and a half and hasn't been in a bed too long, don't rule out giving him the cot back. Following big-boy stay-in-bed rules and coping with a new baby may be more than he can handle right now. But keep telling him how much you enjoy having a big boy or girl and how lucky the baby is to have such a great big brother or sister. Make sure visitors make just as big a fuss about your big guy as your little one.

Give the older child some jobs to do: Let him fetch a nappy, or help wash the baby's toes. Remind him of the safety rules, too –

no touching the face, no throwing things or picking up the baby, and definitely no waking up the baby or going in when she's sleeping.

Retraining

When you experience a sleep disruption, address it promptly. You need to be extra consistent at the first opportunity, both in terms of scheduling and in terms of scaling back your own comforting at bedtime and at night wakenings.

Usually, the briefer and less extreme the disruption is, the easier it will be to overcome. For instance, a twenty-four-hour stomach bug is going to be a lot less difficult to cope with than a week in the hospital, and a napless weekend at a relative's house an hour's drive away will be a lot less disruptive than a two-week holiday abroad. But as long as the regression doesn't last months, it's usually less a matter of relearning a sleep skill than of remembering to use a skill your child already knows.

A child who has a lot of disruptions – for instance, irregular parental schedules combined with frequent illnesses – may have more trouble than a child who goes away for one week a year. You may have to go through the Sleep Lady Shuffle again, but you can probably do it quickly, just one or two nights in each position. Usually you don't even have to do the entire Shuffle; it's enough to just do the last few nights, sitting in the hallway and then doing checks.

If the regression is significant and recurs soon after you've finished the Shuffle, say, a week or two, you may have to go back to the beginning, to sitting beside the cot or bed. But then move very quickly; change positions every night instead of every three nights. Other families just go to the sitting-in-the-doorway stage and progress from there. You may have to endure some crying because the break in the routine amounts to intermittent reinforcement, even if it was unintentional or unavoidable. In general, the longer your child has been sleeping well, the longer he's been well rested, the quicker the transition to peaceful nights. I remember getting an e-mail from an amazed parent who had worked with me six months earlier on both her children's sleep. They had just returned from a vacation, and for the first time ever, both kids slept all night while they were away and didn't miss a beat when they came back home.

Some children conquer their sleep problems and just shake off later disruptions. Others remain highly sensitive to them – and often these are the children who were very alert as newborns and reached developmental milestones early. Babies who have reflux for more than three months often tend to have more long-term vulnerability to sleep disruption. Ilan was one of those very alert children, and Joanne certainly knew all the ins and outs of my sleep system as we worked on this book. Travel didn't disturb him too much; he usually shared her bed in a hotel but returned to his routine at home quite easily. But even a minor illness could throw his sleep off significantly.

One time, he ran a high fever for a whole week. Joanne was so tired, she kept toppling over, finding herself curled up sleeping like a kitten at the foot of his bed. He of course would want her to resume her kittylike pose at 3:00 a.m. the next night, too. She went through countless variants of star and sticker charts, including special glow-in-the-dark star bonuses. Once, she noticed that he always wanted to sign himself in and out of preschool (only adults were allowed to do that), so she started having him 'sign' himself into bed every night! Once he signed himself in, he knew he wasn't allowed to get up and go out again. You'd be surprised how well it worked. He loved that sign-in privilege.

17

Problem Solving and Taking Care of Mums and Dads

After weeks, months, or even years of caring for a baby or child who does not sleep well, you may be more exhausted than you ever imagined possible. You may well be irritable and depressed – and feeling guilty about being irritable and depressed when you are supposed to be blissful about parenthood. You may feel that you can't be the parent you want to be.

In this chapter, I want to help you minimize the stress and maximize the success of my Sleep Lady program. I want to help you get your own sleep back on track after months or years of disruptions that may date back to the pregnancy. As demanding and rewarding as it is to take care of your children, it is also important that you nurture yourself, your spouse or partner, and your relationship.

Problem-Solving Basics

Review the Information

After more than a decade of working with families with sleep problems, I know my system works for almost everyone who tries it *and* sticks with it for at least a couple of weeks. I also know from years of experience that parents want quick fixes, and, in their desperation, they don't even want to read a whole book; they just want a few key paragraphs. You don't have to read this entire book to carry out my system, but if you tried to pick out a few pages that applied to your child and found that you didn't make much progress, please go back and read (or reread) the first four chapters, or first six chapters if you have a newborn. It won't take long, and you'll get a much better sense of how and why the Sleep Lady system works, and what it needs from you: patience, consistency, and faith in your own intuition as a parent. Then review the relevant age chapter.

Eliminate the Possibility of Medical Problems

If you have been utterly consistent in your response to your child's awakenings and you still see scant progress, read Chapter 15, 'Medical Problems,' and consult your doctor. Summarize your sleep log for the doctor, and note if your child has any symptoms of reflux, sleep apnea, or allergies. Even if your child is healthy now, if she had colic or reflux past the age of three months, if she has multiple allergies, or if she is unusually active or alert, it may take longer for you to see results. (Very alert children may need a little extra time during the bedtime and nap routines to prepare themselves for sleep. See my tips for very alert children in Chapter 2, 'Getting Started and Tips for Success.')

Use the Buddy System

Keep in mind my suggestion about finding a 'buddy' to talk to each morning and review how the night went, what you did right, what was not so hot. Your buddy can be your spouse, but you may do better with a friend or a group of friends. It's particularly helpful for single parents.

The buddy system is like stepping on the scale at Weight Watchers: It's easier to stick to the program when you know you will be held accountable. Maybe your buddy will help you realize that you aren't being quite as consistent as you are telling yourself. Maybe you are breaking the rules just a wee bit at 3:00 a.m. when you are so tired it is really easier to give in and nurse her one more time, or hold her hand until she falls asleep, or let her crawl into your bed just this once. If you are doing everything right but still feel tired and discouraged, your buddy might be able to help you see that you really are making more progress than you realize. It's also nice just to know that you aren't alone.

> As Julia, a mother of three whose youngest had sleep difficulties, put it, 'When you are making decisions about sleep, you are already so tired. By 8:00 p.m. I am exhausted, and kids have been placing normal childhood demands on me all day long. My willingness to lay down the law is less evident than when I have more energy and more sleep.' Knowing she had to report to someone in the morning helped Julia summon the energy and determination she knew she needed to stay on track.

Respect Your Own Limits

You may also reach a point in my program where you have solved some but not all of your child's sleep problems, and know that you have reached your own limits. For instance, you might have decided that you can't cope with nap training now, that it's taking you two hours a day to get your nine month old to nap in his cot for thirty minutes at a stretch. Grant yourself permission to give up for now, find an emergency backup way of getting him that daytime sleep, and try again in a few months.

Or you may have reduced your eighteen month old's awakenings from three times a night to three times a week, which is not perfect but tolerable. You may sense that getting her over that last hump, that last need to say 'Hi, Mum' now and then, might be too hard on her, or maybe just too hard on you. Maybe you can take tears at bedtime now, but you can't take too many of them at 4:00 a.m. You know her limits, and you know your own. You'll come back to tackle those remaining awakenings when you feel ready, maybe when she's got more words and can articulate what she needs from you in the middle of the night. You may decide that you aren't ready to give up bedsharing after all, that you'll do what you can to improve the quality of your shared sleep but that you like having your toddler in your bed, even if she does kick you in the head, sleep sideways, and hog the pillow. None of this means you are failing.

Do what's right for you now, and know that you have the tools for change, whenever you are ready to use them. Indeed, even if you have achieved all your sleep goals, if your child has become, as Ellen said of James, 'an Olympic sleeper,' you may still find yourself reaching for this book now and then. Children go through so many different stages, and their sleep, like any complex engine, needs periodic maintenance and an occasional tune-up.

Resolve Sleep Deprivation (Yours!)

Many parents complain to me that they become even more tired when they begin sleep training, and that can tempt them to give up. It's true that you might feel worse before you feel better. Remind yourself that it's a short-term situation, usually a matter of days until you start seeing results. That's because you have to give up all those little tricks you use to get your child back to sleep so that he can now learn to do it himself. So instead of being half awake for two minutes while you fetch a dummy or take him into your bed to nurse, you may be wide awake for twenty minutes helping and soothing a frustrated child, quite possibly a crying, frustrated child, who no longer has his sleep crutch but has not yet learned what to do instead. And once you've been up and around and experiencing the stress that we all feel when our child is in tears, it might be harder to get back to sleep yourself.

Be kind to yourself if this early stage of sleep shaping is difficult. Take naps when you can. Hire a babysitter if that's an option, or arrange some co-op sitting with a friend. Accept all the help you can get from your partner, relatives, and friends, and if you are uncomfortable imposing even on people who care about you, then swap favors instead.

Get to bed early yourself, too, by 10:00 p.m. or earlier, even if you are normally a night owl. I know the temptation is to get the kids down and then run around and pick up the house and answer your e-mail and do a load of laundry and pay the bills, but, really, you are better off going to bed at the first available moment. You'll manage to get the essentials done during the day, and whatever isn't essential can and should wait a few more weeks (or, some would say, eighteen more years). When you're sitting in his hallway at 3:00 a.m., shushing him back to sleep, you may be really glad you had that extra hour or two of sleep.

Work Out a Schedule

Some parents express concern that if they commit to sleep training, they will lose their freedom. To the contrary, I believe they gain freedom: the freedom for them and their children to enjoy themselves and each other without being exhausted, cross, or at their wit's end.

You do lose a little flexibility, particularly for the first two or three weeks, maybe a little longer if your child's nap problems are especially stubborn. For those few weeks, until you get the nap schedule down, you (or your babysitter) will have to be somewhat housebound. And once your child adapts to a nap schedule, you need to respect it. She can't sleep on the run or change her schedule every day to suit yours. But if you lose some flexibility, you will gain a great deal of predictability. You will be able to make plans and enjoy your outings because you'll know when she needs to sleep and when she'll be awake and sociable.

Sleep Lady Tip

I'm amazed at how many baby and toddler activities, gym classes, music classes, and even new mums' groups are so poorly scheduled, smack in the middle of naptime. Don't take a class if it means skipping a nap or gently persuade the school or teachers to consider rescheduling, so the eighteen month olds' class is not at 1:00 p.m., or the six month olds' class isn't at 9:30 a.m. – prime naptime for those age groups.

Once your child is well rested and sleeping well, she'll deal better with an occasional deviation from her schedule. But keep that a rarity, and ask yourself whether it's absolutely necessary, whether you can do what you want within the schedule. Or can you change the schedule? Instead of keeping your child up late for a family gathering, why not ask the family to gather a little earlier? Relatives can be surprisingly accommodating when you make simple and sensible demands. Maybe they'll shift a big family dinner to 5:30 or 6:00 instead of 8:00 – particularly if it means a pleasant evening around the table with no meltdowns. Then you can either get your children back home to bed at a reasonable hour, or after dinner put the kids to sleep at their grandparents' house, enjoy some adult family conversation, and then transfer the kids into the car and home to their own beds. The better they sleep, the more easily they adapt to sleeping in unfamiliar places, or getting themselves back to sleep after they've been moved.

Troubleshooting Emotional Factors

If you are having trouble following my Sleep Lady program, take a step back and ask yourself whether some of your own emotional history may be getting in the way, involving either your own childhood or your marriage. And if you are working outside the home, remember that we all have moments when we second-guess ourselves, when we feel guilty, when we wonder if we should be spending more time with our babies. It's a tricky balancing act, not just when our children are infants but throughout their lives. We aren't helping our children if we try to compensate by letting them sit in our lap for an hour at 3:00 a.m. If you get your child sleeping through the night, you'll have more joy and fewer power struggles the rest of the time.

Separate Your Issues (If Any) from Those of Your Children

As parents, we have to be cognizant of our own fears, problems, and 'stuck' points and how they play out in our children's lives. Our own unresolved issues from our childhood and the parenting we received may color our attitudes about sleep and make it harder for us to be consistent as we embark on a sleep program. Even if we had a relatively happy childhood, we may still react or overreact to our own experiences as we find our way as parents. For instance, an adult who recalls being afraid of the dark as a child may be overly concerned with shielding his own child from being alone in a dark room and may project that fear onto his child.

One mother I worked with felt her own mother had been cold and abandoning. When she had her own baby, she was not able to set any limits whatsoever, equating *no* with *no love*. Not surprisingly, the baby was not a good sleeper. The mother never set any limits around nursing, or any limits around bedtime. Her own unresolved feelings obstructed her child's healthy sleep.

Another woman was so scarred by her girlhood separation fears that she was convinced her own baby couldn't be without her for more than the most fleeting of moments and wouldn't even let her husband form healthy bonds with their baby. Arriving home from work, the father would want to take part in his fifteen-month-old daughter's bedtime routine, both because he wanted to spend time with his baby and because he considerately wanted to give his wife a break after a long day of nonstop child care. But if the little girl cried for even a nanosecond, the mother rushed in, taking the baby from her father and nursing her to sleep.

Sometimes we need professional assistance or therapy to sort out these issues, but usually we just need to be aware of them, to figure out which of our own burdens we are trying to rest on our children's slender shoulders.

Let Them Learn

It is essential to find the balance between 'doing for' our children all the time in an attempt to shield and protect them and not providing enough direction for them and leaving them vulnerable. That's why I urge you to think of sleep training as a form of coaching. Remember, you are giving your child sleep strategies, but he's the one who has to play the sleep game. A coach doesn't 'emotionally damage' his players by letting them go out on the field, even if they make mistakes once in a while. Parents don't damage their children by helping them learn to sleep.

A lot of the parents I work with recognize the many levels on which they struggle with sleep issues. Many say they have tried everything – but acknowledge they have not really given anything a chance to work. Some have not tried anything at all because they are so afraid of emotionally damaging their child. They are afraid of 'breaking their child's spirit' if they impose any limits and structure around sleep.

The Sleep Lady approach gives you a framework for making changes gently and helps you understand why you have to make them. If you understand how and why you are helping your child, you will understand the difference between 'crushing' him, harming him, or making him feel abandoned and making him feel loved. Once you get it, your perspective changes. As you see your child thriving because he's not so sleep deprived all the time, it will become so much easier for you.

> 'If I'm not comfortable with what I'm doing, then I can't live with the crying,' said Sam's mom, Nora, a nurse. 'But if it's something that will work for my kid, then I don't have trouble listening to him cry.'

Postnatal Depression

I see postnatal depression (PND) a lot in the families who come to me with sleep issues. *Exhaustion is a risk factor for depression.* And depression makes it harder to sleep coach successfully, which in turn breeds more exhaustion. I'd like mums and mums-to-be to read this section. I'd like dads and dads-to-be to read it. And the grandparents and best friends, too. Women experiencing postnatal depression (and as we'll see there is a lesser-known version that afflicts men) don't always recognize the signs or may already be too depressed to take action, so it's important for the people who are close to them to be on the lookout.

Postnatal depression is common – 10 to 15 percent of women experience it globally.

Postnatal depression is common – 10 to 15 percent of women experience it globally. Traditionally, postnatal depression was thought to begin in the first month after birth, but now we know it can also occur later in that first year. It's not good for the mum, and it's not good for the baby, who may have more trouble forming a secure bond with a depressed, emotionally flat, unresponsive mother.

Postnatal depression has biological components. Pregnancy hormones plummet, affecting brain chemistry; a history of depression adds to the risk. Exhaustion, stress, and new-mum anxiety play a role. Depression does not mean you are a bad mother, an unloving mother, a failed mother. It does not mean that you will not feel better and enjoy motherhood for many years to come. It does not even mean you will experience a similar depression after every birth (although you are at higher risk).

Check out The Association for Post-Natal Illness (www.apni.org) for resources, Better sleep, exercise, nutrition, and social support can help. You should also have your doctor do a simple test to rule out a thyroid problem. But you may also need therapy, drugs or alternative treatments, support groups, or some combination thereof. Doctors can help you find an antidepressant, if necessary, that you can safely take while breastfeeding. If you find you need a drug that may not be as compatible with nursing, or if you refuse to consider medication while you are nursing, please consider whether the benefits of breastfeeding outweigh the benefits of treating a serious depression that may interfere with your ability to take good care of yourself, your baby, as well as other older children. I'm not saying that breastfeeding isn't healthy and desirable. I'm saying that untreated depression can be very harmful, and you should not feel guilty or inadequate about stopping breastfeeding earlier than you had hoped and planned.

Serious depression can be very harmful, and you
should not feel guilty or inadequate about stopping
breastfeeding earlier than you had hoped and planned.

If you do wean early for medical reasons, do it slowly because the hormonal changes can aggravate depression. (Even if you don't have postnatal depression rapid weaning can give you flashes of depression. I didn't have PND, but I did experience those flashes as I weaned my first daughter, and I wish someone had warned me about that. I weaned my second daughter more gradually and avoided the problem.)

I can't 'fix' postnatal depression in a few pages here, nor should I try. What I want to do is help you recognize the warning signs, understand the difference between postnatal depression and the 'baby blues,' and learn some techniques that you and your family can use to address the sleep and exhaustion aspects.

Getting five or six hours of uninterrupted nighttime sleep is essential – and yes, it's possible even with a breastfed newborn. For more information, I recommend the books of Shoshana Bennett (*Beyond the Blues, Postnatal Depression for Dummies*, and *Pregnant on Prozac*). She's a psychologist who experienced two very severe undiagnosed postnatal depressions herself, and some of what I will share with you here is drawn from her work. She offers phone consultations and can be contacted through www.DrShosh.com.

Baby Blues

Baby blues, that is, brief episodes of mild mood changes, are extremely common the first few weeks after giving birth. You may feel moments of sadness or mood swings, you may cry, and you may feel vulnerable, stressed, or anxious. But the blues are transient. They go away in about two weeks. If sad feelings or anxiety are overwhelming, if you experience any thoughts of harming your baby, or if your symptoms start to interfere with your daily life, get evaluated for postnatal depression.

The Warning Signs of Postnatal Depression

If the baby blues last longer than two weeks, you are in PND territory. Even if the depression is relatively mild, you should get help so it doesn't last for months and doesn't get worse. We all have an occasional stressed-out day, and we all worry about our child's eating and sleeping. But if you have several of these signs and they are severe, oppressive, or obsessive, please listen to the warning bells. Friends and relatives, you be on the lookout, too.

- Excessive worry about the baby's health or schedule
- Loss of appetite or excessive weight gain or loss
- Inability to sleep at night even when the baby is asleep
- Hopelessness
- Very poor concentration
- Anxiety or panic attacks
- Deep sadness or an inability to feel pleasure
- Anger
- A lack of energy even if you got sleep
- Feeling guilty
- Prolonged lack of interest in sex (after you've recovered from labor and delivery)
- Missing doctors appointments (for mum or the baby)

A few other things that friends or relatives should watch for in the mum – or in the baby:

- Requiring another adult to accompany the mum to all doctor appointments (some couples choose to both go – the problem is when there's a palpable anxiety about it)
- Has many physical complaints with no apparent cause
- Poor milk production or other breastfeeding problems (there can be other physical reasons for this, but it's a potential sign)
- Evades questions about herself

- Cries easily
- Seems uncomfortable being with her baby
- Won't let someone else care for the baby
- Expresses concern that the baby does not like her
- Baby having excessive weight gain or loss
- Delays in the baby's cognitive or language development
- The baby has low or decreasing responsiveness to the mother

Parents, and especially mums, are under a lot of pressure in our society. We are bombarded with conflicting advice to do this or to do that, and sometimes we're told we're doing things 'wrong' if we choose not to bedshare, or if we go back to work soon, or if we don't 'wear' our baby all the time. Give yourself a license to be human! If you have the time and inclination to make homemade strained baby food and you feel good about it, more power to you. But a lot of babies eat food out of a jar and grow up happy and healthy.

Postnatal Depression Action Plan

I've already stressed the need to get professional help. Here are some other things you can do on your own:

- **Eat healthy foods.** Avoid caffeine and definitely avoid alcohol, as it's a depressant. Drink plenty of water and eat a healthy, balanced diet with a lot of fruits, vegetables, pulses, and whole grains. Bennett also recommends nibbling on high-protein snacks and drinking whey protein shakes. Consider a multi-vitamin.
- **Exercise.** It doesn't have to be superambitious – walking and stretching are good ways to start. For a severely depressed woman who may be having trouble even getting out of bed, exercise may seem overwhelming. Friends and family should encourage her to at least go outside, stand up straight, breathe deeply, and get some sunshine.

- **Take time for yourself – a few breaks a week, each an hour or two.** Take a walk. Read a book. Meet a friend. Get a manicure. New-mum playgroups, support groups, and baby-mummy yoga classes are great, but they don't count as pure mum time.
- **Sleep!** Getting at least five or six hours of uninterrupted night-time sleep is essential to treat and potentially lower your risk of postnatal depression. Even breastfeeding mums can do this. Here are some tips:

  - If your baby is four to six months old, and the doctor gives you the okay, start sleep coaching now. Have your partner do it if you are too depressed.
  - Split nighttime baby duty so you each get at least one five-hour uninterrupted block of sleep. One of you is 'on' from 8:00 p.m. to 1:00 a.m., and the other from 1:00 a.m. to 6:00 a.m. (adjust these figures to your family's schedule). When you are 'off duty,' sleep in a separate area, and try earplugs, a fan, or a white-noise machine. The on-duty parent can sleep, too, but he or she will be the one who has to wake up to respond to and feed the baby.
  - If you tend to obsess about when the baby will wake up or how long you've been awake, move the clock away from your bed.
  - Consider pumping breast milk so your partner can feed the baby with a bottle of your milk while you get your 'off-duty' sleep. Empty both breasts before bed so you won't wake up painfully engorged.
  - If you are bottlefeeding, alternate nights with your partner to get a full night's sleep. If you can afford it, hiring a night nurse or doula for even a few nights can help.

Depressed Dads

We can't blame fathers' depression on reproductive hormones, but at least one in ten fathers experiences depression after the birth of a child (and not necessarily the first child). Symptoms are different. They are less likely to experience mood swings and more likely to be tense, short-tempered, fearful, angry, and frustrated. They may feel helpless, worry about finances, or have concerns about the family's new interpersonal dynamics. They often have high expectations for themselves and are confused about their new role.

What's the biggest risk factor for a dad to get depressed? When the mum has postnatal depression. A father whose partner is seriously depressed has between a 24 and 50 percent risk of developing depression after the baby is born. The onset is usually after the mother's depression. And when fathers have depression, the children may suffer. Sons in particular are at high risk for behavioral problems in early childhood if their fathers were depressed.

Resolve Marital Tensions

Marital tensions can also make sleep success elusive, and let's face it, sleep deprivation isn't exactly an aphrodisiac. It's hard to be a good parent or attentive partner when one is irritable, impatient, anxious, depressed, forgetful, unfocused, and just plain exhausted. 'I was so tired and so nervous about going back to work when I was so tired,' said Nina, Lydia's mother. 'I got really snappy with my husband, I didn't care what I looked like, and I couldn't be bothered to brush my hair.' Try to recognize that this is transitory and that when you solve your child's sleep problems, many marital tensions may dissipate.

However, as we all know, some marital problems go much deeper than exhaustion. Indeed, I have found that couples with troubled marriages often have a lot more difficulty in solving their kids' sleep issues than those with basically solid marriages that are experiencing temporary exhaustion-induced stress. If two people are constantly at loggerheads, it is difficult to give a child a consistent message, and larger marital power struggles might create a tug-of-war over the child's sleep.

Sleep Lady Tip

It's a vicious circle, because exhaustion, depression, and irritation aggravate marital tensions, and the marital tensions will then prolong the exhaustion, creating more depression and irritation. Seek counseling if you feel that there are longer-term issues that need to be resolved in your relationship.

Work as a Team

In my private practice, I always urge both parents to come in for the consultation, and I would hope that both of you acquaint yourself with my program. Ideally, both of you should read and discuss the first few chapters. But even if only one of you actually reads the book, you both need to talk about it and think about it. You may need to make some decisions as a couple, like how quickly to end cosleeping, or whether you should dreamfeed, or what to do about the dummy. You need to know how you are going to support each other when one of you feels too tired or too discouraged or too upset to stick it out. You need a plan for how you will respond to your child's wakening, a plan you are both comfortable with and will be able to carry out, whether it's 10:00 p.m. or 4:00 a.m.

> *'We needed to bounce ideas off each other, how to tailor this program to Kerry,' said Laurel, whom you met in Chapter 11, 'Two and a Half to Five Years Old.' 'We needed to figure out how to make it work with what Kerry's used to. And we needed the encouragement from each other. Richard was logical, and I was emotional. I guess that's fairly typical, but he helped me look at it more practically.'*

Like Laurel and Richard, you should talk this through before you start working on sleep, not after, or else you may end up undermining or even sabotaging each other. If one of you is trying to teach the child to sleep longer between feedings and the other one

is jumping up with a bottle every two hours, the marital reper-
cussions can get ugly.

Work out the nuts and bolts of the sleep logistics. Review which
parent is responsible for which tasks, and at what times. You can
take turns being on duty at night, and whoever is 'off' can even
go to a quiet room with earplugs. Or you can take shifts, depending
on who functions better at which times and who gets back to sleep
more easily. For instance, one of you could take the 11:00 p.m. to
3:00 a.m. 'get the baby back to sleep' shift, and the other can take
the 3:00 a.m. to 6:00 a.m. shift, if that's the best fit for your
particular internal clocks.

Divide up household errands on weekends, so one of you can
stay home during naps (and maybe nap yourself) and one of you
can do the running around. Alternate weekends, if it suits you.
Remember, this is a shared responsibility, and even if one of you
is a stay-at-home parent and takes on a larger share of sleep-training
responsibilities, you should not have to take on 100 percent. You
can maximize your sleep and minimize your stress if you do this
together. Remember that sleep learning is a partnership between
you and your child, and between you and your spouse or partner.

Spending time on the blame game will prolong your child's sleep
problems and might do long-term damage to your marriage. Make
sure that you are responding to your partner calmly and consistently, not fighting about what to do or whose fault it is that your
child doesn't already know how to sleep. 'This placed a lot of stress
on our marriage. We're still recovering,' one mum said. 'He was
blaming me that the baby didn't sleep. He said it was all my fault,
that I was establishing patterns that the doctor told me not to. But
he didn't help much. He didn't have any solutions. In fact, later
when he did try to help some of the time, by then our daughter
wouldn't even let him put her to bed.'

Another couple, the parents of twins, recalled constant arguments
in the middle of the night as they tried to figure out how to carry
out my program, arguments that lessened as they grew more comfortable with sleep shaping and learned to discuss it at a more civil-
ized time of day. 'We were groggy, and the next thing you know
we were arguing,' the wife said. 'We weren't making good

decisions. We were talking about divorce – even though divorce wasn't in the picture before or after that. It was just a scary time.'

It helps to reward yourself for doing well, as a couple. Getting a good night's sleep in itself may make you feel like you've won the lottery, but beyond that, one of the benefits of a child who knows how to sleep is that you can leave her with a babysitter and take a night out, or maybe let Grandma take her for a slumber party.

Four months after working with me, Adele and Geoff took a day off and left Alex, then nineteen months old, with friends who had a toddler of their own. 'He stayed with them, he played with them, he even napped there. He went to bed, only fussing a little. Then we came, got him into the car, and drove him home, a half-hour drive. He had his eyes open the whole time, glassy-eyed. When we got home, we put him to bed, and he went right to sleep,' Adele said. 'It was such a huge moment of triumph!'

Shape Your Own Sleep

After months of sleep disruption, parents may find their internal clocks are waking them up every few hours, even after the baby has learned to stay asleep. Some parents awake with jolts of anxiety when they don't hear that familiar sound of 2:00 a.m. tears and wonder if the baby has stopped breathing. (It's very common, so don't feel silly.)

Jayne and Paul, whom you met in Chapter 12, 'Whose Bed Is It Anyway?' found their sleep problems, exacerbated perhaps by the extra layer of anxiety that accompanies having a premature baby, lasted far longer than their infant daughter's! 'Cynthia still sometimes cries out in the middle of the night. She gets herself right back to sleep but it would wake us up; we wouldn't be able to get back to sleep,' Jayne said. 'Both of us have become bad sleepers. I used to sleep like a rock; now I'm always keeping one ear out for her. Both of us have a really hard time falling back to sleep. She can cry out once, and we're awake for hours.'

Treat yourselves with the same tenderness you give
your child, and take your own sleep needs just as
seriously as you take those of your child.

Treat yourselves with the same tenderness you give your child, and take your own sleep needs just as seriously as you take those of your child. You've spent a lot of time creating an appropriate bedtime routine for your child; make sure you have one for yourself. Give yourself time to unwind and switch your own gears from wake to sleep, and learn to respect your own sleep windows. It can take one to three months for parents' sleep to get back on track, but if you follow the advice here on sleep regulation, it may go faster:

- Go to bed and wake up at around the same time (and while you have young children you might want to set your bedtime earlier than usual). Even on weekends, try not to modify it by more than an hour. Routines 'condition' us for sleep, psychologically and physiologically, and the conditioned response then makes it easier to fall asleep and stay asleep.
- Give yourself plenty of time to wind down, letting your body and mind become more relaxed and ready for sleep. Listen to quiet music, take a bath, or read a book. Some people find that light stretches, meditation, creative visualization, or progressive relaxation helps. This is the adult equivalent of going to bed drowsy but awake!
- If you need to catch up, rather than tinker too much with your nightly sleep schedule, take naps. But either take a short twenty- to thirty-minute nap or take a longer ninety- to hundred-minute nap so you don't wake up during a non-REM sleep cycle and feel groggy. Before I learned that, I used to set the alarm for one hour and wake up feeling lethargic and lousy, like I needed a major infusion of caffeine.
- Make sure your bed and your bedroom are sleep friendly. Your room should be quiet, dark, and secure, and your mattress, pillows,

and sheets should be comfortable. Sort out any temperature-control issues with your spouse!

- Exercise at least twenty to thirty minutes three times a week, but try to do it in the morning or during the day, not in the evening. If possible, leave at least three to four hours between strenuous exercise and sleep, and you certainly don't want to work out right before you go to bed.
- Try to get some natural light in the afternoon. Go for a walk or sit in a sunny room, and try to get out of the house or at least briefly escape your artificially lit office cubicle.
- Eat dinner at least three hours before going to bed.
- Reduce your caffeine consumption, and don't have any caffeine for at least six to eight hours before bedtime because it stays in your bloodstream. Caffeine doesn't just mean coffee – it means tea, many fizzy drinks, chocolate, and some over-the-counter cold and headache remedies. We become more sensitive to caffeine as we approach our forties.
- Nicotine is a stimulant, so if you haven't stopped smoking, poor sleep is yet another incentive.
- Watch your alcohol consumption. Alcohol may help you fall asleep, but more than three to five glasses, even less for some individuals, fragment our sleep. We wake up more often at night and earlier in the morning.
- To figure out how much sleep you need to function optimally, go to bed at the same time every night for three weeks and don't use an alarm clock in the morning. (Of course, this assumes your children are not human alarm clocks, but you can give it a try.) Even if you can't do this until your kids are older and sleeping better, keep it in the back of your mind and try it when you can; it's quite a useful exercise. I learned that I needed nine hours of sleep. No wonder I made a career out of this!

Withdrawal from Sleep Medication

If you have been taking any sleep medication, either prescription or over the counter, you may experience withdrawal symptoms and a 'rebound' effect when you stop taking it – meaning you may have more trouble going to sleep in the short run before your sleep patterns level out again. This is normal, but give yourself a little extra TLC at bedtime. Talk to your doctor about any specific concerns.

Insomnia

If you suffer from insomnia, it's even more essential that you pay attention to sleep hygiene. If after fifteen minutes or so of trying to sleep you are still wide awake, get up and go to another room. Read, relax, watch television, whatever soothes you. (Actually, it's a good idea to try to get yourself out of the habit of falling asleep with the TV on, but you can tackle that when your sleep is better regulated and you aren't having as much trouble with insomnia.) When you feel tired, go back to bed. Make sure you follow the general sleep rules above; the advice about getting some natural light in the afternoon is especially useful for insomnia.

Sleep Lady Tip

I strongly recommend *The Promise of Sleep*, by Dr William Dement, the Stanford doctor who more or less invented the modern field of sleep medicine. I have yet to come across a more useful volume on adult sleep.

Sleep Apnea

If one person snores, two people can suffer sleep interruption. Dr Dement estimates that nearly 40 percent of the adult population has some sleep apnea, and about half the cases are clinically significant. In addition to snoring, signs of obstructive sleep apnea in adults include pauses in breathing, waking up with headaches, having diffi-culty concentrating, fighting sleep while driving, feeling tired even after eight hours of sleep, and extreme fatigue. Consult your doctor and consider undergoing a sleep study. (Women who are persistently fatigued after pregnancy or as they get older might want to check with their doctors about thyroid hormone levels.)

Trust Yourself as a Parent

For my system to work, you need to have faith in yourself as a parent. This isn't a one-size-fits-all program, so you must trust your intuition and respect your child's individuality. The schedules I give you are guidelines, not decrees, so don't get overly attached to numbers. Watch your child for her sleep cues, and adjust her schedule accordingly. Adapt the program to the realities of your family. Obviously, you can't feed your child dinner at 5:00 and have her in the bath by 6:00 if she is still at child care and you are stuck in traffic. Do the best you can, and don't beat yourself up if you can't be perfect. But please try not to fall into the trap of convincing yourself that your child needs less sleep than average. Chances are that at least part of her sleep problem is that she isn't getting enough sleep as it is.

Many parents have told me that their friends or mothers or mothers-in-law have dismissed my advice, telling them that they are being too rigid or that children don't really need to nap, or that all eight month olds wake up at 5:00 a.m., or that it's normal for eighteen month olds to still wake up twice a night, or that they read something in a magazine in the doctor's office that says you are doing everything wrong. Don't let them deter you. They aren't living your life or parenting your child.

> 'My friends told me it was normal, that kids wake up at night, that you have to lie with them, that all mothers are exhausted,' said Amanda, who got her son, Wes, sleeping well at age four through a combination of Sleep Lady behavioral modification and medical treatment for his sleep apnea. 'But now my son wakes up happy. He isn't tired; he doesn't struggle anymore. And my friends are still having sleep issues with their kids.'

Similarly, you may be one of those parents who read a dozen different parenting books and then can't figure out whose advice to follow. Take a deep breath and listen to your own voice. You know what's right for your child, and you know what you need to do. I believe I give you enough flexibility to make my program fit your needs, your values, and your parenting style. If you like what you've read here, then follow my advice and give it time. If you don't think it will work – well, I disagree, but go ahead and try something else.

Whatever you do, stick with it. Don't do one system for two days, decide it won't work, do something else for another two days, and then complain that nothing works. You'd be surprised at how easily you can confuse even a very young child. Consistency counts.

Remember how Carol, Joshua's mum (in Chapter 9, 'Thirteen to Eighteen Months') thought of herself as a 'major rescuer'? She held Joshua all the time, nursed him all the time – and still felt guilty all the time. 'I still like some of the ideas about attachment parenting, but it messed me up about setting limits; it messed up my boundaries and made me crazy. I was always soothing him, but I wasn't always giving him what he needed. I wasn't doing him any favors by always rescuing him,' she said. 'Sleep is still where Joshua's issues come out; any transition or stress in our lives, any developmental change, we see sleep disturbances. But we can deal with it now. We have a foundation, and he understands it, too. As I rescued him less, he became a more confident child, and that's my mantra now. I say, "Joshua, I know you can do this. I know it's hard, but you can do it." And he does it. Changing how I dealt with sleep led to changes in so many other things. It helped me have a lot more faith in myself as a parent.'

Marcy too came to see herself as 'a very different parent.' Initially loath to let her baby cry, equating it with teaching a child to 'give up' and suffer, she had gone into overdrive every time Ariella whimpered. But by the time she had a second daughter, Peg, she knew the difference between a cry and a crisis. 'Every time Ariella cried, I thought, "She needs me." With Peg, I hear a cry and I think, "She's clean, she's safe, she's warm, she's okay, she'll work it out."' After three years of motherhood, Marcy trusts in her ability to know when something's wrong, when a child is sick, when a child is in need, and then of course she or Doyle goes in immediately. 'I know when a cry means something's up; I know when something's hurting. I can tell the difference. With Ariella, I was the one who created the sleep problems. With Peg, I've set her up for sleep success.'

Carol and Marcy have come to understand that sleep requires learning, and learning may require a few false starts, a few moments of frustration, and even a few tears. We can and should help our children, support our children, comfort our children, but we can't airbrush all sadness, anger, or frustration out of their emotional picture. Luckily, learning isn't only about frustration. It's about pride, achievement, a sense of self-worth – and a good night's sleep. When our babies are newborns, they need us to get them to sleep; they need us to make that magic. But then it's time to pass them the wand, to let them make their own magic. Go ahead and do it now. Good night, and sleep tight.

Appendix

Safe Sleeping Recommendations for Babies

Here are some tips for baby safety. Most of the information is from the American Academy of Pediatrics, First Candle and the U.K. Department of Health. I'd like to emphasize that this advice is primarily for healthy infants. Always talk to your doctor, particularly if your child was premature or has any health problems or unique circumstances. Recommendations have changed over the years as we have learned more about child safety and development, and they may well change again, so revisit safety issues with your doctor frequently. You may see all kinds of contradictory information on parenting and health websites. A good place to sort it all out is the American Academy of Pediatrics parenting corner, www.aap.org/parents.html.

1. 'Back to Sleep.' Always place your baby on his or her back to sleep – both at naps and at night. Side and tummy positions are not safe. This is absolutely essential to reduce the risk of sudden infant death syndrome (SIDS). Once your baby rolls over consistently backward and forward you won't be able to keep him on his back all the time, unless that's his preferred sleeping position, so make sure he has enough room to move around and no unsafe items in his cot. Unsafe items include quilts, loose blankets, pillows, soft or pillowlike bumpers, stuffed animals or toys with pieces that can come off, and soft bedding.

2. Babies should sleep on a firm surface, such as a safety-approved cot mattress, covered by a tight-fitting cot sheet. Never place your baby to sleep on pillows, quilts, sheepskins, or other soft surfaces. Infants should never sleep or nap on adult beds, waterbeds, sofas, or soft mattresses.

3. Be careful about buying secondhand or using hand-me-down cots, Moses baskets, cosleepers, even if they've been in the family for years. Safety standards have changed, and some products have been recalled or taken off the market. Contact the Consumer Product Safety Commission at at www.cpsc.gov. *Consumer Reports* has also reminded parents that cosleepers have not been tested as of this writing.

4. You'll see numerous devices and gadgets on the market designed to maintain sleep positions, but they have not all been tested for safety and efficacy and are not recommended. Generally, avoid them. If you have some specific concern about your child's sleep position or movement, talk to your doctor.

5. Cots should be placed in a warm, dark part of the room, away from windows. Blankets should not dangle from the side of the cot, and wall hangings need to be well out of the baby's reach so he can't pull them down on himself. Keep soft objects, toys, and loose bedding out of your baby's sleep area. Don't use pillows, blankets, quilts, sheepskins, or soft or pillowlike cot bumpers in your baby's sleep area (other than the small blanket you swaddle a newborn in, and that should be away from the face – see Chapter 5, 'The Right Start for Newborns and Infants'), as these all pose a risk of suffocation.

6. At six months, remove all cot mobiles or toys attached to cot sides because once the baby can pull and grab, they become a hazard. I like keeping mobiles away from the cot all the time; use it someplace where she's awake. Make the cot or sleep area 'boring' as well as safe.

7. Do not let your baby overheat during sleep. The room temperature should be comfortable for a lightly clothed adult. Once you stop swaddling your baby, use a sleeping bag or blanket sleeper. If the bedroom is cooler, use two sleeping bags or place one over the pajamas or onesies.

8. Remember that the American Academy of Pediatrics and U.K. Department of Health strongly recommend that you do not smoke around your baby and should not allow anyone else to smoke around your baby. Smoking exposure may increase the risk of SIDS and other respiratory illness.

9. The American Academy of Pediatrics and the U.K. Department of Health recommend you not let your baby sleep in a bed or on a couch or armchair with adults or other children. But it's fine to have an infant close by in your room, particularly in the early months. See my advice on roomsharing in Chapter 12, 'Whose Bed Is It Anyway?' for more information. If you bring your baby in bed with you to breastfeed, put him back in a separate sleep area, such as a Moses basket, cot, cradle, or a bedside cosleeper (infant bed that attaches to an adult bed) when finished. When baby starts to roll and move in his sleep, graduate to a standard cot for better – and safer – sleeping. Beds that are perfectly safe and comfortable for adults or older children can be very hazardous for babies. Soft bedding and other items in the adult bed increase the risk of SIDS and suffocation, especially for young babies. A baby or small child can also fall from the bed or get trapped between the mattress and the structure of the bed (the headboard, footboard, side rails, and frame), between the bed and the wall or nearby furniture, or even between railings in the headboard or footboard. Fatalities have been documented.

If you do choose to have your baby in the family bed, understand all the bed-sharing safety rules and *always follow them*. Parents who do have a baby in bed with them for even part of the night must never smoke or use substances, such as alcohol or drugs (including prescription drugs that make you sleep heavily), that may impair arousal, making them less aware of their baby's needs or position in the bed.

10. Dummies can significantly reduce the risk of SIDS (see www.firstcandle.org). They also soothe infants. Talk to your own doctor or health visitor about when to start – and stop – the dummy. Many doctors advise using a clean dummy when putting the infant down to sleep, although you shouldn't force the baby to take it. If you are breastfeeding, wait about four to six weeks before intro-

ducing the dummy. Many parents stop the dummy after six months, so the baby doesn't get so accustomed to falling asleep with something in his mouth. (Medical advice has changed frequently over the years, so make sure you discuss dummies with your doctor and check back as the child gets older.)

Resource Directory

Books

ADD and Sensory Integration Books

Amen, Daniel G. *Healing ADD: The Breakthrough Program That Allows You to See and Heal the 6 Types of ADD.* Berkley Publishing Group, 2002.

Barkley, Russell A., Ph.D. *Taking Charge of ADHD: The Complete, Authoritative Guide for Parents.* Rev. ed. Guilford Publications, 2000.

Kranowitz, Carol Stock, M.A. *The Out-of-Sync-Child: Recognizing and Coping with Sensory Processing Disorder.* Rev. ed. Perigee Books, 2006.

Miller, Lucy Jane, Ph.D., OTR, and Doris A. Fuller. *Sensational Kids: Hope and Help for Children with Sensory Processing Disorder.* Perigee Books, 2007.

Adult Sleep/Care

Bennett, Shoshana, Ph.D., and Ped Indman, Ed.D., MFT. *Beyond the Blues: Prenatal and Postnatal Depression, a Treatment Manual.* Mood Swings Press, 2002.

—. *Postnatal Depression for Dummies.* Wiley Publishing, 2007.

—. *Pregnant on Prozac: The Essential Guide to Making the Best Decision for You and Your Baby.* GPP Life, 2008. For more information on postpartum depression and Dr. Bennett, visit her Web site, www.DrShosh.com.

Breus, Michael, Ph.D. *Good Night: The Sleep Doctor's 4-Week Program to Better Sleep and Better Health.* Dutton, 2006.

Dement, William C., M.D., Ph.D., and Christopher Vaughan. *The Promise of Sleep: A Pioneer in Sleep Medicine Explores the Vital Connection Between Health, Happiness, and a Good Night's Sleep.* Dell, 2000.

Hauri, Peter, Ph.D., and Shirley Linde, Ph.D. *No More Sleepless Nights: A Proven Program to Conquer Insomnia.* John Wiley and Sons, Inc., 1996.

Bedtime

Bauer, Marion Dane. *Sleep, Little One, Sleep.* Simon and Schuster, 2002.

Bentley, Dawn. *Good Night, Sweet Butterflies.* Atheneum Books for Young Readers, 2003.

Boynton, Sandra. *Snoozers: 7 Short Short Stories for Lively Little Kids.* Little Simon, 1997.

Brown, Margaret Wise. *A Child's Good Night Book.* HarperCollins, 2000.

—. *Goodnight Moon.* Campbell Books 2001.

Dillard, Sarah, illustrator. *Ten Wishing Stars: A Countdown to Bedtime Book.* Orchard Books, 2003.

Fox, Mem. *Time for Bed.* Red Wagon Books, 1997.

Hague, Kathleen. *Good Night, Fairies.* Seastar Books, 2002.

Henkes, Kevin. *Owen.* Greenwillow Books, 1993.

Inkpen, Mick. *Is it Bedtime Yet Wibbly Pig?* Hodder Children's Books, 2005.

Lewis, Kim. *Good Night Harry.* Walker Books, 2004.

McBratney, Sam. *Guess How Much I Love You.* Walker Books, 2001.

McCue, Lisa. *Snuggle Bunnies.* Reader's Digest, 2003.

McMullen, Nigel. *It's Too Soon!* Simon and Schuster, 2004.

Meyer, Mercer. *Just Go to Bed*. Random House Books for Young Readers 1983.

Munsch, Robert. *Love You Forever*. Firefly Books, 1986.

Paul, Ann Whitford. *Little Monkey Says Good Night*. Farrar, Straus, and Giroux, 2003.

Penn, Audrey. *The Kissing Hand*. Tanglewood Press, 2007.

Rathmann, Peggy. *Good Night, Gorilla*. G. P. Putnam's Sons, 2000.

—. *10 Minutes till Bedtime*. G. P. Putnam's Sons, 2001.

Steinbrenner, Jessica. *My Sleepy Room*. Handprint Books, 2004.

Trapani, Iza. *Twinkle, Twinkle, Little Star*. Charlesbridge Publishing, 1998.

Yolen, Jane, and Mark Teague. *How Do Dinosaurs Say Good Night?* Blue Sky Press, 2000.

Bedtime Fears

Holabird, Katharine. *Alexander and the Dragon*. Random House Children's Books, 1988.

Leuck, Laura. *Goodnight, Baby Monster*. HarperCollins, 2002.

Meyer, Mercer. *There's an Alligator Under My Bed*. Dial Books, 1987.

Nadeau, Nicole. *Caillou: Bad Dreams*. Chouette, 2000.

Robbins, Beth. *It's OK! Tom's Afraid of the Dark!* D. K. Publishing, 2001.

Weinberg, Jennifer Liberts. *Slumberfairy Falls*. Random House Books for Young Readers, 2003.

Bedwetting

Bennett, Howard J., M.D. *Waking Up Dry: A Guide to Help Children Overcome Bedwetting*. American Academy of Pediatrics, 2005. You can visit his Web site, www.wakingupdry.com, for his free downloads with practical tips.

Mack, Alison. *Dry All Night: The Picture Book Technique That Stops Bedwetting*. Little, Brown, 1990.

Breastfeeding

American Academy of Pediatrics, Joan Younger Meek, M.D., and Sherill Tippins. *The American Academy of Pediatrics New Mother's Guide to Breastfeeding*. Bantam, 2005.

Gromada, Karen Kerkhoff. *Mothering Multiples: Breastfeeding and Caring for Twins or More!* 3rd ed. La Leche League International Book, 2007.

Huggins, Kathleen. *The Nursing Mother's Companion*. Rev. ed. Harvard Common Press, 2005.

La Leche League International. *Womanly Art of Breastfeeding*. Plume Books 2004.

Mohrbacher, Nancy, and Kathleen Kendall-Tackett. *Breastfeeding Made Simple: Seven Natural Laws for Nursing Mothers*. New Harbinger Publications, 2005.

Newman, Jack, M.D., and Teresa Pitman. *The Ultimate Breastfeeding Book of Answers: The Most Comprehensive Problem-Solving Guide to Breastfeeding from the Foremost Expert in North America*. Rev. ed. Three Rivers Press, 2006.

Pryor, Gale, and Kathleen Huggins. *Nursing Mother, Working Mother*. Rev. ed. Harvard Common Press, 2007.

West, Diana, and Lisa Marasco. *The Breastfeeding Mother's Guide to Making More Milk*. Foreword by Martha Sears, R.N. McGraw-Hill, 2008.

Infant Massage

McClure, Vimala Schneider. *Infant Massage: A Handbook for Loving Parents*. Souvenir Press, 2001.

Reese, Suzanne P. *Baby Massage: Soothing Strokes for Healthy Growth*. Studio, 2006.

Meditation and Guided Visualization for Children

Garth, Maureen. *Moonbeam: A Book of Meditations for Children*. HarperSanFrancisco, 1993.

—. *Starbright: Meditations for Children*. HarperSanFrancisco, 1991.

New Sibling

Ballard, Robin. *I Used to Be the Baby*. Greenwillow, 2002.

Bourgeois, Paulette, and Brenda Clark. *Franklin's Baby Sister*. Kids Can Press, 2000.

Brown, Marc. *Arthur's Baby*. Little, Brown, 1990.

Henkes, Kevin. *Julius, the Baby of the World*. Harper Trophy, 1995.

London, Jonathan. *Froggy's Baby Sister*. Puffin Books, 2005.

Meyer, Mercer. *The New Baby*. Golden Books, 2001.

Dummies

Boelts, Maribeth, and Kathy Perkinson. *Little Bunny's Pacifier Plan*. Concept Books, 2001. Murphy, Jill. *The Last Noo-Noo*. Walker Books, 1997.

Parenting

American Academy of Pediatrics. *Caring for Your Baby and Young Child: Birth to Age 5*. 4th ed. Bantam Books, 2005.

Bowlby, John. *A Secure Base: Parent-Child Attachment and Healthy Human Development*. Basic Books, 1988.

Brazelton, T. Berry, M.D. *Touchpoints: Your Child's Emotional and Behavioral Development, Birth to 3 – The Essential Reference for the Early Years*. 1992. Reprint, Da Capo Press, 2006.

—. *Touchpoints: 3 to 6*. Da Capo Press, 2002.

Dunstan, Priscilla. *The Dunstan Baby Language System on DVD*. www.dunstanbaby.com.

Ernsperger, Lori, Ph.D., and Tania Stegen-Hanson, OTR/L. *Just Take a Bite: Easy, Effective Answers to Food Aversions and Eating Challenges!* Future Horizons, 2004.

Karen, Robert. *Becoming Attached: First Relationships and How They Shape Our Capacity to Love*. Oxford University Press, 1998.

Karp, Harvey, M.D. *The Happiest Baby on the Block: The New Way to Calm Crying and Help Your Newborn Baby Sleep Longer*. Bantam Dell, 2002.

Sammons, William, M.D. *The Self-Calmed Baby: Teach Your Infant to*

Calm Itself—and Curb Crying, Fussing, and Sleeplessness. St Martin's Press, 1991.

Schmitt, Barton D., M.D. *Your Child's Health: The Parent's One-Stop Reference Guide to Symptoms, Emergencies, Common Illnesses, Behavior Problems, Healthy Development.* 2nd ed. Bantam Books, 2005.

Stamm, Jill, Ph.D. *Bright from the Start: The Simple Science-Backed Way to Nurture Your Child's Developing Mind from Birth to Age 3.* Gotham Books, 2007.

Zweiback, Meg, R.N., C.R.N.P., M.P.H. *Keys to Toilet Training.* Barron's Educational Series, 1998.

Transitioning to a Bed

Beck, Sheryl. *Going to My Big Bed! Barney's Little Lessons.* Lyrick Studios, 2002.

Bunting, Eve. *My Big Boy Bed.* Clarion Books, 2003.

Jordan, Apple. *Big Enough for a Bed.* Sesame Workshop. Random House, 2002.

Yoga Books for Children

Baptiste, Baron. *My Daddy Is a Pretzel: Yoga for Parents and Kids.* Barefoot Books, 2004.

Garabedian, Helen. *Itsy Bitsy Yoga: Poses to Help Your Baby Sleep Longer, Digest Better, and Grow Stronger.* Simon and Schuster, 2004.

—. *Itsy Bitsy Yoga for Toddlers and Preschoolers: 8-Minute Routines to Help Your Child Grow Smarter, Be Happier, and Behave Better.* Da Capo Press, 2008.

Music

Ackerman, William. *The Opening of Doors.* Windham Hill Records, 1992.

Baby's First Lullabies. Twin Sisters, 2005.

Disney Baby Lullaby: Favorite Sleeptime Songs for Baby and You. Walt Disney Records, 1992.

Falkner, Jason. *Bedtime with the Beatles: Instrumental Versions of Classic Beatles Songs*. Sony Wonder, 2001.

Golden Slumbers: A Father's Lullaby. Rendezvous, 2002.

Malia, Tina. *Lullaby Favorites: Music for Little People*. Music for Little People, 1997.

Music for Babies. *Sleepy Baby*. Big Kids Productions, 2002.

Parents: The Lullaby Album. Angel Records, 1993.

Solnik, Tanja. *From Generation to Generation: A Legacy of Lullabies, in Yiddish, Ladino, and Hebrew*. Dreamsong Recordings, 1993.

—. *Lullabies and Love Songs*. Dreamsong Recordings, 1996.

Stroman, Paige. *Lullabies to Celebrate Mother and Child*. National Music Marketing/Lullabyland, 2001.

West, Kim, John Judge, and Jim Conley. *The Sweetest Dreams*. Sleep Lady Solutions, 2008.

Web Sites

Amby Baby Motion Bed
United States: www.ambybaby.com
Canada: www.ambybaby.ca
Europe: www.amby-baby-europe.com

American Academy of Pediatrics
www.AAP.org

Arms Reach Co-Sleeper Moses basket
www.armsreach.com

BabyCentre
Pregnancy and parenting website
www.babycentre.co.uk
www.babycenter.com.au

Circle of Security
Early intervention programs for parents and child
www.circleofsecurity.net

Consumer Product Safety Commission
www.cpsc.gov

First Candle Organization: Helping Babies Survive and Thrive
www.firstcandle.org

Halo Innovations
Maker of the SleepSack™ wearable blanket and swaddle
www.halosleep.com

Marpac Sleepmate – sound screen
www.marpac.com/soundscreen.asp
1-910-602-1421, worldwide

The Miracle Blanket
Swaddling blanket
www.miracleblanket.com

Monster Go Away! Spray
www.monstergoaway.com

Mumsnet
Parenting website
www.mumsnet.com

National Childbirth Trust
Charity for parents offering antenatal and postnatal courses, local support and information
www.nct.org.uk

National Sleep Foundation
The Web site of this nonprofit group addresses numerous sleep issues for children and adults and includes the group's new childhood sleep guidelines.
www.sleepfoundation.org

The Tucker Sling
An infant position system
www.tuckersling.com

Breastfeeding Information

Guidelines for Professionals
The Academy of Breastfeeding Medicine
www.bfmed.org

Australian Breastfeeding Association
www.breastfeeding.asn.au

Breastfeeding Made Simple
www.breastfeedingmadesimple.com

International Lactation Consultant Association
www.ilca.org

Jack Newman
www.bflrc.info/newman/articles.htm

Lactation Consultants of Great Britain
www.lcgb.org

La Leche League GB
www.laleche.org.uk

La Leche League International
www.lalecheleague.org

Milk Supply
www.lowmilksupply.org

Nursing Mothers Counsel
www.nursingmothers.org

United States Lactation Consultant Association
www.uslcaonline.org

Information on Postnatal Depression

Association for Post-Natal Illness
www.apnl.org

Medical Education on Postnatal Depression
An educational Web site developed with the support of the National
Institute of Mental Health. Updated information and resources for
care providers and women with PND.
www.MedEdPPD.org

Post and Antenatal Depression Inc.
www.panda.org.au

Postnatal Support International
www.postpartum.net

Photo Credits

Index

cosleeping and, 385
described, 383, 384–8
No-Cry Sleep Solution, The (Pantley),
343
Non-REM sleep, 55, 91, 111, 383,
390, 453
night terrors and, 388
North American Society for Pediatric
Gastroenterology and Nutrition,
397

Out-of-Sync Child, The (Kranowitz),
408
Overstimulation, 11, 58, 94, 95, 96,
100, 104, 143, 183, 205, 216
Overtiredness, 54, 58, 90, 95, 96, 100,
106, 112, 125, 134, 156, 162, 171,
173, 226, 228–9, 249, 262
early risers and, 192, 224, 274, 328
napping and, 194, 197, 201, 358
nightmares and, 384
Owens, Judith, 390

Pantley, Elizabeth, 343
Parenting styles, 20, 25, 89–90, 250,
304, 312, 355, 362, 456
Partial arousals, 56, 91, 111, 115, 123,
188, 226, 388, 389
cosleeping and, 344
intervention at, 123
naps and, 160
whimpering/crying during, 317
Patience, 16, 18–19, 408, 436
Patting, 112, 141, 143, 165, 179, 183,
185, 186, 187
PND *See* Postnatal depression
Positive reinforcement, 295, 301, 308
Postnatal depression (PND), 39, 104
experiencing, 442–4

treatments for, 443, 446–7
Postnatal Depression for Dummies
(Bennett), 444
Potty training, 236, 244–5, 408, 415
sleep patterns and, 294–5
sleep training and, 244–5
Power struggles, 45, 141, 298, 304,
314, 440, 448
Predictability, 58, 67, 123, 173, 207,
211, 236, 237, 246
craving for, 65, 250
routines and, 36
Pregnant on Prozac (Bennett), 444
Preschoolers:
napping and, 246, 302
schedules for, 279, 302–6
sleep for, 252, 283, 322
stalling by, 283
testing by, 310
Problem-solving basics, 435–42
Progressive relaxation, 385, 387, 453
Promise of Sleep, The (Dement), 454

Quiet time, 283, 299, 329–31

Reassurance, 119, 150, 165, 181, 193,
202, 214, 215, 262–3, 291, 313,
349, 363, 380, 385, 430
brief, 317
checks and, 41
maximizing, 11
offering, 11, 17, 42, 109, 111, 114,
117, 140, 200, 218, 219, 237,
243–4, 251, 256, 271, 284, 293,
311, 312, 316, 323, 325, 352,
353, 355, 370, 377, 426
older siblings and, 431
seeking, 235
Reflux, 4, 42, 93, 164, 216, 266, 380,

Photograph: Charles Bethman

Kim West LCSW-C is a mother of two and has been a licenced practising child and family therapist for over seventeen years. She has helped thousands of tired parents all over the world.

THE BABYMOON EXPERIENCE

How to nurture yourself and your baby through pregnancy and the early weeks

Caroline Deacon

A babymoon is a special time out of your everyday life, taken in the first six weeks after your baby is born. It's a time to recover from birth and to get to know and fall in love with your new baby. Traditional societies have long known the benefits of a babymoon, and there are sound biological reasons for this period of adjustment, but in the West most women are pressured to 'get back to normal' as soon as possible after birth.

Caroline Deacon, NCT breastfeeding counsellor and author of *Babycalming*, champions the case for taking a babymoon, advocating a return to a gentler, more nurturing start in life.

Reassuring and entertaining, *The Babymoon Experience* will help you to make the most of this precious time as well as offering practical guidance for a happy and healthy pregnancy and birth. Discover how you can:

- Be in great shape to cope well with birth and recover quickly
- Feel relaxed and in control at every stage
- Approach birth and beyond with confidence
- Prepare for and adjust well to becoming a parent
- Develop a strong bond with your new baby
- Minimise your risk of postnatal depression

Experiencing a babymoon will give you, your new baby and your partner the best possible start in your new life together.

978-0-7499-4247-2

OPTIMUM NUTRITION FOR YOUR CHILD

How to boost your child's health, behaviour and IQ

Patrick Holford and Deborah Colson

Patrick Holford illustrated the connection between nutrition and all aspects of health in his best-selling book *The Optimum Nutrition Bible*.

In *Optimum Nutrition for Your Child*, he reveals how crucial optimum nutrition is for children's general health and development, as well as their behaviour and IQ. He explains why certain foods are so beneficial and why others are damaging, and enables you to identify common problems in children which can be improved or solved with the right foods and supplements.

With invaluable advice on getting children to eat healthy food, food plans and practical tips, this book is the definitive guide for parents.

978-0-7499-5353-9